Synopsis of

OBSTETRICS

SYNOPSIS OF
OBSTETRICS

CHARLES E. McLENNAN, M.D.

Professor of Gynecology and Obstetrics, Stanford University
School of Medicine, Stanford, Calif.

EUGENE C. SANDBERG, M.D.

Associate Professor of Gynecology and Obstetrics,
Stanford University School of Medicine,
Stanford, Calif.

NINTH EDITION

With 220 illustrations, including 2 in color

The C. V. Mosby Company

Saint Louis 1974

NINTH EDITION

Copyright © 1974 by The C. V. Mosby Company

All rights reserved. No part of this book may be reproduced in any manner without written permission of the publisher.

Previous editions copyrighted 1940, 1943, 1947, 1952, 1957, 1962, 1966, 1970

Printed in the United States of America

Distributed in Great Britain by Henry Kimpton, London

Library of Congress Cataloging in Publication Data

McLennan, Charles E
 Synopsis of obstetrics.

 First-5th ed. by J. C. Litzenberg.
 1. Obstetrics. I. Sandberg, Eugene C., 1924-
joint author. II. Litzenberg, Jennings Crawford, 1870-
1948. Synopsis of obstetrics. III. Title.
[DNLM: 1. Obstetrics. WQ100 M164s 1974]
RG101.M17 1974   618.2'002'02   74-1147
ISBN 0-8016-3317-6

GW/M/M   9   8   7   6   5   4   3   2   1

Preface

This and the numerous previous editions of *Synopsis of Obstetrics,* now spanning nearly thirty-five years, have been designed chiefly for the undergraduate medical student who feels a need for a summation of the vast amount of material to be found in the large standard textbooks of obstetrics, to use either as an initial survey of the subject or for a rapid preexamination review. A synopsis may be helpful similarly for the graduate physician reviewing for various state or national qualifying examinations, or one in need of brief and easily located epitomes of current obstetric practice and theory.

With the needs of all such readers in mind, we have made many minor and some major additions and deletions in an effort to have the current text reflect established obstetric practices as well as seemingly meritorious theoretical concepts that have gained acceptance over the past four years. As before, we have tried to emphasize basic principles, omitting wherever feasible the finer details of pharmaceutical treatment and operative or other technical procedures. References to articles in journals have been omitted intentionally, because of our conviction that the usual reader of a synopsis has little time and probably even less incentive to pursue original sources.

Some of the older illustrations have been replaced with newer versions, and a few entirely new figures have been added. We are grateful to Halcyon Harris Cowles for the attractive new drawings and to our secretaries, June Ursem and Mary Ellen Blencoe, for their meticulous preparation of typescript for the revised portions of the text.

Charles E. McLennan
Eugene C. Sandberg

Contents

Synopsis of
OBSTETRICS

1

Ovulation and fertilization

Obstetrics is that segment of gynecology concerned with human reproduction and its immediate effects on the mother. As the merger between obstetrics and gynecology becomes ever more complete in teaching and in practice, obstetrics tends to lose its identity as an isolated discipline and yesterday's obstetrician becomes today's gynecologist, who may be described as a reproductive biologist with some of the skills of the internist, the psychiatrist, the pediatrician, and the surgeon. There is a spreading tendency in academic centers to reverse the order of the words in the traditional disciplinary title "obstetrics and gynecology" in order to emphasize gynecology as the broader and more significant designation, and it is possible that classical obstetrics will one day follow its predecessor, midwifery, into the pages of history.

In its original usage the Latin term *obstetrix* meant "one who stands before" and thus referred to a *midwife* assisting the pregnant woman at the time of delivery. But the concept of obstetrics has been greatly broadened to include conception, placentation, fetal development, maternal physiology, the mechanism of obstetric labor, postpartum changes, and at least a portion of neonatal physiology.

It seems logical to begin this book with a description of the germ cells and the events immediately preceding the union of sperm cell and ovum. We assume that the reader has somewhere acquired a reasonable knowledge of human embryology and anatomy and that a standard description of the female

1

reproductive organs and their development need not be repeated here.

GAMETOGENESIS

The ova of the female and the spermatozoa of the male are collectively known as *gametes*. During fertilization a male and a female gamete unite to form a single cell or *zygote* from which a new individual develops. Germ cells (sex cells), by successive divisions, produce gametes. All other cells of the body not directly concerned with perpetuation of the race are called somatic cells. Primordial germ cells migrate from the yolk sac entoderm to the embryonic genital ridge and enter the mesenchyme of the future ovary. Presumably these cells become the ova in adult life. The suggestion that functioning ova arise later from the so-called germinal epithelium of the ovary has not been substantiated in human beings. Estimates of the number of oocytes at birth vary from 40,000 up to more than half a million.

The sex cells that appear in the epithelium of the ovarian surface descend into the ovarian connective tissue as ovigerous cords, and these break up into egg nests composed of potential *oogonia*. Subsequent development of the ovum and ovarian (graafian) follicle may be outlined as follows:

1. By the seventh fetal month most oogonia have been transformed into primary oocytes in the pachytene stage. Reduplication of DNA in preparation for meiosis occurs in the earliest stages of oogenesis. By the time of birth, primary oocytes have entered the dictyotene, or resting stage, and remain there as tetraploid cells until maturation occurs some 15 to 45 years later. In the resting stage the ovum is about 40 microns in diameter, but by the time of ovulation it has grown to measure between 100 and 150 microns.

2. Adjacent follicle cells arrange themselves around a future ovum, and the entire structure is then a *primary* or *primordial ovarian follicle* (Figs. 1-1 and 1-2).

3. Cells surrounding the oocyte multiply, a cavity known as the *antrum* appears in the follicle, and this cavity contains *liquor folliculi*.

4. The primary oocyte becomes much larger than any of the surrounding follicular cells, and its cytoplasm is dotted with yolk granules.

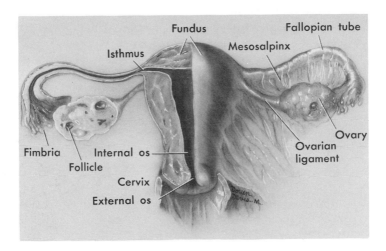

Fig. 1-1. Normal uterus, tubes, and ovaries.

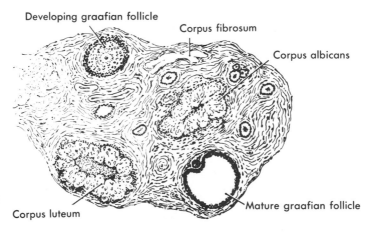

Fig. 1-2. Section of ovary, showing developing and mature graafian follicles, corpus luteum, corpus albicans, and corpus fibrosum.

5. The oocyte (ovum) is surrounded by the transparent *zona pellucida,* which, in turn, is surrounded by a layer of radially elongated follicular cells called the *corona radiata.*

6. As fluid accumulates in the antrum, follicular cells are pushed peripherally to form the *stratum granulosum.* At the point where the ovum lies in the follicular cells, these cells form a mass known as the *cumulus oophorus.*

7. Connective tissue surrounding the mature follicle is condensed into the *theca folliculi,* which is subdivided into *theca interna* (relatively loose vascular tissue) and *theca externa* (densely fibrous layer).

Ovulation. Mature follicles protrude at the surface of the ovary (Fig. 1-2), and the fluid within them is under considerable pressure. Although this fluid pressure may ultimately produce enough ischemia to devitalize an area of ovarian surface through which rupture may occur, the precise hormonal mechanisms underlying this chain of events is not clearly understood. Analysis of the mechanics of ovulation by use of a mathematical and physical model has shown that there is a limit to the pressure that can be achieved by the follicle wall and this falls as the follicle increases in size. A relative increase of the osmotic pressure of the follicular fluid provides a trigger mechanism to effect ovulation in follicles that have reached a critical size. Thus mechanical factors may provide a common pathway for the individual actions of follicle-stimulating hormone (radial growth of follicle), estrogens (increased mass and volume of follicle), and luteinizing hormone (possibly related to increase in osmotically active particles to provide a colloid-loaded system). Moving pictures have been made of ovulation in the rabbit, and these films exhibit an explosive gush of follicular fluid that carries with it the ovum and its *corona radiata* (Fig. 1-3). Presumably the fimbria of the uterine tube comes sufficiently close to the ovary at the moment of ovulation to pick up the liberated ovum and direct it into the ampulla of the tube. However, it is possible for an ovum to find its way into the tube of the opposite side of the pelvis. At least, conceptions have been reported after removal of one ovary and the tube from the opposite side. It is believed that only a single follicle matures about every 4 weeks, whereas other follicles well advanced in their development undergo *atresia.* Occasionally,

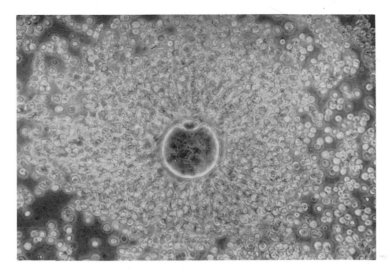

Fig. 1-3. Unfertilized ovum recovered 4 hours after ovulation, showing corona radiata and first polar body. (Mouse, phase contrast, ×80.) (Courtesy Dr. A. H. Gates, Palo Alto, Calif.)

of course, more than one follicle ruptures at approximately the same time and thus a multiple pregnancy may result.

Women usually ovulate about 14 or 15 days before the onset of menstruation or about the middle of the menstrual cycle. A rise in basal body temperature commonly is observed at the time of ovulation, and the temperature remains at the elevated level until menstruation begins or for about 20 weeks if pregnancy occurs. This phenomenon is an indirect indication of ovulation that has been widely used in studying patients with infertility problems.

Corpus luteum. The corpus luteum, so named because of its yellow color when fresh, forms rapidly by conversion of follicular cells to lutein cells, which surround a central mass of blood (Fig. 1-2). This central mass of blood is soon reduced in size, but lutein cells, nourished by rapidly developing capillaries from the adjacent theca, proliferate quickly to form a structure much larger than the original follicle. If the liberated ovum is not fertilized, the corresponding corpus luteum regresses to a small scarred area called a *corpus albicans*. When pregnancy occurs, the corpus luteum continues to flourish for several months and is referred to as the *corpus luteum of pregnancy*.

Polar bodies and chromosomal reduction. Two divisions of the primary oocyte occur in rapid succession at about the time of its liberation from the follicle. Two ootids form at each division; one receives practically all the stored food material of the original cell, while the other receives almost none and soon dies. The ootid that dies is called a polar body. The second maturation division does not occur until the ovum has left the ovary and may not be completed unless the ovum has been penetrated by a spermatozoon.

During maturation the chromosomes are reduced to half the number characteristic of the species (Fig. 1-4). By the process of synapsis, which begins before birth, chromosomes are arranged in pairs. One member of each pair is derived at fertilization from the ovum and the other from the spermatozoon. The first maturation division forms a large secondary oocyte and a small first polar body (Fig. 1-3). When the spermatozoon enters the oocyte, a second polar body is formed and the paired chromosomes separate in such a way that only half of them remain in the egg (reduction division) and half are lost in the polar body. Since the usual number of chromosomes in human cells is 46, maturation reduces the number to 23.

Spermatogenesis. Primordial sex cells extend from the epithelial surface of the male gonad down into its substance and form seminiferous tubules, from the walls of which come *spermatogonia*. The daughter cell of a spermatogonium grows into a *primary spermatocyte* and moves nearer the lumen of the tubule. Further meiotic division produces two *secondary spermatocytes*. Each of these divides into *spermatids*. The first division of the primary spermatocyte is reductional, and the further division into spermatids is equational. Spermatids are transformed to *spermatozoa* in a series of 12 developmental steps. Toward the end of spermiogenesis the spermatid discards its residual cytoplasm. When fully formed, with head, neck, and tail portions, spermatozoa move along the tubal lumen toward the epididymis (Fig. 1-5).

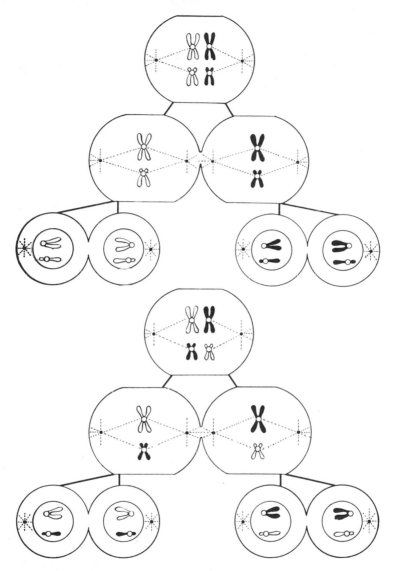

Fig. 1-4. Showing how a premeiotic germ cell with two sets of chromosomes forms four germ cells, each with a single set of chromosomes, by the process of meiosis. Two alternative arrangements of chromosome pairs on the first meiotic spindle are diagrammed.

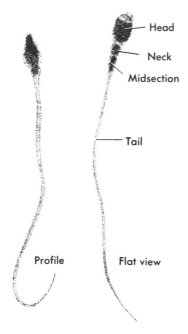

Fig. 1-5. Normal spermatozoon in profile and flat-surface views.

Although spermatogenic cells develop in intimate relation to the surfaces of surrounding *Sertoli cells,* the latter are always separated from adjacent germ cells by distinct intercellular spaces. There is no detectable specialized zone of cytoplasm in the peripheral region of a Sertoli cell that might be involved in the release of spermatozoa.

Fertilization. After semen is placed by any means in the vagina or even near the vaginal introitus, spermatozoa therein make their way in about an hour through the uterus and into the outer thirds of the uterine tubes, where fertilization is thought to occur most frequently. They are assisted in their movement toward the ovum by the cilia of the tubal epithelium, which beat in the direction of the tubal fimbria. Spermatozoa probably retain their fertilizing

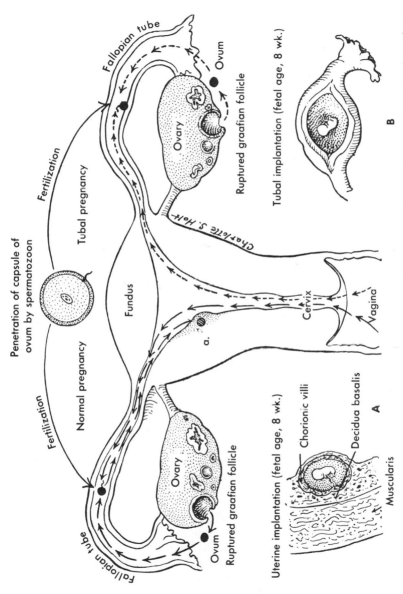

Fig. 1-6. Fertilization of ovum. Note fertilization in the tube and implantation of the fertilized ovum in the endometrium. (From Falls and McLaughlin: Obstetric and gynecologic nursing, St. Louis, The C. V. Mosby Co.)

power in the female genitalia for 1 or 2 days, although motility may persist for longer periods. During coitus an average ejaculate of 3 to 5 ml. with an average sperm count of 120 million per ml. is deposited in the vagina. Thus only one of some 250 to 500 million spermatozoa ultimately is responsible for fertilization. Probably only a few thousand sperm survive to reach the distal portion of the tube and peritoneal cavity. Though tubal peristaltic activity is directed toward the uterus, spermatozoa appear to ascend without difficulty, perhaps aided by tubal fluid moving toward the fimbria. Many aspects of sperm transport in human beings remain to be elucidated. (See Fig. 1-6.)

It has been shown that in certain mammals spermatozoa must be conditioned in some manner by incubation in the female genital tract or in other tissue receptacles before they are capable of fertilization. This process, presumably chemical in nature, has been termed *capacitation*. Whether this is essential in women has not been determined.

Immediately after ovulation the ovum is surrounded by thousands of corona radiata and cumulus cells, but within 12 to 24 hours the zona pellucida is denuded. Probably hyaluronidase in the spermatozoon helps dissolve the intercellular cement of follicular cells. The human ovum dies within a day if it is not fertilized, and fertilization generally occurs less than 12 hours after ovulation (Fig. 1-7).

Few direct observations of fertilization have been made in mammals, and much of our information has come from the study of marine forms in which fertilization occurs outside the mother's body. Although several spermatozoa may penetrate the zona pellucida, usually only a single spermatozoon (of the several hundred million in the ejaculate) enters the ovum, whereupon a change occurs in the surface membrane of the egg that seems to make it impermeable. Only the head and neck of the spermatozoon (now called the *male pronucleus*) enter the ovum, while the tail drops off and disappears.

With the formation of the male pronucleus (Fig. 1-7), the second maturation division of the ovum completes itself, and thus the *female pronucleus* is formed. Chromosomes of the two pronuclei merge to restore the species number, and fertilization is effected. Cell division then proceeds rapidly. Lysis of zona cells

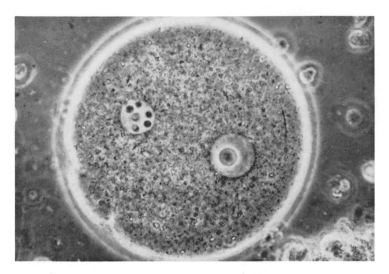

Fig. 1-7. Fertilized ovum 12 hours after ovulation, showing male and female pronuclei, polar body, and a portion of spermatozoon tail. (Mouse, phase contrast, ×320.) (Courtesy Dr. A. H. Gates, Palo Alto, Calif.)

occurs only after cavitation of the developing ovum and after embryonic cells differentiate and trophoblast delineates the shell. It has been postulated that late zona lysis, usually occurring in the uterus, may prevent ectopic implantation or fusion of zygotes to form chimeras.

Sex determination. Mature human ova contain a specialized X chromosome and 22 autosomes, but after the reduction division there are two kinds of spermatozoa—those with an X chromosome and those with a Y chromosome. Thus fertilization may result in either an XX zygote (female) or an XY zygote (male), and the sex of the embryo is determined at the moment of fertilization. Since presumably there are equal numbers of the two kinds of spermatozoa available, there must be some explanation for the unexpected sex ratio at birth of 106 boys to 100 girls (United States, Caucasians). The ratio at the time of fertilization is believed to be very much higher, around 160 male to each 100 female conceptions. It may be that fertilization of ova by Y spermatozoa is much more common than fertilization by X spermatozoa, but no reason for this has been demonstrated.

Many schemes for ascertaining the sex of a fetus in utero have been devised, but at present the only test that is reliable depends on the nuclear *sex chromatin* pattern of fetal cells recovered from amniotic fluid. The sex of embryos may be determined from a study of nuclei in villous stromal cells. It has been predicted that eventually the determination of sex in male will be subject to willful control, probably by the selection of X or Y spermatozoa for fertilization.

One of the two X chromosomes in human female somatic cells becomes condensed in intermitotic nuclei to form the sex chromatin or *Barr body,* which lies adjacent to the nuclear membrane. Its DNA is not used for genetic transcription, in contrast to the euchromatin of the remainder of the chromosomal set. The condensed X is most easily identified in buccal mucosal or vaginal smears appropriately fixed and stained, but is present, of course, throughout all tissue cells. In a normal female at least 20% of well-preserved cells are chromatin-positive in the sense that they possess at least one Barr body. Cells from normal males are chromatin-negative; that is, they lack a Barr body. The presence of a Y chromosome can be established in nondividing cells with quinacrine hydrochloride, a fluorescent compound with great affinity for this chromosome. Since the X chromosome is larger than the Y chromosome, the female has about 3% more genetic material than the male, but the apparent genetic inactivation of the material in the Barr body compensates for this deficiency. Inactivation affects the two X chromosomes at random. Persons with sex chromosome aberrations may possess cells containing more than two X chromosomes, but the additional chromosomes also are inactivated. Thus the number of sex chromatin (Barr) bodies is always one less than the number of X chromosomes in interphase diploid nuclei. Abnormal females who have only one X chromosome have no sex chromatin. Abnormal males with two X chromosomes and a Y chromosome have one Barr body.

Certain cytogenetic defects are produced by an error in cell division known as *trisomy,* a condition in which there are three, rather than two, of a particular pair of chromosomes. Trisomy commonly results from the failure of a pair of chromosomes to separate during the production of oocytes or spermatocytes, and this phenomenon is called *meiotic nondisjunction.* The result is that one cell contains both members of a particular pair of chromosomes and one contains neither. If the cell with an extra chromosome unites with a normal cell, the new individual will have 47 chromosomes, and there will be three instead of merely two members of one particular set of chromosomes. When a cell that lacks a chromosome unites with a normal cell, the resulting individual has 45 chromosomes, or a condition called *monosomy.* It has been estimated that about one child in every 150 live births has some sort of chromosomal abnormality.

If two chromosomes fail to separate during the first cell division after conception, the result is *mosaicism,* in which half the individual's cells are trisomic (with 47 chromosomes) and half are monosomic (with 45 chromosomes). When failure of chromosomal separation occurs even later in embryonic development, there will be three cell types—normal, trisomic, and monosomic. Thus many different sex chromatin patterns have been demonstrated and still others are likely to be discovered. Mosaicism may be produced by other mechanisms, such as anaphase lag (lost chromosome), and may occur in any of the 22 paired autosomes as well as in the sex chromosomes.

The 22 autosomes are assigned Arabic numerals in order of decreasing size. A combination of paired autosomes, plus the associated X and Y chromosomes of a single cell, comprises the *karyotype* of an individual. The visual presentation of such a chromosomal grouping is called an *idiogram.*

2

Implantation and placentation

YOUNG OVUM

As yet few of the earliest cleavage stages of the human ovum have been observed, but it is quite likely that the sequence of events is similar to that seen in monkey ova cultivated in plasma. Studies now in progress on human ova in vitro, however, may eventually provide much of the missing information. It is possible to stimulate follicular development with gonadotropins and obtain fertilizable follicular ova from follicular fluid aspirated from follicles 2 to 3 cm. in diameter under laparoscopic vision. The goal of these efforts, of course, is to culture and inseminate ova outside the host and then implant a dividing ovum in the uterus of a woman with nonfunctioning or absent tubes and have it develop into a normal fetus. At the outset, cleavage divisions occur so rapidly that there is no growth period between succeeding mitoses and therefore no growth of the cell mass as a whole, the individual *blastomeres* becoming smaller and smaller. The result is a solid ball of cells called the *morula*. With rearrangement of blastomeres about a central cavity, the morula becomes a *blastula* or blastodermic vesicle soon after emerging from the uterine tube into the endometrial cavity.

Assuming that ovulation occurs typically on the thirteenth day of the menstrual cycle and that coitus takes place on the same day, fertilization would occur a few hours later in the outer third of the tube. Passage through the tube requires about 3 days, and the blastodermic vesicle remains free in the uterine cavity 4 or 5 days. Some 7 to 8 days after fertilization the zona pellucida disappears and the *trophoblast* (outer cells of the blastocyst) is able to attach itself to the endometrium. During the next day the *trophoblastic villi* burrow into the endometrium, and the embryo finds itself beneath the surface of the uterine mucosa, surrounded by predecidual tissue.

Detailed studies of the physiologic mechanisms by which the trophoblast of the ovum invades the uterine epithelium have been made in rabbits. Apparently a knob of syncytiotrophoblast adheres to the uterine surface over a capillary, and the intervening cells are dissociated by a local rise in pH. Whether the propulsive mechanism that advances the blastocyst resides in the uterus or in the trophoblast has not been elucidated.

Implantation of the human ovum usually occurs in the superior portion of the endometrium, either anteriorly or posteriorly and seldom laterally, and only rarely does it implant so close to the cervix that the placenta subsequently encroaches upon the internal os (placenta previa).

Hertig and Rock studied many early human conceptuses recovered from uteri removed for gynecologic reasons from fertile women whose menstrual and coital histories have been recorded accurately. All the specimens were younger than 16 days, but many were thought to be abnormal in one way or another and exhibited various germ plasm defects. The youngest normal specimen is a dividing ovum in the two-cell stage, found in the oviduct at operation 60 hours after coitus and presumably 3 days after ovulation (estimated from endometrial pattern).

In a 12-day human ovum (Fig. 2-1), the trophoblast is composed of the peripheral *syncytiotrophoblast* and the inner *cytotrophoblast*. The outer masses of cells contain lacunae filled by maternal blood, while the inner cells are preparing to form the future *chorionic villi*. The outstanding feature of such an ovum is the chorionic cavity lined by a membrane continuous with the primitive *entoderm* of the *embryonic disk*. The double-layered disk also contains primitive *ectoderm,* with a primitive *amnion* attached at its edges. Starting on the seventh day, the amnion delaminates in situ from the adjacent cytotrophoblast. Before the entoderm is fully established, the *mesoderm* extends

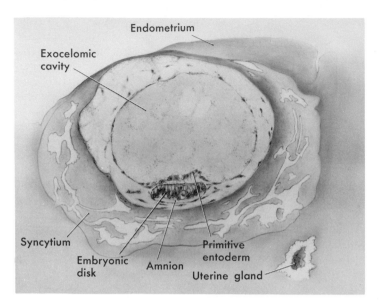

Fig. 2-1. Previllous human ovum near the endometrial surface. Estimated age is about 12 days.

beyond the embryonic disk. Its somatic (outer) portion becomes applied to the trophoblast to form an extranembryonic layer of *somatopleure,* and its splanchnic portion joins the entoderm to form *splanchnopleure.* The cavity thus surrounded by mesoderm is the *coelom* (Fig. 2-2), which at first is entirely extraembryonic.

The cytotrophoblast encircling the chorionic cavity proliferates quickly, comes into contact with maternal blood channels, and sends solid masses out into the syncytium to become the primary chorionic villi. These are observed by the fourteenth day of development.

The establishment of the three "germ layers"—ectoderm, entoderm, and mesoderm—denotes a transition from the developmental period, when more increase in numbers of cells is noticeable, to one in which differentiation of specialized

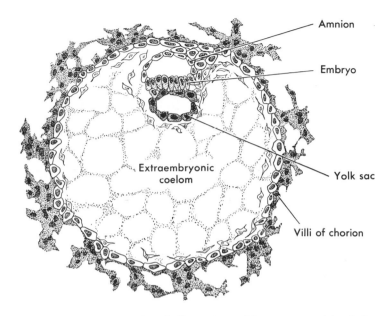

Fig. 2-2. Schematic section of villous stage of human ovum (about six-teenth day).

structures is paramount. The further story of embryology consists of the detailed history of the growth, subdivision, and differentiation of these germ layers. A brief outline is given in Chapter 4, but for details the student should consult textbooks of human embryology (such as those by Arey; Hamilton, Boyd, and Mossman; or Patten).

DEVELOPMENT OF PLACENTA

Mammalian placentas exhibit pronounced differences in various species, and one would be unwise to apply any given information gained from placental study in one species to another, even closely related, species. Grosser's classification of mammalian placentas on the basis of the tissues separating maternal and fetal blood is a helpful concept and should be familiar to all students of obstetrics. In this scheme the human

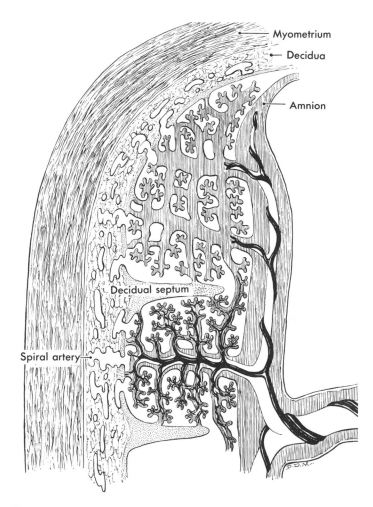

Fig. 2-3. Schematic cross section through segment of mature placenta attached to uterine wall. (See text for details.)

placenta (as well as that of apes, bats, and mice) is hemochorial because fetal chorionic tissues lie in direct contact with maternal blood. Three tissues separate the maternal and fetal blood-streams—epithelium, connective tissue, and vascular endothe-lium of the chorionic villi.

The following descriptions apply only to the human placenta, and its various anatomic portions will be considered separately (Fig. 2-3).

Chorion and intervillous space. Originally a single layer of cells forming the blastodermic vesicle, the portion of the blas-tocyst wall that first comes in contact with the maternal endometrium, grows rapidly to form a *trophoblastic plate.* Cytotrophoblastic buds soon become villi, with mesoblastic cores and outer coverings of syncytiotrophoblast, a cytolytic tissue that invades maternal endometrium. Villi may be ob-served in the human placenta about 12 days after fertilization. It is likely that all three layers of the villus develop from cyto-trophoblast cells. Angioblastic strands appear in the core and pro-duce the endothelium of future blood vessels. At the same time blood cells are formed within the villus, and the vessels of the villus unite with similar channels in the mesoderm around the chorionic cavity. The syncytial lacunae coalesce to form the *intervillous space,* into which some branching villi project, while other villi traverse the space and attach themselves to the endometrium (*fastening* or *anchoring villi*).

Maternal venous sinuses are entered first, but circulation in the intervillous space is not established until about the four-teenth or fifteenth day, when maternal arterioles are invaded. The early embryo is attached to the connective tissue portion of the chorion by the body stalk (abdominal pedicle), the antece-dent of the umbilical cord. Ultimately the embryo's umbilical vessels traverse this stalk and fuse with vessels originating in the chorionic membrane. Thus fetal blood enters the villi, and the mechanism of maternal-fetal exchange is established.

Villi adjacent to the endometrial cavity atrophy because of poor blood supply, and by the third month this portion of the chorion becomes smooth or bald (*chorion laeve*). Villi adjacent to the decidua basalis flourish to form the shaggy or leafy *chorion frondosum* and, eventually, the fetal portion of the placenta.

Thus the chorionic membrane of the gestational sac consists of an inner connective tissue layer, an inner epithelial layer (cytotrophoblast or Langhans' layer), and an outer epithelium (syncytiotrophoblast). Viewed in cross section, a villus shows a similar three-layered structure. The Langhans cells gradually disappear after the sixteenth week, and very few can be found in a term placenta. Most villi are arborescent, ending freely in the intervillous space without reaching the decidua. As the placenta ages, the short stem villi branch repeatedly to form finer subdivisions and increasingly small villi. Each of the main stem villi and its numerous ramifications comprises a *fetal cotyledon*.

The stroma of a young villus contains branching cells separated by much mucoid intercellular material. Later the stromal cells are spindle shaped and closely packed. The so-called Hofbauer cells of the stroma appear to be phagocytes, and they are most numerous in association with defective or infected fetuses. The syncytial cytoplasm has a complex brush border with pseudopodia that presumably engulf particles of maternal plasma and transfer them by pinocytosis to the fetal blood. The trophoblast also serves as an excretory device for numerous fetal waste products. Ultrastructual studies suggest that the syncytium is a differentiated form of trophoblast capable of synthesis of complex molecules and the production of all placental hormones.

Decidua. When conception occurs, the "predecidual" connective tissue cells of the secretory endometrium under the influence of progesterone from the *corpus luteum of pregnancy* become true decidual cells, and the *decidua* begins to develop throughout the whole endometrium. It is called the decidua because it is cast off at the end of pregnancy. It grows much thicker and is thrown into deep furrows, indented with the openings of the uterine glands.

The decidua is composed of three portions (Fig. 2-4). The *decidua basalis* lies at the site of implantation beneath the ovum. The *decidua capsularis* surrounds the growing ovum and excludes it from the rest of the uterine cavity. The *decidua vera* covers the remainder of the uterine cavity. At about the fourth month of gestation the increasing size of the ovum brings the decidua capsularis in contact with the decidua vera, and

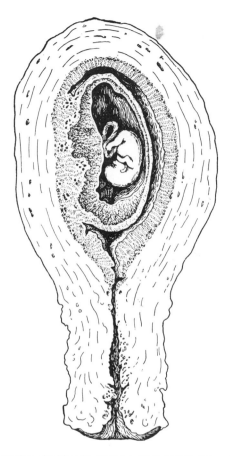

Fig. 2-4. Illustrating decidua in uterus with 2-month fetus. Note decidua vera lining uterine cavity, decidua basalis changing to placenta, and membranes covered with decidua capsularis surrounding the embryo. (Redrawn from Bumm.)

they almost completely disappear, so that at term no evidence of the capsularis can be found.

The decidua consists of three layers: the surface or compacta, the middle or spongiosa, and the basal layer. Early in pregnancy uterine glands may be observed in the compact layer, but they soon disappear, leaving only closely packed oval or polygonal cells with round nuclei. The spongy layer contains hyperplastic endometrial glands separated by small areas of stroma. The basal layer is similar to basal endometrium in the nonpregnant uterus and is the source of endometrial regeneration after labor.

The *decidua basalis* is the area of decidua under the placenta or at the *placental site*. Its spongy portion consists chiefly of arteries and venous sinuses, and at term nearly all glands have disappeared from this area. It contains fetal trophoblastic giant cells that penetrate to various depths, occasionally entering the muscularis. They have also been found floating freely in uterine-vein blood.

Amnion. The amnion begins as a tiny vesicle and then forms a small sac between the cytotrophoblast and the dorsal surface of the embryo; as it enlarges, it completely surrounds the embryo. The amnion and yolk sac, with an intervening embryonic disk, are attached to the chorion by a mesodermal bridge called the body stalk. Growth of the yolk sac ceases after circulation in the chorionic villi is developed.

With advancing size, the amnion comes in contact with the interior of the chorion and obliterates the extraembryonic coelom. The two membranes become adherent but never are intimately fused. The amnion is composed of two layers: an outer layer of mesoderm and an inner layer of ectodermal cells. In a way, it is an extension of the skin of the embryo. Often round plaques 1 to 5 mm. in diameter are seen on the amnion near the attachment of the umbilical cord. These consist of stratified epithelium resembling that of skin and are called *amniotic caruncles*.

Amniotic fluid. The amniotic fluid continuously increases as gestation advances, at least until the thirty-eighth week. At term it normally averages about 1,000 ml. but abnormally may amount to several liters *(hydramnios)*. The reaction of the amniotic fluid is slightly alkaline (pH 7.2). The specific gravity ranges from 1.007 to 1.025, and it contains albumin, urea, uric acid, creatinine, fat, fructose, inorganic salts, epithelial cells, a few leukocytes, various enzymes, and lanugo hairs.

Functions

1. Protects fetus from mechanical injury
2. Prevents adhesions between fetus and amnion

3. Permits free movement of fetus

4. Prevents loss of heat and temperature changes in the fetus

In early pregnancy the fluid is a dialysate of maternal serum across a barrier impermeable to lipids and proteins but relatively permeable to smaller solutes. Thus at first amniotic fluid resembles interstitial fluids in other body spaces. Ultimately this fluid becomes the product of several different exchanges with the fetal circulation. Hypotonic fetal urine is added constantly, and amniotic fluid is swallowed and reabsorbed in the fetal gastrointestinal tract. Free water presumably is removed through another exchange site because the tonicity of amniotic fluid is maintained in a steady state. It may cross the amnion on the fetal surface of the placenta or enter fetal vessels between chorion and amnion. A small net transfer may occur across the chorioamnion into the maternal extracellular space. The water requirements for daily increases in fetal and amniotic fluid spaces are met by a net transfer between maternal and fetal circulations across the placenta. Though there is a large exchange of water between fetus and amniotic sac, there is a very small net transfer of water to the pool of amniotic fluid. Accumulation of excessive amounts of amniotic fluid is caused by a very minor imbalance of transfer rates, whereby a difference of only a few milliliters per hour may lead ultimately to clinical hydramnios. Water and electrolytes are exchanged independently at their own characteristic rates and presumably are in dynamic equilibrium with maternal plasma.

Amniotic fluid obtained by amniocentesis is used for a wide variety of studies concerned with the sex, state of health of the fetus, and its degree of maturity. Cells in the fluid may be cultured for use in the detection of various diseases characterized by enzyme deficiencies or chromosomal abnormalities, and decisions regarding therapeutic abortion may be based on such determinations.

Placenta at term. The placenta is composed of both fetal and maternal tissues. The *fetal portion* consists of the chorion frondosum with villi, and the *maternal portion* consists of the compact decidua basalis.

Villi. The villi of the mature placenta are of two types, free villi and anchoring villi.

Free villi are attached only to the chorionic membrane and float free in the maternal blood of the intervillous spaces. These villi are branched. *Anchoring villi,* relatively fewer in number, are attached at their distal ends to the decidua basalis.

The core of a villus is connective tissue supporting fetal blood vessels. The villi of the mature placenta are covered almost exclusively by syncytium.

Maternal portion. The maternal portion of the mature placenta is mostly compact decidua, with some spongy decidua compressed next to the uterine wall.

It is divided into irregularly shaped lobules or cotyledons. A section through placenta attached to the uterine wall contains, from the inside out, the *chorionic plate* (amnion, fetal vessels, chorion, villi, and placental septa), the *decidual plate* (compact layer), the decidua basalis, and the myometrium. The depressed areas between cotyledons represent fibrous septa of maternal origin (judging from their nuclear sex chromatin). The cotyledons are filled with villi attached to the major villous stalks. A layer of fibrinoid material lies at the level of contact between the trophoblast and decidua. This is called *Nitabuch's layer* and is absent whenever the decidua is deficient.

Physical characteristics. The human placenta at term is a bluish red, round, oval, or irregular disk of spongy tissue 15 to 20 cm. in diameter, 2 to 3 cm. thick, and weighing 500 to 600 grams (Fig. 2-5).

The mature placenta has two surfaces (fetal and maternal).

The *fetal surface* is covered with smooth, glistening amnion, and underneath this cover run the branching vessels that enter and leave the umbilical cord. These vessels dip into the substance of the placenta before reaching its periphery. If they appear to have been interrupted at the placental margin, a *succenturiate* placenta may have been left in the uterus.

The *maternal surface* is the reddish external surface that was attached to the uterus. It is shaggy, with remnants of torn vessels and decidua.

The fetal membranes, both amnion and chorion, merge with the margin of the placenta; the membranes are closely adherent to each other but usually can be peeled apart.

Placental circulation at term. Fetal venous blood flows outward through two umbilical arteries that traverse the cord and then

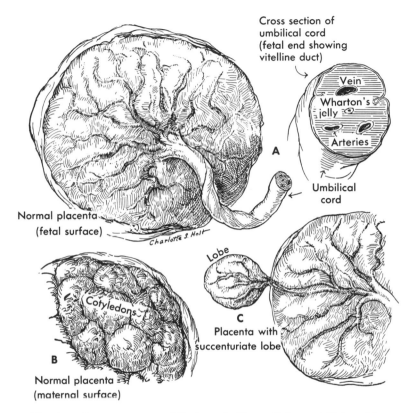

Cross section of
umbilical cord
(fetal end showing
vitelline duct)

Vein

Wharton's
jelly

Arteries

A

Umbilical
cord

Normal placenta
(fetal surface)

Charlotte S. Holt

Lobe

Cotyledons

C
Placenta with
succenturiate lobe

B

Normal placenta
(maternal surface)

Fig. 2-5. Placenta and umbilical cord. (From Falls and McLaughlin: Obstetric and gynecologic nursing, St. Louis, The C. V. Mosby Co.)

through the chorionic plate and into stem villi. Vessels accompany the branching villi and eventually narrow down to capillaries in terminal villi. Oxygenated blood is transported back to the fetus through the umbilical *vein* system. (Note reversal of the usual artery-vein relationship.)

There has been prolonged argument about details of the circulation in the maternal portion of the placenta, and what is written here may not represent the final word. It is now believed by many investigators that numerous spiral arteries of the uterus empty into the intervillous space and that their forceful streams

(70 to 80 mm. Hg pressure) displace overlying villi and produce "lakes" at varying depths in the placental mass. The blood then flows back toward the uterine wall and enters venous exits leading into veins lying more or less parallel with the uterine wall. Apparently this anatomic arrangement provides easy venous closure by uterine contraction and retention of maternal arterial blood in the intervillous space. During uterine contractions, both inflow and outflow are reduced, but the volume of blood in the intervillous space is maintained to provide continual, though reduced, maternal-fetal exchanges. Countercurrent flow, in the usual sense, is precluded by the random distribution of villi in whose capillaries the direction of fetal to maternal flow bears no fixed relationship.

The numerous chorionic villi occupy most of the placental volume and the empty space is relatively small. It is assumed that maternal blood circulates sluggishly in the maze of villi and that its composition changes as it travels from arterial to venous ends of the uteroplacental circulation. Thus the content of respiratory gas in a blood sample from the "intervillous space" will depend on the precise locale sampled by the needle and, particularly, on whether the needle is in the true intervillous space or in an adjacent vessel.

The flow of maternal blood through the placenta per minute exceeds the circulation of fetal blood through the villous system. Pressure within the placental intervillous space rises when the pregnant woman assumes an erect posture, but fetal capillary pressure tends to remain constant at about 20 mm. Hg.

In the main the two circulations are separate, but fetal cells may escape from damaged villi into the maternal circulation. This is assumed to be the basis for Rh and ABO isoimmunization in pregnancy. Various observations also suggest that maternal blood cells and even trophoblastic giant cells can enter the fetal circulation.

Immunologic interactions in the placenta have been studied extensively, but no completely acceptable explanation for survival of the fetoplacental allograft, with its foreign antigens, has been documented. The reason why even less reactivity occurs in successive pregnancies is even more obscure. A recent hypothesis suggests that pericellular sialomucins of the trophoblast present a chemical barrier to immunologically competent cells, but it is obvious that much more investigation of this complex problem is needed.

UMBILICAL CORD (FUNIS)

The umbilical cord or funis extends from the navel of the fetus to the placenta. It transmits fetal venous blood from the fetus through *two arteries* to the placenta, returning arterial blood by *one vein* from the placenta. Venous and arterial blood are more or less mixed in the fetal vessels, but the blood in the arteries is chiefly venous and that in the vein chiefly arterial. Its diameter ranges from 1 to 2.5 cm. and its length from 30 to 100 cm. The right umbilical vein usually disappears early, leaving only the original left vein. A common vascular anomaly is the absence of one umbilical artery, a condition often associated with other severe fetal anomalies, such as esophageal atresia and imperforate anus. The absence of one umbilical artery has been noted in 1% of cords of singletons and in 5% of the cords of at least one twin.

Since the vessels are usually longer than the cord, it has a coiled and twisted appearance. Nodulations on the surface are produced by folded vessels. The cord is covered by adherent amnion, and the interior is a watery material called *Wharton's jelly*. Because of this high water content, the cord dries up quickly after birth.

Resistance to outflow of blood from the cord keeps it distended and facilitates blood flow with minimal friction, despite the relatively great length of cord.

Two embryologic remnants may be found in the umbilical cord upon microscopic examination. The duct or stalk of the umbilical vesicle (yolk sac) may be found in sections through any segment, and remains of the allantois may be found at the fetal end of the cord. The umbilical vesicle persists as an oval sac 3 to 5 mm. in diameter, lying between the amnion and chorion on the fetal surface of the placenta. The intra-abdominal portion of the umbilical duct usually atrophies, but it may persist as *Meckel's diverticulum*.

(For discussion of placental physiology, see Chapters 3 and 4.)

3

Endocrine function in pregnancy

The processes of ovulation, fertilization, implantation, and placentation have been described in the foregoing chapters without reference to their dependency on hormonal initiation and without reference to the concomitant secondary hormone production which has afforded both the biochemical preparation and support for these events. To establish an integrated picture of the entire process, a brief résumé of the variety and activity of these hormones would appear to be a profitable prelude to discussion of endocrine activity following placentation.

HYPOTHALAMIC, ANTERIOR PITUITARY, AND OVARIAN ACTIVITY

A complex interplay between hormonal substances produced by the hypothalamus, pituitary, and ovary are responsible for ovulation. These substances and the products of their activity also provoke other biochemical and histologic effects necessary for the initiation of reproduction. These include facilitation of the transport and maturation of sperm and ovum as well as the preparation of a suitable nutritional bed for the embryo within the uterus.

Follicle stimulating hormone (FSH), a water-soluble glycoprotein produced by the anterior pituitary, initiates and supports ovarian follicular development, maturation of the contained ovum, and production of estrogens.

Luteinizing hormone (LH), a similar glycoprotein produced by the same anterior pituitary cells, acts in conjunction with FSH and provokes ovulation, stimulates conversion of the mature follicle to a corpus luteum, and aids in the maintenance of corpus luteum function.

Nerve endings within the hypothalamus produce a releasing factor, a decapeptide, which initiates the synthesis and release of both FSH and LH from the anterior pituitary. This luteinizing releasing factor (LRF) is transported from the hypothalamus to the pituitary via a unique portal vascular system along the pituitary stalk. Relatively constant levels of pituitary FSH and LH are produced during the preovulatory phase and result in the gradual maturation of a number of ovarian follicles, only one of which typically reaches full development during a single menstrual cycle. A 24- to 48-hour long surge in the release of these hormones occurs at the time of ovulation. The LH surge is considerably greater than that of FSH (Fig. 3-1) and is re-

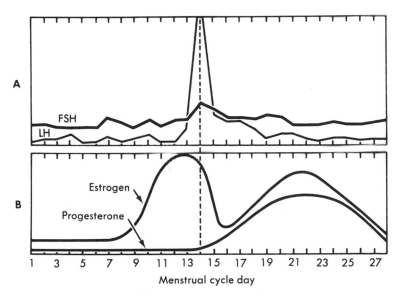

Fig. 3-1. Schematic representation of plasma levels of FSH and LH, **A,** and estrogen and progesterone, **B,** during the menstrual cycle. Ovulation is arbitrarily designated as occurring on cycle day 14.

sponsible for triggering the process of follicular rupture. Circulating levels of FSH and LH thereafter return essentially to preovulatory levels for the remainder of the cycle.

A variable and quantitatively preferential secretion of FSH and/or LH apparently occurs from the single pituitary cell type in response to the single hypothalamic releasing factor. The mechanism whereby this is accomplished is poorly understood. It currently appears that rising levels of 17β-estradiol produced by the developing follicles exert an interrelated negative and positive feedback either on the production of LRF by the hypothalamus or on the sensitivity of the gonadotropin-producing cells of the pituitary to LRF or both. Authorities have long recognized that both endogenous and exogenous estrogens exert a negative feedback action on gonadotropin production by the hypothalamic-pituitary unit. This is considered to develop as a result of both inhibition of hypothalamic LRF release and diminished sensitivity of anterior pituitary cells to the releasing factor. There is current evidence to suggest, however, that as estradiol levels slowly rise during the first half of the menstrual cycle, a change in estrogen feedback sensitivity occurs. A progressive decrease in the negative feedback activity develops in association with a progressive increase in positive feedback action from the same hormone. Positive feedback creates maximal preferential production of LH in response to LRF as well as maximal pituitary responsiveness to LRF in general. The result is the midcycle surge in gonadotropin production and ovulation. Positive feedback effect is rapidly lost thereafter. It does not recur with the postovulatory rise in estrogen levels, possibly because of the negative feedback action of concurrently secreted progesterone, but returns selectively at the preovulatory point in the next cycle.

The ovarian follicle, maturing under the influence of FSH, produces several estrogens, the most potent of these being 17β-estradiol. This estrogen and its oxidative derivative (estrone) are responsible for essentially all physiologic estrogenization, including the development and maintenance of female secondary sexual characteristics, changes in tubal and cervical physiologic condition favoring maturation and transport of sperm and ovum, and the endometrial growth seen during the proliferative phase of the endometrial cycle.

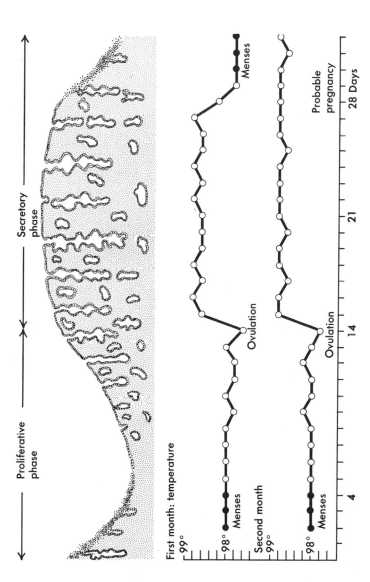

Fig. 3-2. Schematic representation of the endometrial cycle and basal body temperature curves. The corresponding hormonal changes are shown in Fig. 3-1. (From Benson: Handbook of obstetrics and gynecology, ed. 3, Los Altos, Calif., 1968, Lange Medical Publications.)

Ovulation commonly occurs 13 to 14 days prior to menstruation. After ovulation, the mature follicle is converted to a corpus luteum. Progesterone is secreted by the corpus luteum and converts the proliferative endometrium to a progestational (secretory) variety capable of receiving and nourishing a fertilized ovum. Estrogens continue to be produced by the follicular cells, after the cells' conversion into a corpus luteum. When pregnancy does not occur, the corpus luteum expires and, in the wake of falling estrogen and progesterone titers, menstruation ensues (Fig. 3-2).

MENSTRUAL CYCLE

Menstruation is the shedding of secretory endometrium, starting approximately 14 days after ovulation. The day on

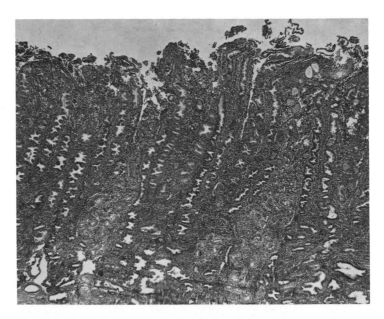

Fig. 3-3. Photomicrograph of progestational endometrium shortly after onset of menstruation, showing absence of epithelial surface and irregular loss of stratum compactum. (×33.)

which menstruation begins is called the first day of the cycle. The duration of bleeding is usually 4 to 5 days, sometimes less, but it may last up to 7 days without being considered abnormal. The intervals between the beginnings of successive menstruations vary a good deal even in the same individual. Although the average cycle for adult women is 28 days, the range is from 21 to 35 days. However, cycles of less than 25 days or more than 34 days are uncommon.

The menstrual cycle is divided into three phases: menstrual, proliferative, and secretory.

The *menstrual phase,* the breaking up and shedding of the compact and spongy layers of the endometrium, is initiated by vasoconstriction in the spiral arterioles (Figs. 3-3 and 3-4).

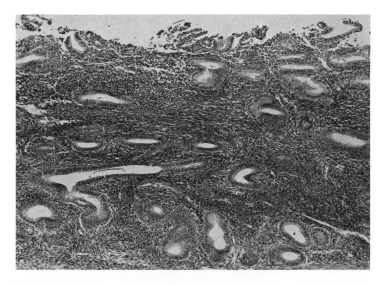

Fig. 3-4. Photomicrograph of endometrium on third day of menstruation. Fragments of stratum spongiosum remain superficial to the denser basal layer. (×95.)

The basal layer and part of the spongiosa remain intact and provide glandular epithelium for regeneration of the surface. Menstrual discharge contains blood, mucus, and fragments of endometrial tissue. The blood usually does not clot because its fibrin has already been destroyed by proteolytic enzymes.

The *proliferative phase,* also called the estrogenic, follicular, or preovulatory phase, is synchronous with the growth of the ovarian follicle or from the end of menstruation to the time of ovulation (Fig. 3-5). Regeneration of the endometrial surface may be completed on cycle day 4 or 5, 1 or 2 days before external bleeding ceases. The mucosa increases in thickness from 1 to perhaps 10 mm. in about 10 days. Narrow tubular glands contain columnar cells with centrally placed oval nuclei. The stroma is dense and relatively avascular. There is active mitosis. As growth continues, the glandular nuclei shift to basal positions, and glands become wavy because of increase in length.

The *secretory phase,* also called the postovulatory or pro-

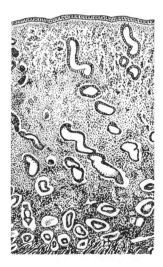

Fig. 3-5. Proliferative endometrium. Simple tubular glands in a young stroma.

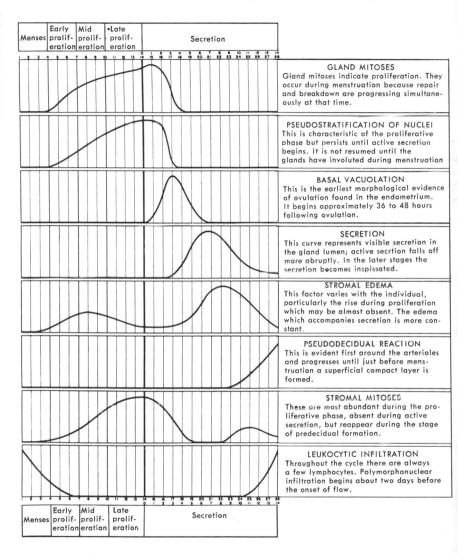

Fig. 3-6. Temporal and quantitative histologic changes seen in the endometrium during the menstrual cycle. (From Noyes, Hertig, and Rock: Fertility and sterility **1**:3, Baltimore, 1950, The Williams & Wilkins Co.)

gestational phase, corresponds to the luteal phase of the ovary. During this time estrogen continues the process of endometrial proliferation, and progesterone produces other histologic changes characteristic of the secretory pattern (Fig. 3-6). Glands become tortuous and the stroma vascular and edematous. The glandular cells bulge with secretion. Eventually three zones are distinguishable: the superficial *stratum compactum,* the intermediate *stratum spongiosum,* and the inner *basal* zone. The endometrium is now ready to receive and nourish the fertilized ovum. If pregnancy does not ensue, hormonal support of the endometrium is withdrawn because of death of the corpus luteum and the bleeding phase begins. Actual vaginal bleeding is preceded by a brief period of ischemia and necrosis, followed by the opening of spiral arteries with extravasation of blood into the superficial tissues.

The precise hormonal or chemical mechanism responsible for menstrual bleeding has not been established. It has been suggested that steroids in some manner control the permeability of lysosomal membranes in endometrial cells. The disruption of the cytoplasmic organelles interferes with the ability of certain enzymes to metabolize catecholamines, and the latter accumulate in sufficient concentration to produce spasm of spiral arterioles in the endometrium. This, in turn, leads to anoxia, necrosis, and dissolution of tissue.

PLACENTAL HORMONES

The syncytiotrophoblast of the chorionic villus produces a luteotropic substance called human chorionic gonadotropin (HCG) (Fig. 3-7). This hormone is excreted in the urine essentially unchanged, and its presence in either plasma or urine forms the basis for the majority of the tests for pregnancy. It is detectable as early as 4 to 5 days after implantation but seldom reaches levels required for most pregnancy tests until 10 to 20 days later. Plasma and urinary concentrations, as measured by biologic tests, rise rapidly, are maximal 60 to 80 days after ovulation, and thereafter fall to roughly one tenth of peak value and remain at this level or decline slowly until parturition. When measured by immunologic tests, however, HCG production falls off only to about one-third of peak value by 120 days after ovula-

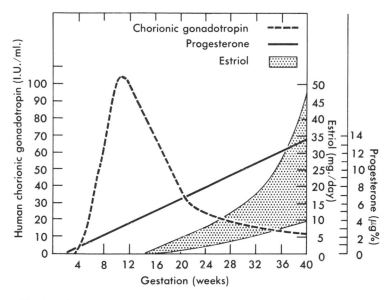

Fig. 3-7. Schematic representation of changes in human serum chorionic gonadotropin (I.U. per milliliter), urinary estriol excretion (milligrams per day), and plasma progesterone (micrograms per 100 ml.).

tion. It thereafter rises slowly to term but never again approximates peak levels. Researchers do not know why its biologic activity seems to decline and its immunologic activity seems to persist after the first trimester. HCG is undetectable in urine within approximately a week after placental delivery. The total lack of dependence on the fetus for its production is shown in the continued excretion of HCG when the placenta is left attached to intra-abdominal structures after fetal removal in an abdominal pregnancy and in the extremely large amounts of HCG excreted by patients with hydatid moles and choriocarcinoma. Large amounts may also be excreted with multiple pregnancy and erythroblastosis.

HCG has biologic and immunologic properties similar to those of LH. It appears to prolong and enhance the activity of the corpus luteum by providing progesterone precursors but does not stimulate the ovaries in higher primates in the sense of producing follicular growth, ovulation, or luteinization. Although the rapidly rising HCG titer in early pregnancy results in accentuated estrogen and progesterone secretion from the ovaries, the greatest secretion of these hormones occurs after the decline in HCG titer and at this time undoubtedly results from fetoplacental steroidogenesis.

Recent studies have disclosed that the syncytiotrophoblast produces other hormones as well. One of these is human placental lactogen, currently termed human chorionic somatomammotropin (HCS). This is a polypeptide that has both lactogenic and growth hormone–like activity in test animals. Radioimmunoassays of this substance demonstrate a gradually increasing titer throughout pregnancy to a peak at term of approximately 10 times early pregnancy levels. HCS production parallels placental weight (which HCG does not) and possibly reflects placental function. However, efforts to employ the assay clinically for this purpose have not yet demonstrated consistent validity. HCS disappears from the maternal circulation within 1 or 2 days after placental delivery and is absent from the serum of nursing mothers. The precise effects of this hormone on the fetal and maternal organisms, its interplay with other substances, and the necessity for its existence have not yet been elucidated. The same is true for the recently demonstrated placental production of human chorionic thyrotropin, a protein hormone immunologically and biologically similar to pituitary thyrotropin. The demonstration of placental production of other analogs of anterior pituitary hormones is anticipated.

The chorioplacental system (in concert with fetal and maternal organs) is also known to produce large amounts of steroid hormones needed during pregnancy. For example, the urinary excretion of estrone, estradiol, and estriol rises rapidly in the latter half of pregnancy. The fetus and placenta are synergistically active in the conversion of both maternal and fetal precursor steroids to maternal urinary estriol. This steroid predominates in pregnancy urine and is normally found in amounts ranging from 4 mg. per day at 18 weeks to 10 to 50 mg. per day at term. Similarly significant elevations are seen in amniotic fluid and maternal plasma as well. These values serve as an index of placental function and fetal well-being and are noted to be depressed with hydatid mole, anencephaly, and fetal death. They may also be depressed with toxemia, prematurity, postmaturity, diabetes, and other conditions if fetal health is compromised. A sudden or progressive fall in estriol levels or a failure of these levels to rise as pregnancy progresses presupposes a deficit in placental or fetal tissue function and suggests that fetal life is in jeopardy. Early termination of pregnancy should be seriously considered under these circumstances. Estriol determinations are not of value in patients receiving large doses of adrenocorticosteroids or those with Rh isoimmunization. Progesterone is also produced by the placenta and is produced in increasing amounts during pregnancy, as noted in both the rising plasma progesterone levels (from less than 1 to 14 μg.%) and in the progressive urinary excretion of pregnanediol (from 5 to 100 mg. per day). Among its other roles, progesterone probably serves as a precursor for fetal steroid synthesis, especially by the adrenal gland. Adrenocortical hormones are apparently not produced by the placenta, although they are known to traverse the placenta quite freely.

The assumption of identical functions by the ovary and by the placenta explains why it is possible in the human being to sacrifice one or both ovaries early in pregnancy without disturbing gestation. This assumption is not true in most laboratory animals in which corpora lutea are essential to maintain pregnancy.

LACTATION

Prolactin or lactogenic hormone is also secreted by the anterior pituitary and its production is modulated by the hypothalamus. This is currently believed to be effected through the action of a prolactin release–inhibiting factor although the activity of a prolactin releasing factor has not been eliminated. Interestingly, thyrotropin releasing factor also has a prolactin releasing effect. Plasma concentrations of prolactin rise substantially and progressively during pregnancy, reach a ten- to twentyfold elevation by the early puerperium, and are elevated even further by suckling. Although the hormone appears to be required for lactation, its mechanism of action is unknown.

During gestation, estrogen and progesterone from the placenta prepare the breast for puerperal lactation. Estrogen stimulates ductal development, whereas progesterone promotes alveolar growth and maturation. It is possible that chorionic somato-mammotropin is also involved in the preparation for lactation, but this has not been established. Blood levels of all three hormones fall abruptly upon placental delivery and before lactation is initiated. This apparently sets the stage for prolactin activity and milk production.

Oxytocin is secreted by the posterior pituitary and promotes expression of milk by causing contraction of myoepithelial cells in the alveoloductal system. Suckling, or the anticipation of such, initiates a reflex that results in oxytocin release and milk ejection or "letdown." Lactation can occur, however, without the presence of oxytocin. These are the rudiments but the precise and integrated neurohumoral mechanisms involved in successful lactation are complex and, as yet, unknown.

4

Fetal development and physiology

FETUS IN VARIOUS LUNAR MONTHS OF PREGNANCY

From a medicolegal aspect it is important that one be able to estimate the approximate age of the embryo or fetus by gross inspection. From the time of implantation until the end of the eighth week when organogenesis is largely completed, the product of fertilization is called an *embryo*. After the end of the eighth week and until the completion of pregnancy, it is called a *fetus* (Fig. 4-1). Major changes occurring in the various periods of pregnancy are listed below. (Pregnancy is assumed to have begun at time of fertilization, and all lengths refer to the crown-rump measurement.)

First two weeks. The youngest human conception studied consisted mainly of the chorionic vesicle, to one side of whose interior aspect was attached the microscopic embryo, a plate-like grouping of cells covered by amnion. The great bulk of the embryo consisted of yolk sac (Chapter 2).

Third week

1. The medullary groove and canal, followed by the head folds, are formed.

2. The abdominal pedicle (beginning of the umbilical cord) comes off the tail end of the embryo.

3. Somewhat later are noted the double heart, cerebral and optic vesicles, and visceral arches and clefts.

4. Limb buds appear on the surface about the twenty-first day.

5. The length of the embryo is 2.5 to 4 mm.

Fourth week

1. The embryo increases greatly in size.

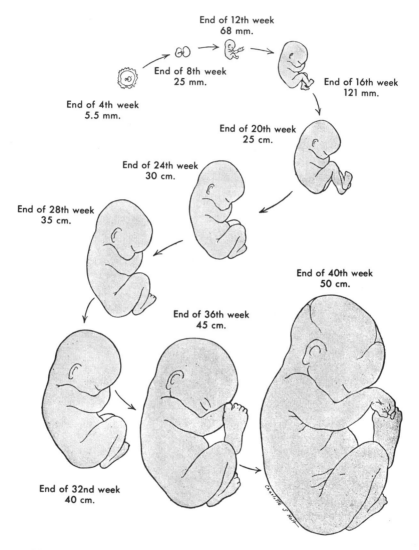

Fig. 4-1. The fetus at different ages. (From Falls and McLaughlin: Obstetric and gynecologic nursing, St. Louis, The C. V. Mosby Co.)

2. It becomes noticeably flexed upon its ventral surface so that the head and tail ends almost touch each other.

3. The rudiments of the eyes, ears, and nose appear.

4. The umbilical vesicle becomes considerably pedunculated.

5. The first traces of all organs become differentiated.

6. The length of the embryo is 7.5 to 10 mm.

Second month (4 to 8 weeks)

1. The embryo is noticeably bent on itself.

2. The visceral clefts and arches are prominent.

3. The extremities are rudimentary.

4. In the seventh and eighth weeks the head becomes disproportionately large because of the development of the brain, while the nose, mouth, and ears are relatively small.

5. The extremities differentiate into their three component parts.

6. The circulatory system between the embryo and the chorion is completed and cardiac pulsations begin.

7. The length of the fetus at the end of the second month is 3 to 3.5 cm.

Third month (8 to 12 weeks)

1. The centers of ossification appear in most of the bones.

2. The fingers and toes are distinct, with soft nails.

3. The external genitalia begin to show definite signs of sexual differentiation. A fetus born at this time may make spontaneous movements if still within the amniotic sac.

4. The length of the fetus is 7 to 9 cm. (2.8 to 3.6 inches), and its weight is about 14 grams.

5. The external genitalia appear in the eighth week, but the sex can be determined only by histologic study of the gonads.

Fourth month (12 to 16 weeks). The length of the fetus varies from 10 to 17 cm. (4 to 6 inches); its weight ranges from 20 to 90 grams. The sex can definitely be determined. Lobulated kidneys are present in their final location, vagina and anus are patent, and meconium has appeared in the intestine. The fetus is quite active.

Fifth month (16 to 20 weeks). A downy covering (lanugo) appears over the entire body, and a small amount of hair appears on the head. The length of the fetus varies from 18 to 25 cm. (7 to 10 inches), and the weight varies from 280 to 300 grams.

Sixth month (20 to 24 weeks)

1. The thin, reddish skin is wrinkled, and fat begins to be deposited beneath it.

2. The head is still comparatively large.

3. If born, the fetus attempts to breathe but never survives more than a few hours.

4. The length varies from 28 to 34 cm. (about 10 to 13 inches), and the weight is about 600 grams.

Seventh month (24 to 28 weeks)

1. The skin is red and covered with *vernix caseosa,* a mixture of epithelial cells, lanugo, and sebaceous gland secretion.

2. The pupillary membrane has just disappeared from the eyes.

3. A fetus born at this time breathes, cries weakly, moves its limbs, but usually dies. Exceptionally, with expert care the baby may survive. The length varies from 35 to 38 cm., and the weight is 1,000 grams or more.

Eighth month (28 to 32 weeks)

1. The skin is still red and wrinkled, and the appearance is that of a "little old man."

2. The length is 40 to 43 cm. (16 to 18 inches) and the weight about 1,800 grams.

3. A fetus born at this time often survives if it has proper care.

Ninth month (32 to 36 weeks)

1. The face has lost its wrinkled appearance as a result of the deposition of subcutaneous fat.

2. The length is about 46 cm., and the weight is 2,500 grams or more by the end of this period.

3. Infants born during this month have a good chance of survival.

Tenth month (36 to 40 weeks)

1. Full term is reached at the end of the tenth month.

2. The length is 50 to 55 cm. (20 to 22 inches), and the weight is about 3,400 grams or 7½ pounds.

3. The skin is smooth and without lanugo, except about the shoulders.

4. *Vernix caseosa* is present over the entire body.

5. The scalp hair is usually dark.

6. The nose and ear cartilages are well developed.

7. The fingers and toes have well-developed nails projecting beyond their tips.

8. In males the testes are usually within the scrotum. In females the labia majora are well developed and are in contact with one another.

9. The skull bones are ossified. An ossification center in the distal epiphysis of the femur appears in nearly all fetuses during early portion of this month, and an ossification center in the proximal epiphysis of the tibia is seen in about 80% at birth.

10. The eyes are uniformly slate colored, and it is impossible to predict their final hue.

HAASE'S RULE FOR LENGTH OF FETUS

The length of the embryo or fetus in centimeters may be approximated during the first 5 months by squaring the number of the lunar month of gestation; after the fifth month, multiply the month by 5, for example:

At the end of the first lunar month, $1 \times 1 = 1$ cm.

At the end of the second lunar month, $2 \times 2 = 4$ cm., etc.

At the end of the sixth lunar month, $6 \times 5 = 30$ cm., etc.

At the end of the tenth lunar month, $10 \times 5 = 50$ cm.

WEIGHT OF NEWBORN INFANT

The average newborn infant weights about 3,400 grams (7½ pounds). Boys weigh about 100 grams (3 ounces) more than girls. Perfectly healthy newborn infants at term may weigh from 2,500 to 5,000 grams (5½ to 11 pounds). Newborn babies rarely weigh more than 11 pounds; although small babies may be at full term, one weighing less than 2,500 grams should be considered premature unless the length exceeds 45 cm. Generally speaking, premature infants weighing less than 1,000 grams or measuring less than 35 cm. in length have little chance of life, although one occasionally survives. Weights vary according to race, size of the parents, age, number of children, and the mother's nutrition during pregnancy.

HEAD OF NEWBORN INFANT

The head of the newborn infant is its most important part because labor is largely the adaptation of the head to the mother's pelvis, through which it must pass.

The face is only a small part of the head. The rest is composed of the skull, which is made up of two frontal, two parietal,

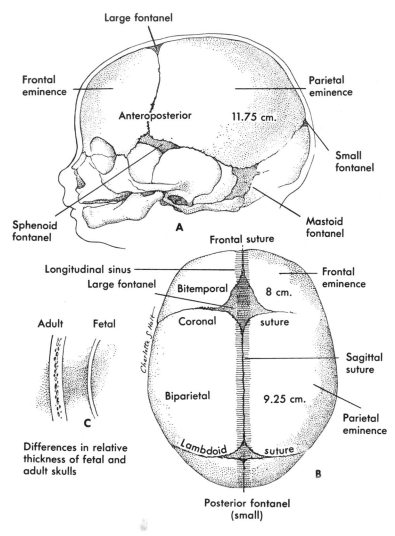

Fig. 4-2. The newborn infant's head. (From Falls and McLaughlin: Obstetric and gynecologic nursing, St. Louis, The C. V. Mosby Co.)

two temporal bones; the upper portion of the occipital bone; and the wings of the sphenoid bone. These bones are separated by the following *sutures* or *membranous spaces* (Fig. 4-2):

1. *Frontal*—between the two frontal bones
2. *Sagittal*—between the two parietal bones
3. *Coronal*—between the frontal and parietal bones
4. *Lambdoid*—between the parietal bones and the upper margin of the occipital bone
5. *Temporal*—on each side between the inferior margin of the parietal and the upper margin of the temporal bone

Where the sutures meet, there is an irregular space closed by a membrane, called a *fontanel*. Although several of these may be outlined, two have special clinical significance and usefulness:

1. The large or *anterior* fontanel (bregma) is a four-sided, lozenge-shaped space at the junction of the sagittal, coronal, and frontal sutures.
2. The small or *posterior* fontanel is small and triangular and lies at the intersection of the sagittal and lambdoid sutures.

There may be *temporal* fontanels at the junction of the lambdoid and temporal sutures.

Palpation and identification of these sutures and fontanels furnish important information during labor in determining the presentation and position of the fetus. Occasionally another lozenge-shaped space, the *sagittal* fontanel, may be found midway between the anterior and posterior fontanels. If this is large, it may lead to error in estimating the degree of flexion of the fetal head.

To estimate the adaptability of the fetal head to the mother's pelvis, one needs to know certain *diameters* and *circumferences*. The following are the average normal diameters most frequently considered in clinical situations:

Transverse (Fig. 4-2)

1. *Biparietal* (B.P.)—9.25 cm.; the greatest transverse diameter of the head from one parietal bone to the other. This is customarily the greatest transverse diameter that must traverse the maternal pelvis.
2. *Bitemporal* (B.T.)—8 cm.; the greatest distance between the two temporal sutures.

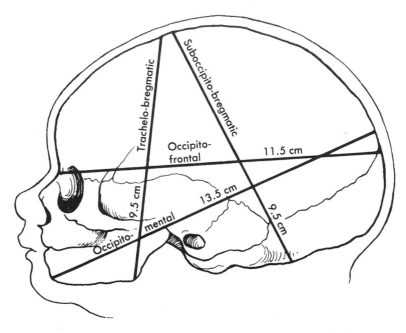

Fig. 4-3. Average anteroposterior diameters of the fetal head.

Anteroposterior (Fig. 4-3)

1. *Suboccipitobregmatic* (S.O.B.)—9.5 cm.; extends from the middle of the large fontanel to the undersurface of the occipital bone, just where it joins the neck. This is the anteroposterior diameter presented to the maternal pelvis with occipital presentations and is the one most commonly seen. With the biparietal diameter it forms a nearly circular plane and presents the smallest possible circumference, 29 cm.

2. *Occipitofrontal* (O.F.)—11.5 cm.; extends from the most prominent portion of the occipital bone to the root of the nose. This is the anteroposterior diameter presented to the maternal pelvis with syncipital presentations and presents a circumference of 34 cm.

3. *Occipitomental* (O.M.)—13.5 cm; extends from the most prominent portion of the occiput to the chin. This is the anteroposterior diameter presented to the maternal pelvis with brow presentations and presents a circumference of 38 cm., the largest of the various planes.

4. *Trachelobregmatic* (T.B.)—9.5 cm.; extends from the anterior junction of the neck and lower jaw to the bregma. This is the anteroposterior diameter presented to the maternal pelvis with face presentations and presents a circumference of 29 cm., essentially identical to that of occipital presentations.

Because of the mobility of the bones of the head at the sutures, the diameters of the head may be altered during labor, thus permitting adjustment of the head diameters to the diameters of the pelvis. This process is called *molding*. Additionally, syncipital and brow presentations usually spontaneously convert during labor to vertex or face presentations to take advantage of the smaller circumferences.

PHYSIOLOGY OF FETUS

Nutrition. Provisions for the sustenance of the ovum from cell division until birth are extensive.

In uterine cavity. While the ovum lies in the uterus several days awaiting completion of the trophoblast so that it can implant itself, its nutriment is provided by the pabulum in the uterine cavity, which is provided by the endometrial secretion.

In endometrium. When the ovum has digested its way into the endometrium, it lies in a little lake (lacuna) of fluid, presumably formed from tissue digested by the trophoblast, which is known to contain a tryptic ferment. It may be assumed that maternal serum and endometrial glycogen continue the nutrition of the ovum.

Nourishment from maternal blood occurs very early when the trophoblast opens up endometrial vessels, and irregular spaces filled with maternal blood are formed—the forerunners of the intervillous spaces of the placenta. Only buds ("rudimentary villi") of future villi are present at this time. "Primitive villi" rapidly develop from the rudimentary villi, but they serve, as yet, only to increase the absorbing surface, for they contain no fetal vessels and nutritive materials are transmitted by osmosis.

Through fetal circulation

1. In the third week of gestation, perhaps earlier, blood vessels form in situ in the chorionic membrane and villi (Chapter 2).

2. At the same time branches of the umbilical vessels approach the chorion and finally fuse with the vessels that have originated in the chorion. Thus the fetal circulation during the fourth week reaches the villi.

3. Hematopoiesis begins in the liver and spleen about the second month, although islands of blood cells may be seen even earlier in the yolk sac. At first all the red blood cells are nucleated, but by the third month only 10% retain their nuclei, and at term the incidence of nucleated erythrocytes is 5% to 8%. Fetal hemoglobin (hemoglobin F) is mixed in varying proportions with the adult type (A) after midpregnancy, but even at term approximately two thirds the hemoglobin is of the fetal type. This amount is advantageous in that fetal hemoglobin, at all levels of oxygen tension, absorbs oxygen more fully and releases it more completely (i.e., has greater oxygen dissociation) than does adult hemoglobin. Essentially complete conversion to adult hemoglobin is accomplished within a few months after birth. Fetal hemoglobin is synthesized primarily in the liver, and ferritin, which is essential in its production, may be found in the liver during the second month.

Fetal circulation. Because the fetus does not derive its nourishment from its digestive tract or its oxygen from its lungs but receives both from the mother's blood by way of the placenta, the fetal blood must be sidetracked to the placenta.

1. From the left ventricle, blood is pumped into the aorta and thence throughout the body, as in the adult.

2. The bypass to the placenta is provided by the two *hypogastric arteries* running from the internal iliac arteries to the umbilicus.

3. Passing through the umbilicus, they become the *umbilical arteries,* traversing the umbilical cord to the chorionic villi of the placenta.

4. After absorbing oxygen and nutritional material from the mother's blood and giving off carbon dioxide and excreted substances, the blood returns to the fetus through the umbilical vein.

5. At the umbilicus the vein divides into a smaller and a larger branch.

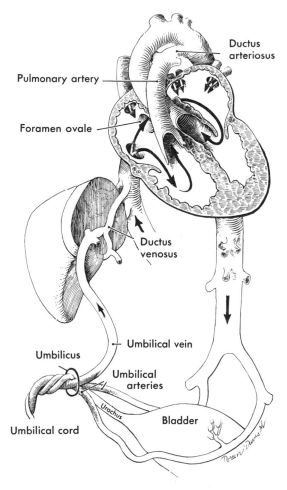

Fig. 4-4. Major circulatory pathways of the mature fetus in utero.

6. The smaller branch carries blood to the liver, through which it circulates, reaching the inferior vena cava through the hepatic vein.

7. The larger branch empties directly into the vena cava through a bypass called the *ductus venosus* (Fig. 4-4).

8. The oxygenated blood from the placenta mixes with the venous blood from the lower extremities in the inferior vena cava, whence it enters the right auricle.

9. A little of it goes to the right ventricle.

10. Most of it, however, is directed by the *eustachian valve* through the *foramen ovale* (an opening between the two auricles).

11. Then the blood goes to the left ventricle and thence is pumped into the aorta.

12. Blood from the head and upper body, by way of the superior vena cava, flows into the right auricle, crosses the stream from the inferior vena cava without appreciable mixing, and enters the right ventricle.

13. Then it is pumped into the pulmonary arteries, but very little blood goes to the nonfunctioning lungs.

14. Most of it crosses by another bypass, the *ductus arteriosus*, to the arch of the aorta and then around the circuit again. Because of the sidetracking through the various bypasses, the blood of the fetus is never strictly arterial (fully oxygenated) or strictly venous, but that in the inferior vena cava is more richly oxygenated than that in the aorta.

15. The relative amount of blood in the placenta diminishes as pregnancy advances, and at term about two thirds of it is in the fetus and one third in the placenta. Intrafetal blood volume at delivery is approximately 80 ml./kg.

Distinctive features of fetal circulation

1. The *ductus venosus* carries arterial blood from the umbilical vein to the inferior vena cava.

2. The *eustachian valve* is a fold that directs the blood in the right auricle toward the foramen ovale.

3. The *foramen ovale* is the opening between the two auricles.

4. The *ductus arteriosus* carries blood from the pulmonary artery to the arch of the aorta.

5. The *hypogastric arteries* run from the internal iliac arteries to the umbilicus, where they become the umbilical arteries.

After birth these structures undergo decided changes. As soon as the lungs expand when the baby breathes, a large quantity of blood goes to the lungs through the normal pulmonary vessels, and none goes through the ductus arteriosus; the ductus arteriosus closes in a minute or two, presumably because of its prominent elastic and muscular tissue. The stimulus for functional closure is the oxygen pressure of the blood passing through it. The effect is reversible in that lowering of blood P_{O_2} may reopen the ductus. Any factor interfering with oxygenation of fetal blood will keep the ductus open and create a "blue" baby. This concept seems to be substantiated by the greatly increased incidence of patent ductus arteriosus in residents of the Andes Mountains.

The ductus venosus is occluded during the first week after birth. The hypogastric arteries carry no blood after the umbilical cord ceases pulsating, and obliteration is complete 3 or 4 days after birth.

As the lungs develop in late fetal life, there is a reduction in interauricular flow and then an abrupt functional closure of this one-way valve at the time of birth when tension in the right auricle is diminished. The valve admits a probe for another 6 to 8 months, but the size of the opening diminishes gradually as the flap is converted into part of the septum. In 20% of adults the fibrous adhesion of the septum is never entirely completed.

Measurements of *fetal blood flow* at various times in pregnancy suggest that it is about 11 ml. per 100 grams per minute. The normal fetal heart rate is 120 to 140 beats per minute and the cardiac output is approximately 200 ml. per kilogram per minute or over three times that of a resting adult. The high cardiac output helps the fetus adapt to the low oxygen tension of its blood while in utero.

Fetal blood is unsaturated with respect to oxygen, having only about two thirds the oxygen saturation of equivalent maternal blood. Thus the fetus appears to live in utero in a cyanotic state. However, fetal hemoglobin content is relatively high (18 grams per 100 ml.), as is the red blood cell concentration (5.5 million per cubic millimeter), presumably in order to increase the store of oxygen in the blood. There is no evidence that the fetus is jeopardized by lack of oxygen. Indeed, there are several other compensatory mechanisms that additionally provide for adequate oxygenation of fetal tissue, such as increased oxygen dissociation of fetal hemoglobin, the inactivity of the fetus, and the relatively great cardiac output.

Carbon dioxide is transferred across the villous membrane even more rapidly than oxygen. Maternal blood has a higher affinity for carbon dioxide than does fetal blood and the partial pressure of carbon dioxide in the umbilical artery is 5 mm. Hg higher than that in the intervillous space.

When the cord is severed and breathing starts, total systemic resistance and arterial pressure rise because the low vascular resistance of the placenta is eliminated. The bradycardia, which appears simultaneously, is probably related to the pressure rise through baroreceptor reflexes. A secondary rise in arterial pressure occurs when blood flow through the ductus arteriosus ceases.

Coagulation factors. Coagulation factors II, VII, IX, XI, and XII are low in fetal blood at delivery and diminish further during the first few days of life unless vitamin K is prophylactically administered. Fibrinogen and platelet values are also slightly depressed. Factor VIII will also be low in male infants with hemophilia.

Leukocyte count. A polymorphonuclear leukocytosis (to 45,000 per cubic millimeter) is present at birth. Within 1 week the count falls approximately 50% while the concentration and absolute number of lymphocytes and monocytes rise progressively and significantly.

Fetal respiration. Rhythmic respiratory movements have been observed in the latter months of pregnancy, and debris from amniotic fluid may be found in fetal lungs. Respiration at birth is believed to be a continuation of intrauterine respiratory activity, demonstrable as early as the twelfth week of pregnancy, rather than an abrupt transition from an apneic state.

Pulmonary surfactants, phospholipids capable of diminishing alveolar surface tension, are required to prevent alveolar collapse on respiratory expiration and are thus required for extrauterine existence. Pulmonary functional maturation is directly proportional to the maturation of the biochemical pathways for the synthesis of these substances, especially lecithin, which is the principle surface active component. A substantial increase in the synthesis of this material begins at approximately 36 weeks of gestation and is reflected by a sharp increase in its amniotic fluid concentration. By quantitative comparison of the amount of lecithin (L) in amniotic fluid to that of sphingomyelin (S), another pulmonary phospholipid, a highly useful clinical prognostication can be made regarding extrauterine fetal respiratory adaptability. Respiratory distress in the newborn is very uncommon when the quantitative amniotic fluid L/S ratio exceeds 2.

The fetal respiratory system is very sensitive to many analgesic and anesthetic drugs and is depressed by most agents that are given orally or subcutaneously for relief of maternal pain during labor. By their effect on maternal respiration, these drugs diminish the placenta's oxygen supply and thus act as a double threat to the fetus at delivery.

Fetal gastrointestinal activity. Amniotic fluid is swallowed by the fetus as early as the twelfth week of pregnancy, and near term the fetus swallows approximately 450 ml. of amniotic fluid each day. Digestive enzymes are present in the second trimester, and meconium (colored by bile pigments) is found in the intestines of the fetus in the second half of pregnancy. Meconium is often passed into the amniotic sac if intrauterine asphyxia occurs.

Liver and pancreas. The liver is relatively much larger in the newborn infant than in the adult. It acts as a storage depot for carbohydrate and iron. Near term the glycogen content of the fetal liver increases to double or treble that present in the adult organ. Biliary function is present as early as the fourth month of fetal life.

Insulin is produced by the fetal pancreas as early as the thirteenth week and increasingly thereafter. The precise role of fetal insulin is unknown, but it probably contributes to fetal carbohydrate metabolism inasmuch as fetal insulin levels are known to rise in response to hyperglycemia.

Renal function. The kidneys are capable of functioning during fetal life, but renal function is not essential for fetal growth. Fetuses without kidneys survive until term, but inasmuch as fetal urinary function contributes to amniotic fluid volume, oligohydramnios is common with urinary tract aplasia or obstruction. Urinary function also contributes to amniotic fluid composition. Fetal renal maturity can be assessed by quantitating nitrogenous products within the amniotic fluid, for example, creatinine. Nearly all fetuses beyond 36 weeks' gestation show amniotic fluid creatinine levels above 1.8 mg.%.

Enzyme activity. Enzyme systems required for extrauterine existence under usual circumstances are fully functional during the final trimester. The maximal rate of synthesis of some enzymes, however, is insufficient to meet the challenge of certain unusual events. Enzymatic glucuronidation by the fetal liver is limited, for example, and any abnormal amount of fetal hemolysis, as with Rh isoimmunization, will frequently lead to high plasma levels of unconjugated and thus unexcretable bilirubin, often with deleterious results to the fetus or newborn unless treated.

Enzyme activity in amniotic fluid cells has been increasingly investigated in recent years and several fetal metabolic diseases caused by enzymatic deficiencies have been diagnosed in utero. These include Tay-Sachs disease, Lesch-Nyhan syndrome, galactosemia, metachromatic leukodystrophy, Niemann-Pick disease, methylmalonic aciduria, type 2 glycogen storage disease, mucopolysaccharidosis, lysosomal acid phosphatase deficiency, and adrenogenital syndrome. Numerous others have been diagnosed or are potentially diagnosable with extension of this approach.

Immunologic status. Maternal immunoglobulins IgA and IgM do not traverse the placenta although IgG does so freely by both simple diffusion and active transport. The fetus is thus passively protected to the extent of the variety and quantity of maternal IgG antibodies. A degree of active protection is also afforded, as demonstrated by the capacity of the fetus to produce various immunoglobulins as early as the fifth month. IgM in fetal or newborn sera signifies fetal response to previous intrauterine infection, the identity of which may be determined by appropriate antibody studies. Passive immunity may persist for several months after birth. Colostrum, though rich in antibodies, does not serve as a source of passive immunity for the human fetus, since enteric antibody absorption is minimal.

PHYSIOLOGY OF PLACENTA

Late in pregnancy only the syncytium and stroma of the villi separate the maternal blood in the intervillous spaces from the fetal vessels in the villi. The total surface of all villi has been estimated as 15 square meters and the total length of all villi as 30 miles. The surface area of the human placenta exchange membrane at term approximates that of the small intestine in the adult. The thickness of the membrane at term is about 0.002 mm.

Gases and substances in solution pass into the fetal circulation by *osmosis*. However, the syncytium does not serve merely as a dialyzing membrane, since colloids and other substances must be changed by the syncytial membrane before they can be transmitted.

The permeability of the placenta has been studied, using deuterium oxide as a tracer substance. At the peak of permeability, around the thirty-fifth week of gestation, the enormous quantity of 3.6 liters of water per hour crosses the placenta to the fetus (Flexner). It has been estimated that this is about 3,000 times more water than is incorporated in the growing tissues.

Internal secretions. The synthesis of chorionic gonadotropin, chorionic somatomammotropin, and chorionic thyrotropin by the syncytiotrophoblast has already been mentioned. Estrogens and progesterone also are elaborated by syncytium, but there is no substantial evidence that adrenocorticosteroids originate in placental tissue. The trophoblast secretes various enzymes, notably oxytocinase.

Transfer mechanisms. As noted previously, the intervillous space is always full of blood, and the pressure in this space is 5 to 10 mm. Hg when the uterus is relaxed or around 40 mm. Hg when contracted. Thus the pressure is below that in endometrial arteries and in fetal capillaries. Transfer of substances into fetal vessels is achieved, then, against an appreciable gradient of hydrostatic pressure.

Diffusion. One must assume that simple diffusion operates in the case of oxygen, carbon dioxide, electrolytes, water, anesthetic gases, steroids, drugs, and many other substances of molecular weight less than 500.

Selective transfer. The concentration of some substances (for example, ascorbic acid) is higher in fetal blood than in maternal blood; thus the placenta is not merely a semipermeable membrane. Immune globulin G is readily transported across the placenta despite its great molecular weight, 160,000. The placenta may transfer fatty acids and cholesterol, but much fetal fat is likely to be synthesized from carbohydrate.

Pinocytosis. Projections from the surfaces of trophoblastic cells engulf particles of maternal plasma and transfer them intact across the cell to a fetal vessel. It is believed that complex proteins, fat, and immune bodies are transferred in this fashion.

Leakage through defects. Clearly, fetal blood elements may enter the maternal circulation through villi damaged by infarction, fibrinoid degeneration, increased fetal intracapillary pressure, or infection. Fetal-maternal transfusion usually occurs at the time of placental separation and delivery, regardless of the stage of gestation. Although the volume of transfused fetal blood is usually small, it is adequate in many situations to immunologically sensitize the maternal organism to foreign blood components (for example, the Rh factor). Conversely, there is at least some evidence that maternal antibody-making leukocytes and platelets may be transferred from mother to fetus, and interesting possibilities for the development of immune phenomena have been suggested on the basis of these observations. If such maternal cells could colonize in the fetus, they might engage in graft versus host reactions to produce "autoimmune" reactions.

Minerals and vitamins. Values for sodium, potassium, and magnesium are about the same in maternal and fetal blood, but fetal blood has more calcium and phosphorus. Iron crosses the placenta from mother to fetus very rapidly (in less than an hour). Vitamin A and carotene seem to be transmitted through the placenta very slowly, whereas thiamine and ascorbic acid pass rapidly. It is uncertain whether vitamin D is transmitted to the fetus, but vitamins E and K probably pass the barrier.

The placenta is permeable to large numbers of pharmaceutic agents, such as the sulfa drugs, morphine, ether, barbiturates, various antibiotics, thiouracil, and many others. Bacteria are transmitted infrequently and then, presumably, as the result of a bacterial lesion in the placenta. Viruses, however, seem to traverse the placenta easily.

Enzymatic detoxification. The placenta appears to provide an additional protective mechanism for the fetus, in that various potentially disturbing amines such as epinephrine, norepinephrine, serotonin, and histamine are rapidly deaminated enzymatically during passage.

SEX OF THE FETUS

Fetal sex may be determined during the second and third trimesters using amniotic fluid obtained by amniocentesis. Fetal cells may be examined for nuclear sex chromatin or Barr bodies by simple staining, for the Y chromosome by fluorescence microscopy, and (for greatest precision) by cell culture and preparation of a chromosomal karyotype. These tests may be used to predict the existence of sex-linked fetal abnormalities prenatally, and the karyotype may be used for the intrauterine diagnosis of certain autosomal defects of the fetus as well.

5

Maternal physiology

The obvious gross anatomic changes that occur in a pregnant woman are accompanied by numerous physiologic changes involving all the organ systems. These variations from the normal, nonpregnant state are traditionally described under the heading *maternal physiology,* but the phrase necessarily includes biochemical and anatomic phenomena, as well as strictly physiologic events.

CHANGES IN REPRODUCTIVE SYSTEM

Uterus

Size. To accommodate the growing fetus, the uterus must increase enormously. It becomes more than four times longer than the uterus of a nonpregnant woman. Its dimensions at term are about 30 × 25 × 20 cm., and its capacity is over 4 liters (only 2 ml. prior to pregnancy).

Weight. The weight of the uterus increases from about 30 to 60 grams before pregnancy to 1,000 grams at term. The enlargement is caused not only by hypertrophy of the muscle fibers but also by formation of new muscle fibers (hyperplasia). All other tissues of the uterus are also much increased, for example, the connective and elastic tissues to enhance the strength and elasticity of the walls and the mesenchymal tissue between muscle bundles. To nourish these growing tissues, as well as the fetus, the blood vessels must enlarge, and at the placental site they become large blood spaces—the placental and uterine sinuses. The augmentation of the nerve supply is illustrated by the enlargement of the cervical ganglion by 50% or more.

Uterine enlargement in early pregnancy results at least partially from elevated hormone levels as is shown by the fact that the uterus increases slightly in size even if the pregnancy is extrauterine.

After the third month mechanical enlargement from the growing fetus becomes increasingly more prominent. Up to this time the walls have been thick, but after this the walls stretch and gradually become very thin, diminishing to 0.5 cm. or less by the fifth month.

Muscular arrangement. The muscle bundles lie in three more or less distinct layers.

1. An *outer* hoodlike layer covers the fundus.

2. An *inner* layer lies next to the endometrium and forms circular bundles around the entrance to the fallopian tubes and the cervix.

3. The *middle* layer, much thicker than the other two, forms dense masses of muscle, with fibers interlacing in a sort of figure-eight pattern. Contraction of these fibers will constrict blood vessels—a most important fact.

Changes in shape and consistency. Until about the sixth week of pregnancy the uterus remains piriform and then becomes ovoid near the end of the second month. After 3 months it is rather spherical and remains so until the middle of pregnancy. As the fetus elongates, the ovoid shape of the uterus returns, but toward the end of gestation the transverse fundal diameter increases, and thus a more or less piriform shape is restored.

Pregnancy produces considerable softening of the uterus. In some instances this seems to involve at first only one side of the uterus—presumably the tissues near the site of implantation. Often the isthmus becomes unusually soft between the sixth and eighth weeks (Hegar's sign). By the fourth month the uterus feels like a sac containing fluid, but later some degree of solidity is restored as the fetal parts become readily palpable through the thinning uterine wall.

Position of uterus during pregnancy. As soon as pregnancy occurs, anteflexion increases in a previously anteflexed uterus, but no substantial locational change is noted in a retrodisplaced organ. Until the fourth month the uterus remains in the pelvis, but then it ascends into the abdomen, displacing intestines laterally. As its greatest height it nearly reaches the liver.

The uterus during pregnancy is quite mobile, as is shown by its normal tipping to one side or the other, usually to the right. It also normally twists to the right—dextroversion.

Contractility. Irregular, painless contractions begin in the first trimester and become more frequent as pregnancy progresses. During the last few weeks of pregnancy they are quite noticeable as a rule and may be confused with real labor. There are other low-intensity rhythmic contractions that may be detected throughout pregnancy only with suitable manometric devices, and these occur with a measurable frequency of 60 to 180 per hour.

Vascular system. Uterine and ovarian arteries increase in diameter, length, and tortuosity during pregnancy. Venous channels are enormously enlarged, and huge sinuses develop at the placental site. Dilated veins become numerous in the broad ligaments. The venous reservoir may prevent external pressure from raising local resistance to the point at which uterine bleeding might be produced. Uterine blood flow per unit weight of uterus, fetus, and placenta is fairly constant throughout pregnancy and approximates 10 ml. per 100 grams per minute. But when calculated for the entire pregnant uterus, blood flow increases progressively throughout pregnancy. Uterine contractions reduce uterine blood flow in proportion to their intensity and duration. As far as is known, only the kidneys and possibly the extremities share with the uterus in absorbing the increased cardiac output of pregnancy.

Cervix. Increased vascularity discolors and softens the cervix, and these changes have been suggested as signs of pregnancy. Endocervical clefts (Fluhmann) (Figs. 5-1 and 5-2) enlarge and secrete large amounts of mucus, some of which accumulates as a plug in the cervical canal. This mucus plug is often expelled in early labor, and its expulsion is usually accompanied by modest bleeding from the disrupted vessels in the fragile supporting architecture ("bloody show"). Hyperplasia and hypertrophy of the muscle and connective tissue occur to some extent, more noticeably in the connective tissues. In a multiparous woman at term, the external os may be so large as to admit two fingers easily.

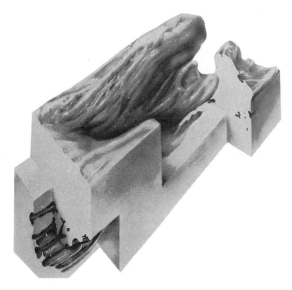

Fig. 5-1. Cervical cleft with associated tunnels. (From Fluhmann: The cervix uteri and its diseases, Philadelphia, W. B. Saunders Co.)

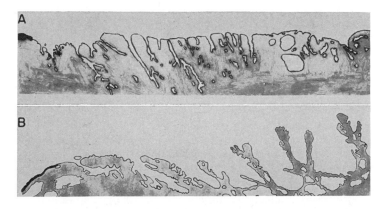

Fig. 5-2. Panoramic views of cervix uteri traced from photographs of microscopic sections. **A,** Normal cervix. **B,** Cervix during late pregnancy. Note widening of clefts and tunnels in pregnancy. (From Fluhmann: Amer. J. Obstet. Gynec. **78:**990, 1959.)

Basal cell hyperactivity and "reserve cell" proliferation are common at the squamocolumnar junction and even more superiorly in the cervical canal. These changes must not be confused with the pattern of carcinoma in situ.

The cervix during pregnancy often appears "eroded" (noticeably reddened) because there is an eversion or proliferation of endocervical tissue. This is not an ulceration, however, because the surface is fully covered by columnar epithelium that has been stimulated to exuberant growth, presumably by estrogen.

Tubes and ovaries. The tubes and ovaries during pregnancy hang down alongside the uterus, almost parallel to its long axis. Their blood supply is greatly increased and their veins are enormously distended. Under endocrine influence no ovarian follicles mature during pregnancy and ovulation ceases. However, the corpus luteum last formed before conception persists as the "corpus luteum of pregnancy," but its bulk diminishes after the middle of gestation.

Patches of decidua are found on and in ovaries quite regularly and occasionally on the posterior serosal surface of the uterus. Decidua-like cells may be seen at times in the mucosal portion of a tube.

Vagina. In common with all other pelvic structures, the vagina is much more vascular, which gives it a violet color deepening to a purplish hue as pregnancy advances (Chadwick's sign of pregnancy). Secretion is more profuse. It is creamy, whitish, and highly acid (lactic acid from the intraluminal bacterial lysis of glycogen contained within desquamated epithelial cells). All tissues hypertrophy, especially the elastic tissue, and the vagina becomes greatly distensible in preparation for childbirth.

Vaginal smears taken in the first trimester of pregnancy have a characteristic pattern, containing wrinkled and clumped precornified cells as well as so-called navicular cells. No true basal cells are seen, and only rarely are parabasal cells observed. Experienced cytologists usually have no difficulty in discerning smears compatible with the pregnant state, and under some circumstances cytologic examination may be a helpful diagnostic device.

Pelvic joints. In some pregnant animals the pelvic joints separate. Although this does not happen in women, the joints do become slightly movable. This pelvic instability, associated with postural lordosis occasioned by the increasingly protruding abdomen, frequently leads to a change of gait and to skeletal muscle strain. Resultant and recurrent episodes of joint and muscle discomfort are common. Subluxations may occur.

Abdominal wall. Stretching breaks the elastic fibers in the deeper layers of the skin, causing the "striae of pregnancy." Overstretching also results in separation of the rectus muscles (diastasis recti), sometimes even to the extent of herniation of the uterus.

The depressed umbilicus becomes flush with the skin surface or even protrudes beyond it, and the midline skin becomes pigmented *(linea nigra)*.

Breasts. Tenseness, tenderness, and tingling of the breasts are common in the first 2 months of pregnancy. Breasts become larger after the second month, and alveolar hypertrophy may produce a sensation of nodularity. Veins become prominent just under the skin and striae may appear.

Nipples increase in size and become more pigmented and more erectile. *Colostrum* may be expressed after the third or fourth month. The areolae around the nipples in brunettes become very dark, but those of blondes are usually quite pink. Numerous small areolar elevations, the *tubercles of Montgomery,* are hypertrophied sebaceous glands; nests of them encircle the periphery of the areola. The understructure of the epidermis of the nipple is as elaborate as that of the volar skin or the rima ani. Perhaps this reflects a morphologic adaptation to the excoriating attrition of suckling.

CHANGES IN OTHER ORGANS AND SYSTEMS

Circulatory system

Blood volume. Both plasma and red cell volume rise progressively during pregnancy with total blood volume increasing by 25% to 40%. This normal hypervolemia of pregnancy minimizes the effect of hemorrhage at delivery, provides the volume required for the enlarged uterine vascular system, and reduces the potential effects on the mother and fetus of impaired venous return and positional reductions of cardiac output. Prepregnancy volumes are restored within 1 to 3 weeks after delivery.

Blood proteins. The concentration of serum albumin falls significantly as pregnancy advances, and there is a minor drop in gamma globulin and an increase in beta globulin and fibrinogen. The reduced concentration of total plasma proteins in pregnancy probably is not a major factor in water retention.

Cell counts and hemoglobin. Hematocrit values tend to decrease during pregnancy because of the relative increase in plasma volume. The concentration of red cells is diminished, but the total mass of circulating red cells is increased. Hemoglobin concentration drops as pregnancy advances, although obviously the total *amount* of hemoglobin increases. White cell counts average around 10,000 per cubic millimeter during the prenatal period and are even higher during labor and in the early puerperium.

Blood coagulation. Various coagulation factors increase in concentration as pregnancy advances. It is assumed that the altered in vitro tests of clotting are paralleled by in vivo changes that create a state of hypercoagulability. Factors VII, VIII, IX, X, and XII are increased as are prothrombin (factor II) and fibrinogen (factor I). Factor V is apparently unchanged, but factors XI and XIII are decreased. The prothrombin time and the partial thromboplastin time are both mildly reduced as pregnancy progresses. The platelet count is stable. Systemic fibrinolytic activity appears to be decreased during pregnancy.

Thrombosis is uncommon during pregnancy despite the increase in the coagulation factors and the decrease in fibrinolytic activity. Oddly, as the hypercoagulability state is being reversed after delivery, thrombosis becomes more common.

Blood pressure and pulse. Arterial blood pressure tends to drop, especially during the second trimester, but may rise toward prepregnant levels as term is approached. Venous pressure remains normal in the upper extremities but rises appreciably in the lower extremities after the end of the first trimester. This elevation is not as great if the venous pressure is recorded while the patient is lying on her side rather than in the supine position, in which vena cava compression by the enlarged uterus is increased. Varicosities may become very prominent in the legs, thighs, and vulva, and even on the lower abdominal wall. Pulse rate usually is elevated, the average value being about 84 per minute.

Heart. Cardiac output begins to rise by the end of the third month and increases about 30%, with an appreciable decline in the last 8 weeks of pregnancy. Cardiac output is increased significantly during labor, however, and even more so with fetal explusion. The apparent cardiac enlargement probably results from upward movement of the diaphragm, possibly to some extent from cardiac dilatation and also from an increase of interstitial and pericardial fluid. Electrocardiograms may show left axis deviation, variously explained as caused by left ventricular hypertrophy or to changes in position of the heart. The great increase in cardiac work during pregnancy is mitigated to some extent by the diminished viscosity of the blood, which results in diminished resistance to flow.

Respiratory system. Although the diaphragm becomes elevated, there are increases in anteroposterior and transverse thoracic diameters, so that vital capacity actually is *increased* slightly during pregnancy. Lung compliance is unchanged, but pulmonary resistance is reduced and airway conductance is increased. Thoracic breathing predominates, respiratory rate increases, and minute volume of respired air increases. Nasopharyngeal mucous membranes may become edematous and hyperemic. Voice changes are attributed to these effects in the larynx.

Dyspnea occurs in about 60% of pregnant women, but its mechanism is obscure and it is rarely severe or incapacitating. It is probably related to the hyperventilation that invariably accompanies pregnancy and presumably promotes desirable gas exchange at the placenta. Dyspnea usually occurs when alveolar carbon dioxide tension is at a minimum, regardless of the absolute level of ventilation or breathing reserve.

Urinary tract. *Ureteral dilatation* during pregnancy, more common on the right side but often bilateral, has been explained on several bases. Hypotonia of ureteral musculature and hypoperistalsis have been attributed to excessive progesterone. In addition, there is increased angulation of the ureter adjacent to the cervix and possibly an element of compression by the uterus or the distended ovarian vein at the level of the pelvic inlet. Dilatation of the kidney pelvis is common, and this may favor the development of pyelonephritis.

Urinary frequency is common early in pregnancy because of bladder compression by the enlarging uterus and again late in pregnancy if the fetal head enters the pelvic cavity. Urinary frequency has been attributed also to hyperemia of the bladder mucosa, associated with pelvic venous congestion.

Glomerular filtration rate and renal blood flow are *increased* 30% to 50% above pregravid levels throughout the latter two thirds of pregnancy. Plasma creatinine and urea decline as a consequence. Tubular reabsorption of various ions, particularly sodium, must be increased in order to avoid depletion of essential substances. A gradual cumulative retention of 500 to 800 mEq. of sodium occurs. Plasma aldosterone, renin, renin substrate, and angiotensin increase significantly during normal pregnancy but decline with toxemia.

Digestive tract. Salivation may become excessive during pregnancy, although this is not a common complaint. Aberrations of the sense of smell and taste may occur. Perverted appetites may produce unusual cravings for certain foods or for items not ordinarily ingested for nutritional purposes (pica). Nausea, vomiting, and anorexia are common in the first trimester and may persist to some degree throughout pregnancy. Constipation is common, and gastric emptying time is prolonged, because of diminished peristaltic activity. Hypochlorhydria is very common. Regurgitation of gastric secretions into the lower esophagus is frequent and results in retrosternal discomfort (heartburn). Emptying time of the gallbladder is increased, and the bile passages become hypotonic and dilated. These changes, plus hypercholesterolemia, may favor the formation of gallstones. Changes in liver function are not well defined, but it is certain that the ability of liver cells to remove certain test materials from the bloodstream is dimished in pregnancy.

Bones and teeth. Pelvic joints during pregnancy become more mobile because of ligamentous softening. Widening of the joint space at the symphysis pubis may be demonstrated radiographically, but seldom does this produce any difficulty in locomotion.

Maternal calcium from the long bones may be partially depleted to provide fetal requirements late in pregnancy unless the maternal diet contains sufficient calcium to supply up to 0.4 gram daily to the fetus. Calcium in teeth is fixed, and demineralization does not occur. Any accentuation of caries results from changes in the oral bacterial flora and the lack of good hygiene rather than decalcification. Edema of the gums and gingivitis are often seen during pregnancy but usually subside spontaneously after delivery.

Skin. Pigmentation is increased in the nipples, areolae, and vulva, as well as along the lower midline of the abdomen (*linea nigra*) and around the umbilicus. Brownish deposits may occur in the skin of the face and forehead—the so-called "mask of pregnancy" or *chloasma,* but these changes disappear after delivery. Striae may form over the abdominal wall, buttocks, and breasts. Many women develop vascular spiders on the face, neck, thorax, and arms, as well as palmar erythema. It has been suggested that these are transient responses to elevated estrogen levels. Sweat glands and sebaceous glands become more active.

Endocrine glands

Thyroid gland. Slight enlargement of the thyroid gland (adenomatous hyperplasia) is common in pregnant women, but this has no clinical significance. Increased renal iodine clearance during pregnancy results in reduced plasma-inorganic iodine levels, with compensatory increase in thyroid activity. This leads to enlargement of the thyroid gland. Such changes are detectable by the end of the first trimester but disappear within 6 weeks after delivery.

The basal metabolic rate increases throughout gestation, reaching values of +15% to +20% in the last trimester. The apparent reason is simply addition of the fetal to the maternal oxygen consumption.

Protein-bound iodine, butanol-extractable iodine, and total thyroxin are all increased in pregnancy while the red cell tri-iodothyronine uptake is diminished. These changes are the result of a two- to threefold increase in the concentration of serum thyroxin–binding globulin, a glycoprotein having electrophoretic mobility with the alpha globulins. The peak is reached by the eighteenth to twentieth weeks of gestation. The concentration of free thyroxin, the metabolically active fraction, remains unchanged, and the patient remains euthyroid. Free serum thyroxin is consequently the most reliable means of evaluating thyroid status in pregnancy. Radioactive iodine uptake is distinctly increased, but administration of radioiodine is absolutely contraindicated in pregnancy as it may result in congenital fetal hypothyroidism.

Parathyroid glands. Parathyroid glands increase in size during pregnancy. Elevated values of parathormone are found between the fifteenth and thirty-fifth weeks, when fetal requirements for calcium are great. Tetany has been observed in pregnant women, and this may be relieved by giving calcium and parathormone.

Pancreas. The maternal islets of Langerhans are enlarged and there is hyperinsulinemia in normal pregnancy, which is particularly accentuated in the last trimester. Fasting blood glucose levels are somewhat diminished but essentially stable throughout, demonstrating the well-known reduced sensitivity to insulin, especially in late pregnancy. It has been suggested that extra insulin is secreted in response to increasing amounts of chorionic somatomammotropin, which is known to oppose the action of insulin. Additionally, peripheral tissues may lose their ability to use insulin during pregnancy. Regardless, it is apparent that homeostasis requires significantly increased insulin secretion and patients with minimal pancreatic reserve, adequate for nonpregnancy stresses, may develop a diabetic glucose tolerance curve during pregnancy, or even frank diabetes. Glucosuria during pregnancy, however, is more commonly the result of increased glomerular infiltration, possibly coupled with a minimal reduction in tubular reabsorption, than it is of diabetes. Nonetheless, it should be investigated in each instance.

Hypophysis. The anterior lobe of the pituitary gland enlarges, and in rare instances it presses on the optic chiasm to produce temporary hemianopsia. Characteristic large granulating cells ("pregnancy cells") appear in the anterior lobe. In addition to thyrotropic and adrenotropic hormones that regulate metabolic processes in pregnancy, the anterior lobe produces *prolactin* to effect the secretion of milk. It is believed that the production of gonadotropins in the pituitary is inhibited or at least limited during pregnancy. Pituitary somatomammotropin (growth hormone) levels are significantly reduced but possibly compensated for by the abundant placental secretion of chorionic somatomammotropin. The posterior lobe does not hypertrophy.

Adrenal glands. The adrenal cortex hypertrophies and there is a noticeable increase in urinary corticoid excretion. Aldosterone production shows a threefold rise after the third month, but nearly all of it is in the conjugated form.

The total plasma cortisol level is significantly elevated, but over 90% is protein bound (to transcortin and to albumin) and is physiologically inactive. Levels of unbound cortisol increase slightly during pregnancy, however, and may contribute to the lower eosinophil counts, pigmentation, striae, and variation in carbohydrate metabolism seen during pregnancy. The rate of metabolism (half-life) of cortisol is substantially diminished and the rate of secretion is essentially unchanged.

Plasma progesterone is apparently also bound by transcortin, and increasingly so to term.

Ovaries. The function of the ovaries has been discussed to some extent in previous chapters. Ovaries are essential for the maintenance of pregnancy in the first month or two, but their secretory activities are assumed by the placenta fairly early in human gestation, and the placenta becomes the chief source of estrogens and progesterone.

Only rarely does the ovary containing the corpus luteum of pregnancy become so large as to be mistaken for an ovarian neoplasm.

METABOLISM

In general, pregnancy has a favorable effect on metabolism. Essential food elements tend to be retained and good health is the rule, except perhaps for a brief period in those women who develop excessive nausea and vomiting in the first trimester.

Weight gain. The usual total weight gain is in the range of 20 to 25 pounds, with about 3 pounds being added in the first trimester and 10 to 11 pounds in each of the other two trimesters. In the last trimester the usual weekly increment is about 0.9 pound, but there are wide individual variations. A loss of 1 or 2 pounds may occur just prior to labor, but this is not a reliable prognostic sign.

The fetus, placenta, amniotic fluid, and the increased weight of uterus, breasts, and blood account for about 14 or 15 pounds. The remainder is largely extravascular fluid and extrauterine fat and protein storage.

Protein metabolism. The fetus accumulates little nitrogen in the first half of pregnancy, but nitrogen retention rises progressively thereafter to an average total storage of 60 grams at term. The mother stores large amounts of nitrogen, which can be accounted for in the fetus, uterus, breasts, and increased blood components. Nitrogen excretion in the urine diminishes as pregnancy advances, and the percentage of ammonia is relatively increased. Creatine appears in the urine in small amounts.

Carbohydrate metabolism. (See Pancreas, p. 70). Glucosuria is common in pregnant women because of a lower renal threshold. Fetal use of carbohydrates and increased metabolism of pregnancy lowers the antiketogenic substances. At the same time, maternal lipids are increased and alkali reserve reduced, so that ketosis is easily produced. Thus the management of diabetes during pregnancy may be difficult. Lactose may be present in urine late in pregnancy and during lactation. It should not be mistaken for glucose.

Fat metabolism. Pregnancy is accompanied by a significant degree of lipemia. Plasma neutral fat is more than doubled, and there is roughly a 25% increase in phospholipids and free cholesterol. The surplus of fatty substances presumably is required for fetal development and for lactation, although these materials are accumulated far in advance of the time they are needed.

Nonesterified fatty acids are elevated late in pregnancy, perhaps indicating impaired carbohydrate metabolism. Fat metabolism in the mother and in the fetus is poorly understood.

Mineral metabolism. An average daily intake of 1.2 grams of calcium by the mother provides an ample supply for fetal needs. Serum calcium values remain within normal limits throughout pregnancy. More than half the fetal calcium is deposited in the last month, and during this period some of the maternal longbone calcium reserves may be withdrawn.

It has been estimated that 800 mg. of iron are needed during pregnancy for fetal and maternal hemoglobin synthesis and tissue growth. Approximately half of this is permanently lost from the maternal organism upon delivery. Demand is greatest in the last half of pregnancy, averaging 6 to 7 mg. per day. It is difficult to meet these needs from maternal stores and from dietary iron even though gastrointestinal absorption of this mineral is increased during pregnancy. Consequently, and because iron deficiency is the most common cause of pregnancy anemia, many physicians believe that all pregnant women should take iron supplements regularly.

Serum phosphorus values are unchanged in pregnancy, while serum copper levels increase substantially. The reason for the latter is unknown.

Water metabolism. Increased retention of water during pregnancy may explain:

1. Weight gain in excess of that from the gestational products
2. Diuresis after delivery, resulting in flaccid skin
3. Postpartum decreases in the circumference of extremities

Various studies have shown increases in extracellular water of 2 to 3 liters. The precise explanation for this phenomenon is obscure.

SEXUAL PHYSIOLOGY

According to Masters and Johnson, the normal pelvic vasocongestion of pregnancy elevates the baseline of sexual tension throughout pregnancy and fully 80% of pregnant women note an increase in sexual interest, anticipation, and fantasy, especially in the midtrimester. As a consequence, the achievement of orgasm is easier and some women become orgasmic or multiorgasmic for the first time while pregnant. Detumescence occurring after orgasm is slower and the period of postorgasmic satiation is shorter. Coital frequency is not necessarily increased, however, as availability, fear of inducing miscarriage or injuring the fetus, physician proscription, and many other elements may serve as tempering influences. Indeed, Solberg et al. noted that as pregnancy progressed there was a linear decline in coital activity for the majority, but not all, of the women in their recent retrospective study. Mutual manual and oral-genital activity also progessively declined and, contrary to the findings of Masters and Johnson, so did orgasmic activity and sexual interest.

Orgasm during pregnancy is accompanied by palpable uterine contractions and occasionally by prolonged uterine spasm. The incidence of orgasmic induction of labor, membrane rupture, or fetal circulatory embarrassment is wholly unknown but is probably low. Coital proscription in pregnancy, if advocated on this basis, should be accompanied by masturbational proscription as well in that the intensity of orgasm is usually greater with masturbation than with coitus.

6

The diagnosis of pregnancy

Although the diagnosis of pregnancy is usually quite simply determined by a history and physical examination, it may offer unusual and sometimes insurmountable problems, for example, in the presence of tumors. This is particularly true prior to the second missed menstrual period. The emotional consequences of misdiagnosis are enormous in some women, and for this reason the physician must be cautious about basing a diagnosis on equivocal evidence. If early confirmation of a suspected pregnancy is demanded, biologic test or an immunologic assay for chorionic gonadotropin should be arranged.

SYMPTOMS AND SIGNS OF PREGNANCY

Although the unquestionable positive signs of pregnancy appear after the fourth lunar month (16 weeks), there are many probable or presumptive signs and symptoms that will lead the physician to make a diagnosis of pregnancy before that time.

Presumptive signs of pregnancy

More details of the presumptive signs and symptoms may be found in Chapter 5. Although these signs and symptoms are not conclusive, they do offer presumptive evidence of pregnancy; they are valuable evidence, but *never proof.*

Cessation of menstruation. Although absence of menstruation is the most common early sign of pregnancy, no reliance can be placed on this symptom until 10 or 15 days have elapsed after the day on which menstruation had been anticipated. Obviously there are many conditions other than pregnancy that may be associated with interruption of normal menstrual rhythm. Fear of pregnancy apparently may influence the hypothalamic-hypophyseal system and result in amenorrhea. Likewise, it is common to implicate change of climate or altitude, various infections and metabolic diseases, or nervous disorders in delaying menstruation.

Lassitude and somnolence. Lassitude and somnolence are obviously very nonspecific symptoms but are exceedingly common and exceptionally pronounced in early pregnancy.

Nausea and vomiting. Nausea and vomiting are only suspicious symptoms, but they occur so frequently that they are considered signs of pregnancy.

Breast changes. Tingling, enlargement, increased pigmentation, secondary areolae, veins, more prominent follicles of Montgomery, and striae are indications of pregnancy.

Discoloration of vagina and cervix (Chadwick's sign). Color changes in the vagina and cervix from pink to bluish, increasing to a deep purplish hue as pregnancy advances, are signs.

Leukorrhea. The quantity of vaginal secretion usually increases because of increased production of cervical mucus, increased vaginal transudation as a result of pelvic vasocongestion, and greater exfoliation of vaginal epithelium stimulated by estrogen. In extreme cases late in pregnancy the volume of cervicovaginal fluid may require the wearing of a perineal pad.

Abdominal striae. Abdominal striae are not invariably present in pregnant women.

Linea nigra. A line of pigmentation in the lower midline of the abdomen, ascending as pregnancy progresses, is an indicative sign.

Frequency of urination. Frequency of urination is common before the uterus ascends into the abdominal cavity.

Probable signs of pregnancy

Changes in consistency of uterus

1. *Softening of the uterus* is a probable sign of pregnancy (Fig. 6-1). The first softening of the uterus is at the site of implantation. Braun von Fernwald (1907) called attention to the fact that the characteristic elastic consistency of the uterine body was unilateral, accompanied by an enlargement of the

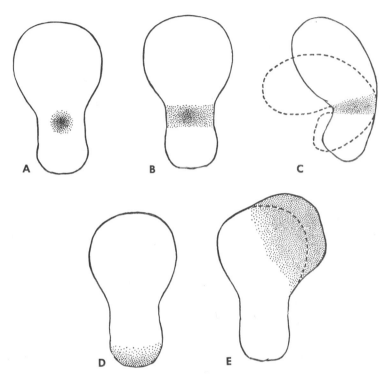

Fig. 6-1. Early signs of pregnancy caused by softening of the uterus (dotted areas indicate softening). **A,** Ladin's sign. **B,** Hegar's sign. **C,** MacDonald's sign, illustrating ease of flexing the uterine body and cervix together caused by softening between them. **D,** Softening of tip of the cervix. **E,** Braun–von Fernwald's sign, unilateral softening and enlargement at the site of implantation.

softened side, with an apparent groove between the soft and the hard side. This is one of the earliest physical signs of pregnancy and is not difficult to elicit. It may be found earlier than Hegar's signs.

2. *Hegar's sign* is a softening between the cervix and the body of the uterus, detectable about the sixth week of gestation (Fig. 6-2).

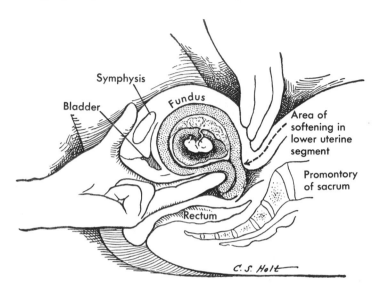

Fig. 6-2. Hegar's sign of pregnancy. (From Falls and McLaughlin: Obstetric and gynecology nursing, St. Louis, The C. V. Mosby Co.)

3. The earliest evidence of *Ladin's sign* is a soft spot, occurring at the sixth week in the midline at the junction of the body and the cervix.

4. *MacDonald's sign* is based upon the unusual ease of bringing the fundus and cervix toward each other, undoubtedly dependent on the softening found in Hegar's sign.

5. *Softening of the cervix* may occur by the end of the first month. This sign is not reliable, however, since the cervix may remain hard throughout pregnancy.

Changes in size of uterus

1. Enlargement of the uterus during the childbearing age is always presumptive of pregnancy until another cause can be definitely established.

2. During the first 2 months the uterus is in the pelvis.

3. In the third month the fundus may be felt above the symphysis pubis.

4. It is rare for the uterus to be palpably enlarged prior to 6 weeks after conception.

Changes in shape of uterus

1. At the very beginning the uterus maintains its piriform shape.

2. Soon it is enlarged on one side.

3. This enlargement gradually extends to the whole uterine body.

4. Then the form of the uterine body becomes globular.

5. Thereafter the growth is upward and the shape is elongated.

Contractions of uterus. *Braxton Hicks' sign* of pregnancy is characterized by intermittent, painless contractions that begin almost as soon as implantation occurs and continue at irregular intervals throughout gestation. They may be felt by bimanual examination, but they are not infallible signs of pregnancy since any irritation may cause them (myoma or hematometra).

Enlargement of abdomen. Enlargement of the abdomen begins when the uterus can be felt above the symphysis pubis in the third month. In the presence of other presumptive signs, abdominal enlargement makes the diagnosis of pregnancy probable.

Quickening. "Feeling life" is a probable sign, but the patient may be deceived by peristaltic movements of the bowel or by her imagination. If, however, the physician can feel fetal movements by abdominal palpation, the evidence is positive (see following discussion).

Positive signs of pregnancy

Palpation of fetus. Palpation of the fetus is a positive sign of pregnancy.

Seeing or feeling active or passive fetal movements

1. Active movements are a positive sign of pregnancy only when felt by the physician through the abdominal or vaginal wall.

2. Ballottement consists of eliciting passive fetal movements per vaginam by the examining finger by tapping fetal parts upward and then feeling them drop back upon the finger.

Seeing fetal skeleton. After the sixteenth week the fetal skeleton may be demonstrated by x-ray examination. Prior to this stage of pregnancy, intestinal shadows and the dense sacrum interfere with fetal identification, but occasionally an oblique view may show fetal bones as early as the twelfth week. Radiologic efforts to diagnose early pregnancy should be avoided whenever possible to minimize gonadal damage and genetic abnormalities.

Hearing fetal heart sounds. Unfortunately fetal heart sounds cannot be detected through a stethoscope (Fig. 6-3) until the eighteenth or twentieth week of gestation. The rate varies from

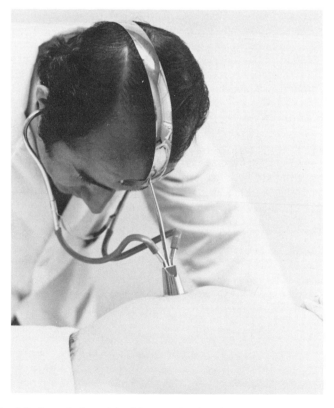

Fig. 6-3. Auscultation of fetal heart using head stethoscope (fetoscope).

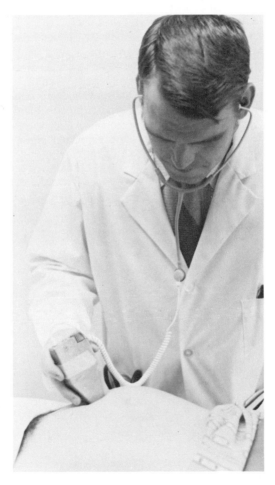

Fig. 6-4. Doppler or ultrasonic auscultation of fetal heart.

120 to 140 beats per minute. To make sure that one is not hearing the mother's rapid heart, the mother's radial pulse should be counted while listening to the fetal heart. When the fetal heart is first detectable, it is best heard immediately above the symphysis pubis; thereafter the point of maximum intensity varies with the different fetal positions and presentations. Usually it is best heard over the infant's back.

The use of the fetal electrocardiogram to demonstrate fetal life is becoming popular in medical centers with special equipment for this purpose. The accuracy of the fetal electrocardiogram increases rapidly after the seventeenth week of pregnancy, but as yet this is far from being a standardized procedure.

An electronic instrument incorporating a hand-operated transducer that simultaneously transmits and receives ultrasound is capable of consistently detecting fetal blood flow and

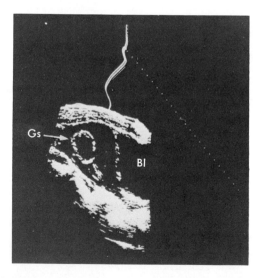

Fig. 6-5. Ultrasonic visualization of the intrauterine gestational sac **(Gs)** 6 weeks after last menstrual period. Bladder **(Bl)** at right. (Courtesy Dr. Louis Bartolucci, San Francisco.)

thus fetal heart rate by the twelfth week (Fig. 6-4). This operates on the Doppler principle, wherein sound reflected from a moving object returns altered in frequency. The method is simple and harmless and the instrument is commercially available without restrictions.

B-scan ultrasonography may also be employed without risk to the mother or fetus. The gestational sac may be visualized within the uterus as early as 5 to 6 weeks after conception (Fig. 6-5).

Other uterine sounds

1. The *funic souffle* is a hissing sound synchronous with the fetal heart rate, and presumably results from the movement of blood within the umbilical vessels. It is only rarely audible.

2. The *uterine souffle* or *bruit* is a soft, rushing sound synchronous with the maternal pulse and located over a uterine artery. These bruits do not indicate the site of placental implantation.

3. Movements of the fetus may be heard by auscultation.

4. Fetal diaphragmatic contractions may occasionally be heard more or less rhythmically, but they are synchronous with neither fetal nor maternal heartbeats.

5. Movements of maternal bowel gas and fluids may be mistaken for fetal sounds.

Biologic hormone tests of pregnancy. Biologic hormone tests all depend on the conclusion of Aschheim and Zondek (1928) that urine of pregnant women contains considerable chorionic gonadotropin, which, when injected subcutaneously, will cause ovulation phenomena in the ovaries of animals. These have been almost totally replaced by immunologic tests having greater sensitivity, specificity, reliability, and speed and are mentioned only for historic interest.

Aschheim-Zondek test. Immature mice are injected with the test urine frequently for 48 hours. Approximately 100 hours after the first injection, the ovaries are examined for hemorrhagic follicles or corpora lutea.

Friedman test. Test urine is injected into the marginal ear vein of a mature, isolated female rabbit. If the woman is pregnant, 16 to 48 hours later the ovaries will show hemorrhagic and ruptured follicles with luteinization.

Rat hyperemia test. Immature female rats are given a single subcutaneous injection of test urine and the normally pale ovaries are grossly inspected for hyperemia 16 to 24 hours thereafter.

Clawed toad (Hogben) test. Urine is injected into the dorsal lymph sac of the South African clawed toad *(Xenopus laevis)*. The test is positive if an extrusion of ova occurs within 4 to 18 hours.

Male frog or toad test. Urine injected into the dorsal lymph sac of the male frog or toad (many species have been used) will result in the extrusion of spermatozoa within 2 to 5 hours if the woman is pregnant.

For some tests, the urinary gonadotropin may be concentrated on kaolin prior to injection and the concentrate employed to increase sensitivity and reliability. Serum may also be used.

Immunologic tests. In 1960 Wide and Gemzell in Stockholm introduced an immunologic assay for human chorionic gonadotropin. They used a system that included red cells of sheep coated with HCG and an anti-HCG serum made in rabbits. The presence of HCG in the pregnancy urine being tested *inhibited* hemagglutination, because a "positive" urine blocked the ability of the antiserum to agglutinate the red cells. In a sense, then, a lack of reaction in the test tube was equated with a positive test for pregnancy.

Several immunologic procedures using either urine or serum and based on hemagglutination, precipitin tests, or complement fixation have been developed commercially in recent years. In some tests latex particles are used in place of animal erythrocytes. Several of the tests offer a reliable result within 5 minutes, and because they are simple, specific, relatively inexpensive, and packaged for office use, these procedures have essentially replaced the biologic assays. They are 95% to 99% accurate. Falsely negative results will occur if chorionic gonadotropin titers are below the level of the tests' sensitivity. Falsely positive results may occur when luteinizing hormone levels are elevated in that the test antibody cross-reacts with this hormone.

A radioimmunossay for chorionic gonadotropin has recently been developed, but for pregnancy testing it does not offer significant advantages over the other immunologic methods.

Pharmacologic tests for pregnancy. The abrupt withdrawal of exogenously administered progesterone or other short-acting progestogen may precipitate endometrial bleeding in an amenorrheic patient. If there is no response within 2 to 5 days to a single injection of progesterone or to a short course of oral progestogens, that is, no withdrawal bleeding, pregnancy may be a likely explanation. On the other hand, uterine bleeding does not prove conclusively that the patient is not pregnant. Various dosage patterns of the progestational steroids have been recommended.

Perhaps the best that can be said of such tests is that they are harmless devices that may be used pending reexamination in a dubious case, and the patient may receive psychic support from the thought that something specific is being done to resolve her dilemma.

SYNOPSIS OF SIGNS AND SYMPTOMS BY LUNAR MONTHS

First lunar month (1 to 4 weeks)

1. Amenorrhea beginning with implantation and lasting throughout pregnancy
2. Breast changes
3. Urinary frequency
4. Lassitude and somnolence
5. Chorionic gonadotropin test positive
6. Increase in vaginal secretion
7. Braun von Fernwald's sign (unilateral softening and enlargement of uterus) frequently present

Second lunar month (5 to 8 weeks)

1. Same as first month
2. Braun von Fernwald's sign always present
3. Hegar's sign
4. Ladin's sign
5. Soft cervix tip
6. "Morning sickness"
7. B-scan ultrasonographic visualization

Third lunar month (9 to 12 weeks)

1. Same as first and second months
2. Uterus above symphysis pubis

3. Nipples more deeply pigmented, secondary areolae
4. Chadwick's sign—cyanosis of vagina and cervix
5. Secretion (colostrum) in breasts
6. May be less morning sickness
7. Increased anteflexion of uterus
8. Breast changes more noticeable
9. Ultrasonic auscultation

Fourth month (13 to 16 weeks)
1. Uterus prominent above symphysis
2. Ossification centers visible by x-ray examination
3. Ballottement
4. Elastic softness of entire uterus
5. Nausea and vomiting less or absent

Fifth month (17 to 20 weeks)
1. Uterus approaches the umbilicus
2. Intermittent painless contractions of uterus
3. Fetal heartbeat heard or detectable by electrocardiography
4. Secondary areolae very distinctive
5. Quickening

Sixth month (21 to 24 weeks)
1. Abdominal striae
2. Uterus at or above umbilicus
3. Fetal movements palpable

Seventh month (25 to 28 weeks). The uterus is three finger-breadths above the umbilicus.

Eighth month (29 to 32 weeks). The uterus is three finger-breadths below the xiphisternum.

Ninth month (33 to 36 weeks.) The uterus is two fingerbreadths below the xiphisternum.

Tenth month (37 to 40 weeks)
1. The fundus of the uterus drops back to the ninth month level because the presenting part partially enters the pelvis.
2. Urinary frequency returns for the same reason.

DIFFERENTIAL DIAGNOSIS OF PREGNANCY

Certain conditions may be confused with pregnancy.

Myomas
1. Menses are not absent.
2. The tumors are usually firm and hard.

3. They do not have the characteristic elastic softness of the pregnant uterus.

4. They usually do not steadily increase in size like the pregnant uterus. A short wait will reveal a soft growing mass if the woman is pregnant.

5. The detection of a myoma in a pregnant uterus is usually easy, but the discovery of pregnancy in a myomatous uterus is difficult or impossible by physical examination.

6. If the condition is solely myomatous, the pregnancy test will be negative; if the condition is pregnancy, it will be positive, and after the fourth month the positive clinical signs of pregnancy will be found.

Ovarian cysts

1. In early pregnancy a cyst is easily differentiated from the uterus.

2. Later it may hide behind the enlarged uterus, or the cyst may obscure the uterus.

3. The probable signs of pregnancy may render the differentiation clearer, and the positive signs will settle the question.

4. Here again the pregnancy test will make the diagnosis certain.

Piskacek's sign. When implantation of the ovum occurs high in the funnel of the cornu of the uterine cavity, near the beginning of the intramural portion of the fallopian tube, the unilateral enlargement is exaggerated and bulges so far out laterally that it feels almost like a tumor on the wall of the uterus and may be mistaken for a soft myoma, ectopic pregnancy, or an ovarian cyst. Careful examination will show it to be a part of the uterus, and its characteristic elastic softening will indicate intrauterine pregnancy. Piskacek of Vienna first described it, hence its name. This phenomenon is simply an exaggeration of Braun von Fernwald's sign of pregnancy because of the place of implantation near the uterine horn.

Pseudocyesis (spurious pregnancy). Pseudocyesis may have all the subjective symptoms of pregnancy, especially in women near the menopause or in young women greatly desiring pregnancy. *Objective signs* may be present, such as the following:

1. Increased abdominal size that is really caused by fat, tympanites, or ascites.

2. Absence of menses attributable to approaching menopause in older women or desire for conception in young women.

3. Movements interpreted by the patient as fetal movements but really caused by gas, imagination, deception, or psychosis.

Careful examination or a pregnancy test will correct the error. The greatest difficulty lies in convincing the patient that she is not pregnant. Psychiatric consultation should be obtained.

Hematometra. Hematometra may be caused by an imperforate hymen or stenosis of the vagina or cervix. Breast changes will be absent, the cervix will not be soft, and the pregnancy test will be negative, but amenorrhea and an enlarging uterus may be momentarily confusing.

DISTINCTION BETWEEN FIRST AND SUBSEQUENT PREGNANCIES

Distinction between first and subsequent pregnancies may present a medicolegal problem. Ordinarily term pregnancy and vaginal childbirth leave indubitable evidence (Table 1). On the other hand, in very exceptional cases, signs may be entirely absent.

DIAGNOSIS OF LIFE OR DEATH OF FETUS

1. In the early months the diagnosis of fetal death is very difficult. However, as time proceeds, either the uterus will not grow or will decrease in size.

2. In later months the diagnosis of fetal death is easier because fetal movements cease.

3. Examination will show that the fetus is dead:

(a) When the uterus ceases to grow or becomes smaller

(b) When there are retrogressive breast changes

(c) When there are no fetal heart sounds by either conventional or ultrasonic auscultation and no fetal electrocardiographic tracing can be obtained

(d) When there are no fetal movements perceived

4. Several examinations over a considerable time will be required as a rule. Occasionally, however, the diagnosis can be made by palpating the macerated head with its loose bones, which gives the sensation that they are contained in a flabby

Table 1. Differential diagnosis of previous pregnancies

Never pregnant before	Pregnant before
Abdomen unrelaxed	Lax, flabby, even pendulous
Uterus firm	Uterus not quite so firm
Breasts firm, with no striae	In addition to striae of present pregnancy, cicatrices of striae of past pregnancies also seen; breasts less firm
Labia majora usually in apposition	Gaping
Hymen torn in several places	Hymen replaced by *carunculae myrtiformes*
Vagina narrow, marked by well-defined rugae	Wider; rugae less prominent, "stretched out"
Cervix, although soft, will not admit tip of finger until near end of pregnancy	Admits tip of finger to internal os; scars of previous lacerations may be felt
Presenting part during last 4 or 6 weeks of pregnancy is "engaged" unless there is disproportion	Usually does not "engage" until onset of labor

bag. X-ray examination is valuable, often showing overlapping of the bones of the skull (Spalding's sign), abnormal flexion or extension of the spine, collapse of the vertebral column (Fig. 6-6), collections of gas in the fetal heart and vessels, and the lack of fetal deglutition of intra-amniotic contrast material. Additionally, amniotic fluid, which is usually clear and colorless, will be deeply stained and muddy within a few days after fetal demise. Ultrasonography can also be used to detect fetal death. Pregnancy tests will not often be of aid as they frequently remain positive for many weeks after fetal death.

DURATION OF PREGNANCY

1. The duration of pregnancy is not exactly known in most instances.

2. Labor usually occurs from 270 to 290 days or an approxi-

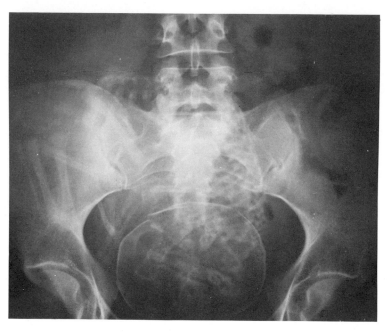

Fig. 6-6. Roentgenologic evidence of intrauterine fetal death with overlapping of skull bones, severe angulation of vertebral column, and total collapse of structural support. (Courtesy Community X-Ray Division, Stanford University Hospital, Stanford, Calif.)

mate average of about 280 days from the first day of the last menstruation (10 lunar months of 28 days each).

3. Exceptionally the pregnancy may seem to last abnormally long but only because the date of ovulation is not known.

4. When the *ovulation* date was determined from basal body temperature records in a large group of women, labor began, on the average, 267 days later.

Estimation of probable date of delivery

1. There is no perfectly reliable method for determining exact date of delivery.

2. The method most commonly employed for its estimation is to determine the date of the first day of the last menstruation,

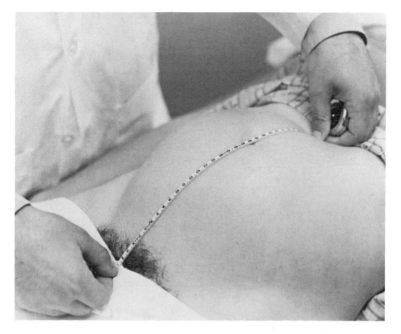

Fig. 6-7. Measuring the length of the uterus with a tape measure.

count back 3 months (ahead 9 months), and add 7 days. This
will, of course, give only the approximate expected date of labor.
An unavoidable error of 2 weeks either way may occur.

3. Counting 5 months (22 weeks) from the date of "quickening" or "feeling life" is useful but not totally reliable.

4. The level of the fundus with respect to various fixed points
is only roughly reliable.

(a) At the fourth month it is three or four fingerbreadths
above the symphysis.

(b) At the fifth month it is two or three fingerbreadths below
the umbilicus.

(c) At the sixth month it is at the umbilicus.

(d) At the seventh month it is three fingerbreadths above
the umbilicus.

Table 2. Spiegelberg's measurements of linear surface distance from symphysis to fundus at different stages of gestation

28 weeks	26.7 cm. above symphysis
32 weeks	29.5 to 30 cm. above symphysis
36 weeks	32 cm. above symphysis
40 weeks	37.7 cm. above symphysis

Table 3. The Ahlfeld table of length of fetus

1 cm.	equals	1 month
4 cm.	equals	2 months
9 cm.	equals	3 months
16 cm.	equals	4 months
25 cm.	equals	5 months
30 cm.	equals	6 months
35 cm.	equals	7 months
40 cm.	equals	8 months
45 cm.	equals	9 months
50 cm.	equals	10 months

(e) At the eighth month it is three fingerbreadths below the xiphoid process.

(f) At the ninth month it is two fingerbreadths below the xiphoid.

(g) At the tenth month it sinks to its level at the ninth month.

The previous measurements are only approximate statements. Spiegelberg proposed measuring the linear surface distance from the symphysis to the fundus with a tape measure (Fig. 6-7), and he prepared a table giving the normal distances at various stages of gestation (Table 2).

MacDonald's rule is a modification of Spiegelberg's table. MacDonald estimated that the distance from the top of the fundus to the symphysis, in centimeters, divided by 3.5 would equal the lunar month of pregnancy. The rule applies only after the sixth month of gestation. Thus at term the distance should be 35 cm.

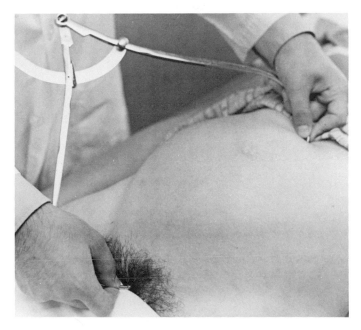

Fig. 6-8. Measuring the length of the uterus (fetus) with a pelvimeter.

Ahlfeld's rule is based upon the actual measurement of the crown-rump length of the fetus by placing the ball of one arm of a pelvimeter against the presenting part and the other arm against the top of the fundus (Fig. 6-8). This measurement is roughly one half the crown-heel length of the fetus. Therefore, when the measurement is multiplied by 2, and 2 cm. is subtracted to allow for the thickness of the abdominal wall, the total or crown-heel length of the fetus is obtained.

Dividing this figure by 5 gives the age of the fetus in lunar months. When the fetus is under 5 months, the square root is taken. See Table 3 (Ahlfeld table).

A simpler method of producing Table 3 is to square the months up to the fourth and multiply the month by 5 after that (*Haase's rule*) (see Chapter 4).

7

Prenatal care

The proper care of the prospective mother during the entire period of pregnancy is quite as important in its health and life-saving function as is expert care during the delivery.

During gestation the step from health to ill health is a short one. Seemingly slight abnormalities, which at other times appear to be of little consequence, during pregnancy may quickly become grave complications, threatening the welfare or even the life of the mother and child. For these reasons the pregnant woman should have her activities carefully and constantly supervised by a competent physician. She should engage the services of a physician as soon as she *suspects* that she is pregnant.

The physician must keep complete and accurate records, especially of blood pressure, urinalysis, and weight, and give explicit instructions to the patient (preferably printed). The patient's manner of living should be changed as little as possible, however, lest she gain the impression that normal pregnancy is an illness. When classes for prospective mothers and fathers are available in the community, attendance at these may be most helpful, especially for the woman experiencing her initial pregnancy. An increasing number of instructional obstetric films are available for purchase or rent by individual physicians for group instruction, and several are available in instant-change cartridges for individual-patient office viewing. Patients should be warned against accepting advice from friends and be encouraged to discuss even their most minor concerns with their physicians.

The chief aims of prenatal care are as follows:

1. To ensure and protect maternal health both before and after delivery
2. To minimize complications that may arise in the course of pregnancy
3. To permit the planning of a safe delivery
4. To reduce perinatal mortality and morbidity to the lowest possible values

HISTORY

Ample time must be set aside to obtain a detailed history of the prenatal patient's medical experiences prior to the onset of pregnancy, as well as to obtain the details of the present pregnancy. Although the history may be quite short for a young nullipara who has always been in good health, considerable time may be required to elicit all of the pertinent details from a patient with a complicated medical background or from one who has had many previous pregnancies.

The *menstrual history* is particularly important because much of the planning for the pregnancy and delivery is related to it. The most recent episode of bleeding may not necessarily have been a genuine menstrual period; therefore, the physician should inquire into the details of the episode, its timing in relation to the previous period, and its relationship to probable dates of ovulation and conception. Later in pregnancy the date of quickening should be related to the date of onset of the last period (LMP) to confirm the accuracy of the date from which the expected date of confinement (EDC) has been calculated. Quickening usually occurs between the seventeenth and nineteenth weeks of gestation. Many women are frightfully casual about menstrual dates, and a good deal of memory searching may be required to elicit a figure that has some semblance of reliability.

More or less standard outlines for prenatal historical data are widely used and should be available to all physicians practicing obstetrics. Usually the same printed form may be used to record the data for the initial physical examination and for all subsequent prenatal examinations. Needless to say, the form should be filled out *completely* and *accurately*.

The date of marriage, especially of a primigravida, should be recorded because it may be a clue to the patient's attitude toward the pregnancy—not only the unplanned but also the pregnancy appearing rather late in the marital career. The unmarried patient will have special problems and often the physician will wish to seek the counsel of a social worker to ensure that the best possible arrangements are made for both mother and infant if the pregnancy is to be continued.

Designation of childbearing experience. A *primigravida* is a woman pregnant for the first time, whereas a *primipara* is one who has delivered a viable infant. A *multipara* is a woman who has had two or more deliveries. Pregnancies and deliveries may be designated numerically in conjunction with the terms *gravida* and *para*. For example, a woman who has had three abortions and one term pregnancy is gravida 4, para 1.

Past obstetric history may be shown simply by a series of four digits separated by dashes, as for example, 5-1-2-6. The first figure is the number of term infants delivered, the second is the number of premature infants, the third is the number of abortions, and the last is the number of children living. This is a concise way to express much factual information and is a device now widely used in teaching clinics.

FIRST EXAMINATION

Every pregnant woman should be given a complete and thorough physical examination, including:

1. A general examination of heart, lungs, etc.

2. Determination of the condition of breasts and nipples

3. Measurement of the following diameters of the pelvis (Chapter 9):

(a) Diagonal conjugate (may not be feasible if the head is fixed or engaged)

(b) Intertuberous (transverse diameter of outlet)

(c) Posterior sagittal of the outlet especially when the transverse diameter of the outlet is 8 cm. or less

4. Examination of the inner contours of the bony pelvis with special reference to the sacrosciatic notch, the pubic arch, the prominence of the ischial spines and the distance between them, the sacral contour, and the length, mobility, and angulation of the coccyx. (This evaluation may be best performed in

the last weeks of pregnancy when the tissues are supple and the examination least uncomfortable.)

5. Examination of the pelvic organs (bimanual) for the condition of the uterus and its adnexa, abnormalities, tumors, etc., *including cytologic smear* and *cervicovaginal* and *anal cultures* for gonorrhea

6. Abdominal palpation

7. Blood pressure

8. *Blood examination,* including tests for syphilis, hemoglobin or hematocrit value, Rh status, blood group, antibody screen, and rubella antibody titer

9. *Urine examination* for protein, sugar, and sediment (clean, midstream specimen)

10. *Weight*

Instructions (preferably written) should be given to the patient at the first visit and at each subsequent visit, according to the conditions found.

INSTRUCTIONS TO PATIENT

1. Consult the physician (bring a specimen of urine at each visit) at regular intervals—once a month during the first 6 months and then every 2 weeks until the last month, when weekly visits arc desirable.

2. Also report at once any abnormality, however slight.

3. *Notify* the physician *at once* if any of the following symptoms occur:

(a) Scanty or bloody urine

(b) Severe and continuous headaches

(c) Disturbance of vision

(d) Swelling of feet, ankles, hands, or face

(e) Any bleeding from vagina or escape of watery fluid

(f) Occurrence of pain

(g) Chills and fever

4. *Take moderate exercise* in the open air, but do not get too tired. *Excessive work or exercise is just as harmful as none.*

DIET IN PREGNANCY

Judging from the great increase in size of some maternal organs and the growth of the fetus, it seems fair to assume that the intake of certain essential nutrients should increase during pregnancy. Despite many careful dietary studies, no absolute requisites have been established, and one can deal only in generalities and recommendations when discussing the diet of the normal pregnant woman. Obviously, special diets must be planned for those who initially are overweight, malnourished, or suffering from some medical disorder requiring nutritional therapy.

There is no need to increase the *caloric* intake more than 10%, although many pregnant women find this difficult to avoid because of increased appetite. An intake of 2,000 to 2,400 calories a day should be ample. If weight gain exceeds a pound per week, some revision of the diet usually is desirable.

1. *Proteins* are nitrogenous tissue-building foods (found in meats, milk, cheese, egg yolk, liver, chicken, whole grain cereals, beans, peas, and fish). A high protein intake is desirable and the Food and Nutrition Board of the National Research Council has advised an allowance of 65 grams daily during pregnancy.

2. *Carbohydrates* are starchy foods (potatoes, cereals, rice, beans, peas, etc.). They are energy foods but must not be eaten in excess. Recommended intake is 150 to 200 grams daily.

3. *Fats* are energy foods also and contain certain vitamins. Butter, for example, has a high vitamin A content. Fats should be eaten sparingly.

4. *Minerals* are important during pregnancy. More than a dozen minerals are essential to human nutrition. For the pregnant woman the principal ones required are as follows:

(a) and (b) *Calcium* and *phosphorus* (approximately 1.2 grams per day of each) are demanded for the mother's health plus unusual requirements for fetal skeletal growth and development (including teeth). The calcium requirement is better supplied by consuming cheese (215 mg. Ca/oz.), yogurt (285 mg. Ca/cup), fish (30 to 125 mg. Ca/oz.), leafy vegetables (150 to 250 mg. Ca/cup), and a pint of milk (580 mg. Ca) daily than by taking medicinal salts of calcium by tablet. Relative lactose intolerance may be present in patients unaccustomed to milk ingestion for monetary or other reasons. The resulting nausea and vomiting may be overcome by small gradual incremental increases in milk consumption. The phosphorus in milk is supplemented by protein, of which it is a constituent. Vitamin D is the chief regulator of calcium and phosphorus metabolism.

(c) *Iron* demands during gestation are great because of the additional requirements of the infant. Eighteen mg. of dietary iron are recommended daily. Iron is furnished by meat, liver, eggs (yolk), oysters, fruits, nuts, raisins, and leafy vegetables (for example, spinach, broccoli, etc.). Experts claim that 30 to 60 mg. of additional elemental iron should be given daily in medicinal form.

(d) *Iodine* (125 micrograms [μg.] recommended daily) is usually sufficiently supplied if seafood is eaten once a week, except in endemic goiter areas (away from the sea), where iodine in the table salt may be used.

5. *Vitamins* are better obtained from foods than pills. By eating the proper foods, adequate vitamins are obtained. Vitamin supplements are very seldom necessary.

Vitamin A (6,000 IU recommended daily) is supplied by whole milk, butter, eggs, green, leafy, and yellow vegetables, fish liver oils, and coarse cereals. Vitamin A deficiency interferes with fetal growth, predisposes to abortion, and is said to predispose to infections in the mother. Butter is the best source of vitamin A.

Vitamin B and *B complex* including thiamine, riboflavin, niacin, pyridoxine (1.1, 1.8, 15, and 2.5 mg. recommended daily, respectively) and others are supplied by whole-grain breads and cereals, lean meats, vegetables (especially beans, peas, and lentils), and fruits. Folic acid requirements are substantially increased in pregnancy and many investigators believe that a folic acid supplement of 0.1 to 1.0 mg. should be given to pregnant women daily to prevent megaloblastic anemia. Oral Dilantin therapy will reduce folic acid absorption.

Vitamin C (ascorbic acid) is best supplied by citrus fruits, raw vegetables, and tomatoes. A 65 mg. intake is recommended daily.

Vitamin D (400 IU recommended daily) is the regulator of calcium and phosphorus metabolism but *unfortunately* is not found widely in natural foods. It is found in fish liver oils, milk, and egg yolk in small amounts. It is usually sufficiently supplied in a normal diet. However, some patients may require supplemental vitamin D, if sunshine is lacking.

Vitamin E (30 IU recommended daily) helps to maintain pregnancy in some animals. It is found in wheat germ oil. Its value in preventing human abortion is not firmly established.

Vitamin K is the antibleeding factor necessary for maintaining prothrombin blood levels and clotting time. Vitamin K is obtained by extraction from alfalfa or by chemical synthetic preparation. It should be given directly to the baby after birth.

Finally, in everyday, understandable terms, the daily diet should consist of the following:

1. Milk, 1 pint (low fat)
2. Cheese, 1 ounce
3. Eggs, 1
4. Butter or margarine, 1½ squares at each meal
5. Meat or chicken, moderate serving twice daily
6. Vegetables (leafy) twice daily, potato at one meal
7. Coarse, whole grain cereal, moderate serving one meal
8. Whole grain bread, 1 slice at two meals
9. Orange, 1; grapefruit, ½; or tomato juice, 6 ounces daily
10. Liver and fish once a week
11. Medicinal iron in form of ferrous sulfate

During the first 3 months less food than usual may be eaten because of nausea and vomiting. By the second trimester the dietary program just listed can be fully followed, and in the final trimester, a little tapering off may be permitted, especially if there is a tendency to overweight. Weighing at every prenatal visit will detect excessive gain, at which time the physician can determine whether it is caused by overeating or occult edema (an early sign of toxemia).

A bizarre appetite for unusual foods or materials (pica) may develop during pregnancy. Excessive ingestion of ice or frost (pagophagia) has frequently been associated with iron deficiency anemia as have occasional instances of ingestion of clay, dirt, starch, and other items. In the main, however, pica is not associated with any specific abnormality and is poorly understood. It generally is not detrimental to mother or fetus if a noxious chemical or parasites are not ingested.

DRUGS IN PREGNANCY

The vulnerability of a developing embryo or fetus to various chemical agents given to the mother has been demonstrated repeatedly. Despite the possible or proved teratogenicity of numerous pharmaceuticals, many pregnant women still receive a wide spectrum of potentially hazardous antidotes for every conceivable symptom or complaint, particularly during the first trimester. Some of the more undesirable substances are noted in the following paragraphs:

Cytotoxic drugs cause abortion if given early in pregnancy and cause a variety of malformations if used later.

Androgens and certain *progestogens* have produced masculinization and labial fusion in the female fetus.

Antithyroid drugs of the thiouracil group interfere with thyroxin synthesis and fetal goiter may develop. Radioactive iodine may lead to congenital hypothyroidism. Suppression of fetal thyroid may lead to mental deficiency.

Streptomycin may cause acoustic nerve deafness and various skeletal anomalies in an infant whose mother receives long-term treatment for tuberculosis. *Tetracyclines* discolor the infant's teeth and produce hypoplasia of dental enamel. *Nitrofurantoin* may produce hemolysis in the newborn if given to the mother near the time of delivery. *Novobiocin* and long-acting *sulfonamides* may lead to fetal hyperbilirubinemia, and *chloramphenicol* may lead to fetal death, if administered near term.

Coumarin derivatives may produce fatal hemorrhage in the fetus or newborn infant; heparin appears to be a safe anticoagulant because it does not readily cross the placenta.

Sedatives, hypnotics, and tranquilizing drugs have been implicated in various kinds of fetal damage. *Thalidomide* is definitely teratogenic and causes phocomelia (incomplete development of arms and legs), hearing loss, or even fetal death. *Phenobarbital* in excessive amounts leads to neonatal bleeding, *meprobamate* to general retardation of development, and the *phenothiazines* may produce hyperbilirubinemia and thrombocytopenia.

Salicylates in high dosage near term may lead to fetal blood coagulation defects and neonatal bleeding.

Morphine, heroin, methadone, and other addictive narcotics may lead to premature delivery and addiction, respiratory distress, and death of a newborn.

It has recently been established that maternal ingestion of *diethylstilbestrol* is associated with an increased incidence of vaginal and cervical adenocarcinoma in female offspring 8 to 26 years after delivery. Furthermore, at least one third of these individuals exhibit additional benign stigmata of such exposure in the form of effluent vaginal adenosis, and anatomic aberrations of the vagina and cervix. No abnormalities have yet been detected in the male offspring.

Much remains to be learned about the deleterious effects of drugs given to pregnant women, either intentionally to treat maternal symptoms or inadvertently before the existence of pregnancy has been recognized. In general, drug therapy in pregnancy should be restricted to the most urgent situations. New and experimental drugs, as well as all potential teratogens, must be carefully excluded.

It is unwise to succumb to the clinical philosphy that "it can't hurt and it might help," when groping for a therapeutic agent, at least until the former has been assured.

COMMON COMPLAINTS IN NORMAL PREGNANCY

Abdominal pain, usually minor and transient, is common in mid- and late pregnancy. Specific causes rarely are identified, though it is common to ascribe such discomfort to traction on the round ligaments or to intestinal compressions and displacements. Women with such pain should be examined carefully to exclude the possibility of appendiceal or gallbladder disease, partial placental separation, urinary tract infection, or premature labor.

Backache is very common, perhaps because of relaxation of pelvic joints. The usual remedies are analgesics, a firm mattress over a bed board, local heat and massage, and exercises designated to eliminate lumbar curvature. Herniation of an intervertebral disk as well as skeletal and renal abnormalities may develop during pregnancy and should be considered when evaluating this complaint.

Constipation is common because intestinal smooth muscle

activity is lessened by steroid hormones and because intestines are displaced by the enlarging uterus. The patient should make a serious effort to evacuate the bowels at the same time daily, increase the bulk and roughage in her diet, use laxative fruits freely, and increase her fluid intake and her exercise.

If medicinal aids are required to promote intestinal function, bulk laxatives, stool softeners, or one of the older standard remedies such as milk of magnesia or cascara may be tried. Although mineral oil is effective in some patients, it has been condemned on the ground that it prevents absorption of fat-soluble vitamins. Suppositories or enemas are rarely required.

Cramps in legs may occur suddenly when the patient is recumbent, usually precipitated by shortening of leg muscles ("pointing the toes" movement). It is claimed that leg cramps are provoked by excessive dietary phosphorus, but efforts to prevent them by reducing the intake of meat and milk, absorption with aluminum hydroxide, and adding calcium lactate to the diet have not been universally successful.

Headaches are common and most often are associated with emotional tension. Refractive errors and toxemia should be ruled out, and mild analgesics and sedatives should be tried before resorting to neurologic consultation unless the headache is accompanied by visual or neurologic symptoms.

Leukorrhea has already been noted as a presumptive sign of pregnancy. This complaint must be investigated, particularly if there is associated pruritus, to be certain that the vaginal discharge is not caused by trichomoniasis or candidiasis (moniliasis). If only the physiologic secretions are found, the treatment is frequent washing of the genital area and thorough drying and dusting with bath powder. Douching is generally unnecessary and not recommended.

Syncope or faintness are related to vasomotor instability and postural hypotension, particularly after prolonged standing or sitting in a warm area. Attacks may be diminished by deep breathing, vigorous leg motion, avoidance of rapid changes of position and elastic stockings.

Nausea and vomiting occur to some extent in about 75% of pregnant women. Although it may recur sporadically in later pregnancy, it is commonly confined to the first 2 or 3 months of gestation. It is usually intermittent rather than constant and may be accentuated, or appear, at any time. Its etiology is unclear, but authorities believe that rising estrogen and gonadotropin levels as well as emotional factors may be involved. Only rarely is the vomiting severe and intractable and only rarely is the situation grave enough to require hospitalization and treatment for resultant dehydration, starvation, alkalosis, and electrolyte depletion. This syndrome of *hyperemesis gravidarum* was more common in past decades but has largely passed from the obstetrical scene in this country. Severe vomiting may, on occasion, be attributable to hyperthyroidism, chronic poisoning, intestinal obstruction, carcinoma of the stomach, and other gastrointestinal abnormalities. Obviously, these must be considered and excluded.

Treatment for the typical nausea and vomiting of pregnancy usually rests with time, frequent small feedings, avoidance of any initiating situations, emotional support, repeated verbal reassurance of the temporary nature of the symptom, antiemetic drugs, and possible mild sedation. No one of the antiemetic drugs consistently appears to be more efficacious than the others, but one may be more effective than another for a given patient. Trials with different agents may be necessary before the most appropriate drug is found. Rarely do any give total relief, but reduction of symptoms to tolerable limits is usually achievable.

If the nausea is recurrent at relatively specific times, initiation of medication before its onset will accentuate effectiveness. Nausea noted upon awakening may be treated by taking medication at bedtime the night before, and that which develops shortly after arising may be treated by taking medication upon awakening, allowing 10 to 15 minutes for absorption before arising.

Edema, varicose veins, and *hemorrhoids,* as well as *urinary disturbances* and *heartburn,* are described in Chapter 22 in conjunction with medical and surgical problems complicating pregnancy.

MINOR PRENATAL QUESTIONS

Bathing in tubs need not be restricted in pregnancy, since the water does not enter the vagina.

Clothing should be comfortable, loose, and suspended from the shoulders. Constricting bands about the waist or circular garters must not be worn.

The *breasts* and *nipples* require no special treatment. If the breasts are large and heavy they need only a supporting, never a constricting, brassiere. Special treatment of the nipples in anticipation of nursing has not been shown to be of value.

Sexual intercourse is generally permissible throughout pregnancy but should be avoided if vaginal bleeding or uterine cramping is present. The potential effects of coitus and orgasm have been discussed in Chapter 5.

Dental care is permissible during pregnancy, contrary to older beliefs. Obviously prophylactic antibiotic therapy should be used to prevent bacteremia whenever dental abscesses are disturbed.

Smoking in moderation does not appear to be detrimental to most pregnancies, although there is some evidence that women who smoke bear lighter weight infants than those who do not. This lower birth weight, however, is not associated with any increased incidence of prenatal or neonatal mortality, or major anomalies. Smoking should be severely curtailed or stopped by pregnant women with chronic respiratory irritation, indigestion, or asthma.

Alcohol, used in moderation for social purposes, apparently exerts no harmful effect on the course of the pregnancy or on the fetus. Alcohol may stimulate the appetite and is itself a source of calories and thus should be avoided by patients trying desperately to limit their weight gain.

Travel in itself does not cause abortion or premature labor, but lengthy trips should not be undertaken for frivolous reasons because the patient may be far from competent care if an obstetric emergency arises. While one is away from home, it may be impossible to maintain a suitable diet, and there is always a risk of accident involving both mother and fetus. For necessary long trips air travel is recommended because it diminishes the time during which the patient is out of touch with obstetric care.

The use of *drugs* during pregnancy should be discouraged as much as possible. Teratogenesis clearly is related to the taking of certain pharmaceutic agents early in pregnancy, but information about harmful compounds is far from complete. The greatest danger of inducing malformations is in the first trimester, including the weeks prior to the patient's awareness of her pregnancy. For this reason women of childbearing age, and particularly those making a serious effort to conceive, should avoid all self-medication. Likewise, physicians should prescribe drugs for this group only when clear indications can be documented, and accurate records of what is taken must be kept.

Immunizations in pregnancy are generally acceptable, although pregnancy is currently considered to be a contraindication for vaccination against rubella, measles, and mumps. Viral infection of the fetus is feared in these instances. Although there is little benefit to be derived from wholesale immunizations during pregnancy, pregnant women should be immunized against poliomyelitis routinely and against influenza in the event of an epidemic, as pregnancy increases susceptibility to these diseases.

SUBSEQUENT OFFICE EXAMINATIONS

1. General condition—inquire carefully
2. Special examination if symptoms indicate
3. Blood pressure
4. Blood examination (PCV and/or antibody titer) if repetition indicated
5. Urinalysis
6. Weight—taken at every visit to detect excessive weight increases that may indicate occult edema, one of the earliest signs of toxemia
7. Abdominal examination—height of uterus, fetal position, and fetal heart rate
8. Rectal or vaginal examination, as indicated, to determine presenting part and status of cervix. (In the final month the degree of effacement and dilatation of the cervix may suggest that labor is imminent, and this information is needed to make a decision about induction of labor.)

Several weeks before the expected delivery date, the patient must be given explicit information about detection of incipient labor, premature rupture of membranes, how to get in touch with the physician day or night, and when to present herself at the hospital. Much anxiety can be avoided by making specific plans to cover any contingency.

During the last trimester the question of infant feeding should be discussed, and it seems desirable to decide prior to delivery whether the mother will attempt breast nursing. If a pediatrician has been selected well in advance, his views should be sought by the prospective mother.

Likewise, the various methods of analgesia and anesthesia available to the patient should be explained at least briefly and a tentative plan noted on the prenatal record. Generally speaking, it is unwise to promise any particular system of pain relief, lest conditions during the labor be unfavorable for it. The patient should be persuaded that the obstetrician and anesthesiologist jointly will provide the best possible management and that she should have faith in their judgment.

All pregnant women have concern, if not outright anxiety or fear, regarding the potentiality of miscarriage, malformations of the fetus, pain and death with labor and delivery, ineptitude at infant care, and a tremendous host of lesser items involved with vanity, self-image, aging, change in social role, family pressures, finances, marital relationships, etc. Although the majority of these anxieties cannot be resolved by the physician and must be handled by the patient, the obstetrician can greatly ease her psychologic burdens by initiating a discussion of these anxieties as routine prenatal occurrences and by counseling and reassuring her or by directing her to information or supportive services within the community. Minimalization of the patient's anxieties will make the pregnancy immensely happier for patient, family, and physician.

ASSESSMENT OF FETAL MATURITY AND INTRAUTERINE STATUS

It is often desirable in the last month or two of pregnancy to be able to assess the weight and maturity of the fetus in utero and, consequently, its potential to successfully accommodate to extrauterine existence. This is particularly true in instances of anticipated elective induction of labor or repeat cesarean section, and in situations in which fetal extraction at the earliest safe moment is desired to avoid the continued consequence of an abnormal environment (for example, maternal diabetes, toxemia, placental insufficiency, etc.). Many methods have been developed, none of which are infallible. Taken cumulatively, or in combination, however, they have considerable value, and because of their importance in the management of high-risk pregnancies, new and more sophisticated methods are constantly being sought.

History and physical examination. An accurate menstrual history can be of prime importance with the consideration that the average gestational duration is 267 days from the *time of conception*. Inaccuracies in determining the latter are manifold, but the more regular the menstrual interval, and the more secure the date of the last menstrual period, the greater the reliability of the estimate. The availability of the basal temperature chart exhibiting clear-cut evidence of the time of ovulation in the cycle of conception is extremely helpful.

If one assumes that quickening normally occurs between the eighteenth and twentieth weeks, that ultrasonic auscultation will usually reveal fetal heart activity at the tenth to twelfth weeks, and that the fetal heart may be heard with the fetoscope at approximately the twentieth week, the appearance of these may be correlated with the historical calculation. Frequent examinations during the tenth to twentieth weeks will be required for these assessments but may well be rewarded in subsequent months.

Correlation of the fundal height with that anticipated at various times in gestation, as noted in the last chapter, may be of use, but there are numerous aspects, even apart from wide individual variation, that can distort this measurement (for example, volume of amniotic fluid, parity, twins, diabetes, toxemia, etc.). Nonetheless, close attention to clinical details and repeated thoughtful evaluation during pregnancy may ultimately be more important in decision making than the assessments that follow.

X-ray examination. Roentgen evaluation of fetal osseous development has been of modest aid in past years when other assessments were unavailable. Although several presumed correlations have been described, including attempts to

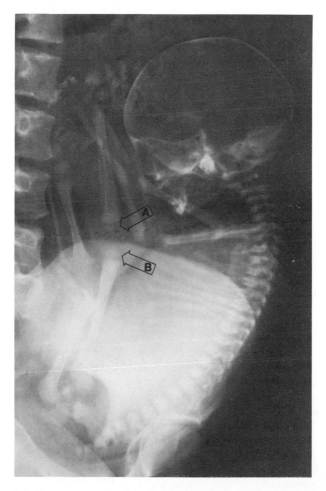

Fig. 7-1. Roentgenogram of term fetus (in frank breech presentation) demonstrating proximal tibial, **A,** and distal femoral, **B,** epiphyses. (Courtesy Community X-Ray Division, Stanford University Hospital, Stanford, Calif.)

approximate the fetal biparietal diameter, the most frequently utilized have been visualization of the distal femoral epiphysis at approximately 36 weeks of gestation and visualization of the proximal tibial epiphysis at 38 weeks (Fig. 7-1).

Ultrasonic scanning. Roentgen evaluation has been largely superseded in the more modern centers by safer and more reliable ultrasonic scanning. The fetal biparietal diameter can be determined by A-scan ultrasonography with an accuracy within 1 mm. The fetal weight may then be estimated with a standard deviation of ±500 gm. by the use of the following formula:

$$\text{Weight in grams} = \text{Biparietal diameter} (\times 1,060) - 6,575.$$

Accuracy can be significantly improved by averaging the result of this method with that obtained by determining the anteroposterior (AP) and transverse diameters of the thorax and applying the following formula:

$$\text{Weight in grams} = 1,000 \times \frac{\text{AP diameter} \times \text{transverse diameter}}{2} - 7,170.$$

This method may also be used serially to follow fetal growth rate, as there is no known adverse effect from ultrasonography on either the fetal or maternal organism.

Amniotic fluid examination. Evaluations of several constituents of amniotic fluid, obtained by direct amniocentesis, are currently being used for assessment of fetal maturity. Each assesses the functional maturity of a different fetal organ, much as the appearance of the fetal heartbeat was used to assess maturity of the fetal cardiac system. These are most useful during the final months of gestation and have shown considerable reliability, especially when used in combination.

1. *Bilirubin pigment.* The optical-density deviation at 450 mμ normally declines progressively in the last trimester and is less than 0.01 at time of fetal maturity.

2. *Lipid cells.* Skin maturity is assessed by estimating the percentage of amniotic fluid cells that are derived from fetal skin and consequently contain fat and become orange upon staining with nile blue sulfate or oil red O. When more than

20% of the cells contain lipid, the gestation is considered to be beyond 35 weeks.

3. *Creatinine.* Fetal renal maturity is assessed by measuring the concentration of creatinine. After the thirty-sixth week this is greater than 1.8 mg.%. If maternal renal disease coexists, amniotic fluid creatinine concentration may be abnormally high, but fetal maturity can be predicted if the concentration is more than treble that of maternal plasma.

4. *Lecithin-sphingomyelin ratio.* Lung maturity is assessed by determining the ratio of lecithin to sphingomyelin (Chapter 4) after chromatographic separation and colorimetric quantitation of these amniotic fluid phospholipids. Respiratory distress in the newborn rarely occurs when the ratio is greater than 2.

Progression of the lecithin-sphingomyelin (L/S) ratio to mature levels is accelerated in instances of maternal hypertension, toxemia, placental insufficiency, and other states associated with fetal stress. In these circumstances fetal lungs mature faster than with normal pregnancy and fetal survival is greater than for unstressed fetuses of similar weight. Membrane rupture is also associated with an accelerated rise in the L/S ratio, but this rise is not associated with an increased rate of pulmonary maturation.

Progression of the L/S ratio to mature levels is delayed with diabetes, and consequently fetuses of diabetic mothers have lower than normal L/S ratios for gestational age.

Variations on this test include the direct quantitation of lecithin (wherein maturity is associated with a lecithin phosphorus concentration of greater than 0.1 mg.%) and a rapid bedside "form test." In the latter, mature levels of phosphatide are believed to be demonstrated by the formation of small stable bubbles at the meniscus 15 minutes after vigorous shaking of a mixture of amniotic fluid, normal saline, and 95% ethanol (1:1:2).

Amnioscopy. Transcervical amnioscopy may also be used to assess fetal intrauterine status by observing the amniotic fluid for the presence of meconium. This method has not been noted to be highly reliable, but the notation of greenish discoloration prior to labor is considered to be an unfavorable prognostic sign associated with depressed fetal oxygenation. With fetal death, the fluid is brown and murky. The procedure is cumbersome and occasionally leads to bleeding or rupture of the membranes. Identical information can be obtained by the observation of fluid obtained by amniocentesis.

Estriol quantitation. The concentration of estriol in maternal urine or plasma is an index of the functional capacity of the placenta as well as certain fetal organs, especially the liver and adrenal glands. Although estriol levels rise progressively in late pregnancy (Chapter 3), they cannot be used as a direct assessment of fetal maturity because of the placental component in their formation. They are employed as an index of fetoplacental integrity and the intrauterine status of the fetus.

Estriol levels fail to rise in certain circumstances, such as molar pregnancy, anencephaly, placental sulfatase deficiency, and early fetal death. In late pregnancy they fall slowly or abruptly with fetal death and in circumstances in which fetal survival is imperiled (such as toxemia, diabetes, postmaturity and other states associated with placental insufficiency). Frequent serial determinations are essential, as single determinations do not give adequate reliability and the trend is usually more important than the absolute value.

Oxytocin stress test. The oxytocin stress test is used to assess fetal intrauterine status in late pregnancy or, more specifically, the functional reserve of the placenta and the potential of the fetus to survive the rigors of labor. While the patient is under close observation and the uterine contractions and fetal heart rate are being constantly monitored electronically, dilute oxytocin solution is intravenously administered until uterine contractions occur at 3-minute intervals. The development of fetal distress in the form of abnormal fetal heart rate patterns (Chapter 12) implies embarrassment of the fetal circulatory system resulting from decreased fetal oxygenation. This most often occurs because of placental insufficiency or because of occlusive cord complications induced by uterine contractions. Fetuses without this response customarily survive further gestation or labor without incident, but intermittent reassessment is required.

8

Postures of the fetus
in the uterus

TERMINOLOGY

An exact knowledge of the many different postures in which the fetus may be found in utero is necessary for accurate diagnosis, for a clear understanding of the mechanism of labor, and for the proper conduct of parturition. Certain terms are used to designate different phases of these postures. Unfortunately, some of these terms are confusing, and considerable differences of opinion have developed over their usage. The common descriptive words are *attitude (habitus), presentation, presenting part, lie, position,* and *variety.*

Attitude (habitus). There is general agreement that attitude or habitus means the posture of the baby in relation to itself, with no regard for the relation of the fetus to the mother. In the normal attitude the baby's back is arched, the head flexed, the chin touching the chest, the arms folded across the chest, the thighs flexed on the abdomen, the knees flexed, with the legs crossed, and the feet flexed on the legs.

Presentation. Most textbooks use the term "presentation" in two different and confusing ways: (1) it may mean the relation of the long axis of the fetus to the long axis of the mother and in this sense there are two presentations, the longitudinal and the transverse (when the baby lies crosswise); (2) it may mean the part that is "presented" to the mother's pelvis, for example, vertex or breech. The confusion that arises from giving the terms "presentation" and "presenting part" two different meanings may be avoided by using them synonymously.

Presenting part. The presenting part is the most dependent portion of the fetus at the inlet of the pelvis and therefore that part with which the examining finger first comes in contact. The presenting part is designated by its characteristic anatomic landmark. For example, a vertex presentation is spoken of as *occipital* because normal flexion of the head on the trunk dictates that the occipital portion of the skull will be most dependent. If the head is deflexed so that the fetal face is lowermost, the chin *(mentum)* is the landmark. When the breech is presenting, the prominent anatomic part is the *sacrum*.

Lie. Lie designates the relation between the long axis of the mother and child, that is, longitudinal lie or transverse lie.

Position and variety. Position denotes whether the presenting part of the fetus (for example, occiput) lies adjacent to the right or to the left side of the maternal pelvis. Variety further defines the position by denoting whether the presenting part is situated adjacent to the anterior, the lateral (transverse), or the posterior portion of a particular half of the maternal pelvis. Thus there are six varieties of position, three on each side of the pelvis.

PRESENTATION AND POSITION

There is no single term to designate both presentation and position, but by usage, the separate terms "position" and "presentation" are employed when both are meant. When one wishes to diagnose the position and presentation, he asks himself two questions:

"What part is presenting?" and "Where is it in relation to the mother's pelvis?" If the vertex presents and if it is in the left anterior quadrant, the presentation and position are left occiput anterior, usually designated by the three capital letters L.O.A.

POSTURES OF FETUS
Longitudinal lie
Cephalic (head) presentation
Vertex (occipital). In the vertex or occipital presentation the head is completely flexed (Fig. 8-1).

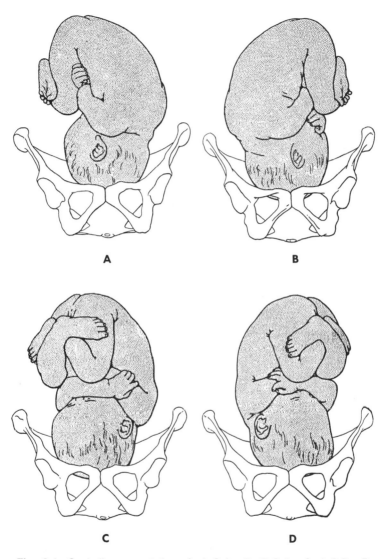

A **B**

C **D**

Fig. 8-1. Cephalic presentation. **A,** L.O.A.; **B,** R.O.A.; **C,** L.O.P.; **D,** R.O.P. (Redrawn from Bumm.)

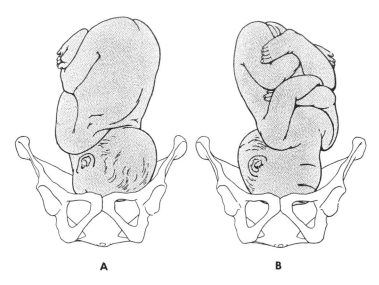

A **B**

Fig. 8-2. Face presentation. **A,** R.M.P.; **B,** L.M.A. Note complete extension of the head. (Redrawn from Bumm.)

Face (chin). When the face or chin presents, the head is completely extended (Fig. 8-2).

Bregma (sincipital). In the bregma presentation the head is midway between flexion and extension.

Brow (frontal). In the brow presentation the head is partially extended (Fig. 8-3).

The bregma and brow presentations are often transitory, becoming vertex or face presentations, according to the degree of flexion or extension during labor. However, they may persist.

Breech presentations

Complete breech. In the complete breech presentation the thighs are flexed upon the abdomen and the legs upon the thighs (Fig. 8-4).

Frank breech. In the frank breech the thighs are flexed upon the abdomen and the legs extended over the chest with the feet near the chin.

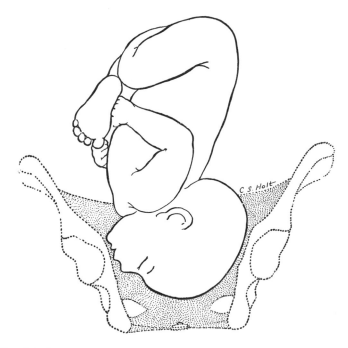

Fig. 8-3. Brow presentation. Note partial extension of the head. (From Falls and McLaughlin: Obstetric and gynecologic nursing, St. Louis, The C. V. Mosby Co.)

Footling. In the footling presentation one or both feet are in the pelvis below the fetal buttocks.

Knee presentation. The flexed knee is in the pelvis when the knee presents.

Transverse lie

In the transverse lie the shoulder is the presenting part, with the back anterior or with the back posterior (Fig. 8-5).

POSSIBLE POSITIONS OR PRESENTATIONS

The initial letter of the name of the presenting fetal part is used to distinguish the presentation, and the initials of the pel-

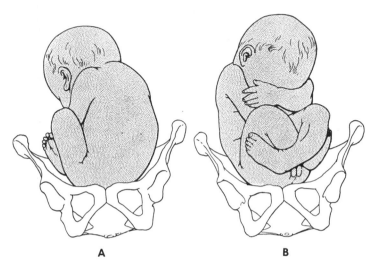

Fig. 8-4. Complete breech presentation. **A,** L.S.A.; **B,** R.S.P. (Redrawn from Bumm.)

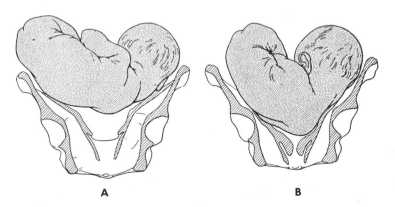

Fig. 8-5. A, Transverse lie, shoulder presentation. **B,** Impacted shoulder presentation. (Redrawn from Bumm.)

vic quadrant in which it lies are used to designate the position. Therefore, three initials are employed to distinguish each presentation and position. The initials used are as follows:

L.	Laeva or left
D. or R.	Dextra or right
A.	Anterior
P.	Posterior
T.	Transverse (for example, when the occiput is directed toward the right or left but is neither anterior nor posterior)
O.	Occiput
M.	Mentum (chin)
S.	Sacrum (buttocks)
Sc.	Scapula (shoulder)

The various positions and presentations are vertex (occipital), face, breech (sacral), and shoulder (acromial or scapular). A brow (forehead) presentation is usually temporary and changes during labor to face or vertex. There are six positions or varieties in which every presentation may lie—right or left anterior or posterior, and right or left transverse.

Vertex (occipital) presentations
1. Left occiput anterior—L.O.A.
2. Left occiput transverse—L.O.T.
3. Left occiput posterior—L.O.P.
4. Right occiput anterior—R.O.A.
5. Right occiput transverse—R.O.T.
6. Right occiput posterior—R.O.P.

Face presentations
1. Left mentum anterior—L.M.A.
2. Left mentum transverse—L.M.T.
3. Left mentum posterior—L.M.P.
4. Right mentum anterior—R.M.A.
5. Right mentum transverse—R.M.T.
6. Right mentum posterior—R.M.P.

Breech (sacral) presentations
1. Left sacrum anterior—L.S.A.
2. Left sacrum transverse—L.S.T.
3. Left sacrum posterior—L.S.P.

4. Right sacrum anterior—R.S.A.
5. Right sacrum transverse—R.S.T.
6. Right sacrum posterior—R.S.P.

Modifications of the breech presentation, such as prolapse of a foot or feet ("footling" or "double footling") and knee, are named according to the location of the sacrum, without consideration of the prolapsed part.

Shoulder (acromial or scapular) presentations. It is difficult, if not virtually impossible, to differentiate the various shoulder presentations by clinical examination alone, and nothing is gained by doing so. On the basis of radiologic examination one may determine whether the presenting scapular region lies toward the mother's right or left side and whether the fetal back faces anteriorly or posteriorly. Thus a particular presentation might be designated, for instance, R.Sc.P.

INCIDENCE OF VARIOUS PRESENTATIONS AND POSITIONS

Authorities do not agree as to the exact frequency, but there is very general agreement as to the relative incidence of the various presentations and positions.

Vertex. About 95% of all presentations at or near term are vertex. Approximately two thirds of these occur in the *left position* and one third in the *right position*. At the onset of labor, the fetal head is in the transverse position in over 60% of patients (L.O.T. or R.O.T.). The straight anteroposterior positions (O.A. and O.P.) are unusual, whereas the various intermediate positions (for example, L.O.A. and R.O.P.) are seen rather often.

Face (chin). Face presentations occur in 0.5% to 1% of patients.

Breech. Breech presentations occur in 3% to 4% of patients.

Shoulder. Shoulder presentations occur in 0.5% to 1% of patients.

Reasons for the incidence of the various positions are largely speculative; although the accommodation theory seems reasonable, it has not been completely explained.

DIAGNOSIS OF PRESENTATION AND POSITION

The diagnosis of presentation and position involves abdominal palpation, vaginal or rectal examination, auscultation, and x-ray examination (in certain doubtful cases).

Abdominal palpation—Leopold's maneuvers

First maneuver. The first of Leopold's maneuvers is to determine what fetal parts are in the fundus uteri (Fig. 8-6).

1. Ascertain the outlines of the uterus. (Stand facing the patient's head.)

2. *Palpate the fundus* gently with the palmar surfaces (not

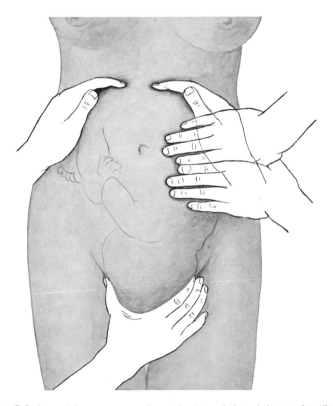

Fig. 8-6. Leopold's maneuvers for palpation of the abdomen for diagnosis of presentation and position of the baby—two hands palpating the breech (or head) in the fundus uteri; two hands palpating the back (or small parts) on the left side; one hand (Pawlik's grip) palpating the head (or breech) at the pelvis.

the tips) of the fingers of both hands to determine *which pole of the fetus is upward.* The breech is large, irregular, and rather soft, whereas the head is hard, round, freely movable, and ballottable.

Second maneuver. The second Leopold maneuver is to determine what fetal parts are on each side of the abdomen.

1. Place the palmar surfaces of the fingers of both hands on each side of the abdomen (both hands side by side, alternately on one side and then the other), making gentle, deep pressure.

2. *One side feels like a hard resistant plane—the back.*

3. *Resistance is less on the other side.*

(a) There is a cystic feeling, that is, like palpating a cystic mass.

(b) Several nodules may be felt—the fetal small parts. It is easy to locate the back on one side and fetal small parts on the other in moderately thin women; often it is very difficult in tense or obese patients.

After locating the back or fetal parts, determine whether they are anterior or posterior.

Third maneuver. The third Leopold maneuver is performed by *facing the patient's head* and by grasping the lower portion of the abdomen between the thumb and fingers to determine what is between them (Pawlik's grip).

1. If the presenting part is not engaged, a movable body will be felt.

2. If it is the head presenting, it will be a hard, round ballottable body; if it is the breech presenting, a large irregular, softer mass will be felt.

3. Determine the "cephalic prominence," that is, on which side of the abdomen the head is more prominent (an obstetric, not an anatomic, term).

4. *If the cephalic prominence is on the side opposite the fetal back and on the same side as the small parts, the head is flexed and a vertex presents. If it is on the same side as the back and opposite the fetal small parts, the head is extended; therefore the face or brow presents.* When the "cephalic prominence" is very prominent, the face presents; when it is less prominent, the brow presents.

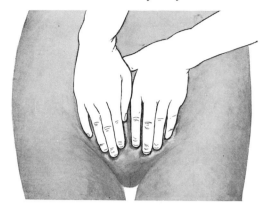

Fig. 8-7. Palpating above symphysis pubis with both hands to determine position of the presenting part.

Fourth maneuver

1. Facing the patient's feet, *make deep pressure with the fingers of both hands, one on each side, in the direction of the axis of the superior strait* (Fig. 8-7).

The information thus obtained depends to some extent on how far the head has descended into the pelvic cavity.

2. If the head presents, the fingers of one hand will come in contact with a hard, round body first—the cephalic prominence—while the other hand descends deeper into the pelvis before reaching the less prominent part of the head.

3. Here, as in the third maneuver, if the cephalic prominence is on the same side as the small parts, the vertex presents and if it is on the side with the back, the face or brow presents.

4. In breech presentations the information obtained by this maneuver is less definite. However, by alternately palpating the fundus and the area just above the symphysis pubis, the head can be located.

Vaginal examination

During pregnancy, vaginal examination may be inconclusive because of the intervening cervix and rather thick lower segment; but in labor, effacement and dilatation of the cervix occur, permitting more accurate palpation.

Important landmarks may be distinguished.
1. The various sutures of the head
2. The different fontanels
3. In face presentations, the chin, nose, supraorbital ridges, orbits, mouth, and eyes
4. In breech presentations, the sacrum, ischial tuberosities, and sometimes the anus or external genitalia

First maneuver. Separate the labia. Insert one or two fingers into the vagina up to the presenting part to determine whether it is a vertex, face, brow, or breech.

Second maneuver. If the vertex presents, sweep the fingers over the fetal head from the pubis toward the sacrum. The fingers will necessarily cross the sagittal suture by this maneuver (Fig. 8-8).

Third maneuver. Trace the sagittal suture in both directions to determine the location of the small and the large fontanels. The location of the small fontanel in one of the four quadrants

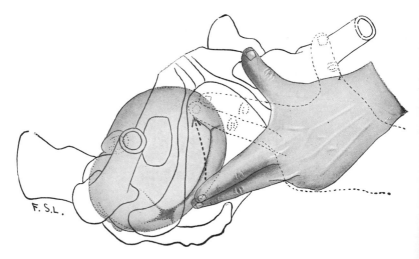

Fig. 8-8. Vaginal palpation of sutures. Note sweep of the fingers across the sutures. (From Stander: Williams obstetrics, New York, D. Appleton-Century Co.)

of the pelvis will determine the position—left, right, anterior, posterior, or transverse (Fig. 8-9).

Fourth maneuver. Note extent of dilatation and effacement of cervix, station of presenting part, and change in station and dilatation created by firm downward pressure on uterine fundus.

Auscultation

1. Auscultation is not always reliable, but in connection with palpatory findings the point of maximum intensity of the fetal heart may be of great diagnostic value, even if not decisive.

2. The heart sounds are usually heard best through the back in vertex and breech presentations.

3. The heart sounds are usually heard best through the chest in face presentations.

4. In cephalic presentations the heart is heard best about midway on a line from the anterior superior spine of the ilium to the navel. In posterior positions the point of maximum intensity is near the flank.

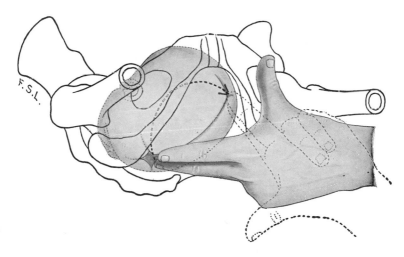

Fig. 8-9. Vaginal palpation of the fontanels. Note sweep of the fingers from the large to the small fontanel. (From Stander: Williams obstetrics, New York, D. Appleton-Century Co.)

5. In breech presentations it is best heard usually about the level of or above the navel.

6. The point of maximum intensity may be particularly misleading in posterior positions because the flexion of the head may be imperfect (which is common in posterior positions), and therefore the thorax may be pushed forward anteriorly toward the abdominal wall where the fetal heart will be heard best, leading to the mistaken diagnosis of an anterior position. Even in normal positions the heart may be best heard on the side opposite the back, especially if the physician forgets that the normal dextroversion and tipping of the uterus toward the right (sometimes toward the left) may be exaggerated, causing a dislocation of the usual point of maximum intensity of the fetal heart.

7. *Although auscultation often gives most valuable supplementary aid in determing the position of the child, the physician must not fall into the error of relying upon it alone.*

X-ray examination

X-ray examination is a valuable diagnostic aid, especially in obese women or in nervous patients with rigid abdominal walls. Because of the potential hazards of roentgenologic examination already described (Chapter 6), x-ray films should not be made unless there is serious doubt about fetal position and about the possibility of disproportion between the fetus and the maternal pelvis.

B-scan ultrasonography can offer evidence regarding fetal presentation and position without these hazards and is to be recommended.

9

The normal pelvis

Inasmuch as the mechanism of birth consists of a succession of adjustments and readjustments of the fetus to the varying diameters of the mother's pelvis, through which it must pass, obviously an understanding of this process is impossible without an accurate knowledge of the bony pelvis and its soft parts.

The ancient belief that childbirth was made possible by a separation of the pelvic bones was dispelled in 1543, when Vesalius first accurately described the bony pelvis as a firm, unyielding osseous ring. The eighteenth century had dawned before the obstetric significance of the pelvis was thoroughly studied by Van Deventer (1701), whose studies included deformed as well as normal pelves. The first accurate treatise in English describing the pelvis from the obstetric standpoint was by Smellie in 1752. His method of measuring the anteroposterior pelvic diameter is used to this day.

ANATOMY OF BONY PELVIS

The pelvis is composed of the two innominate bones, the sacrum, and the coccyx. The innominate bones are joined securely at the symphysis pubis and are even more securely attached to the sacrum at the sacroiliac synchondroses (Fig. 9-1).

The *true pelvis,* lying below the pelvic brim and marked by the linea terminalis, is important in the mechanism of labor; the false pelvis has scarcely any obstetric significance.

The *pelvic canal* is a passage of irregular shape and size that varies at different levels and is larger at its middle than at its inlet or outlet; therefore, the diameters at these different planes

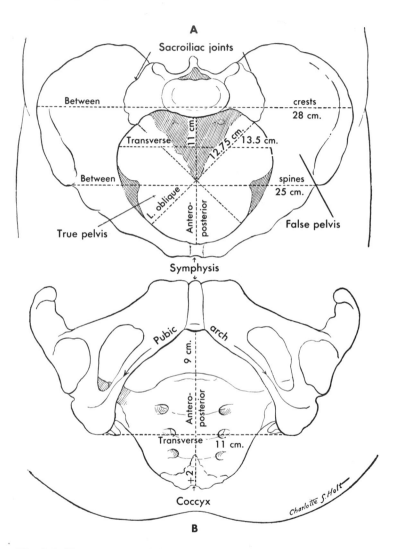

Fig. 9-1. Measurements of the normal female bony pelvis. (From Falls and McLaughlin: Obstetric and gynecologic nursing, St. Louis, The C. V. Mosby Co.)

must be known to understand the mechanism and possibilities of labor.

Plane of inlet (superior strait)

Anteroposterior or conjugate diameters

1. The *true conjugate* or conjugata vera (11 cm. or more), also called the anatomic conjugate, extends from the upper margin of the symphysis pubis to the sacral promontory.

2. The *obstetric conjugate* is the shortest distance between the posterior surface of the symphysis and the sacral promontory. It is a few millimeters shorter than the true conjugate. *This is the most important measurement of the inlet* because it determines whether or not the presenting part can enter the true pelvis.

3. The *diagonal conjugate* (12.5 to 13 cm.) extends from the lower border of the symphysis to the promontory. Its great importance arises from the fact that the obstetric conjugate cannot be directly measured in the living patient; therefore, the easily measured diagonal conjugate is determined, and the obstetric conjugate is estimated by subtracting 1.5 to 2 cm. from the measurement of the diagonal conjugate (Fig. 9-2).

Transverse diameter of inlet (13.5 cm.). Although the transverse diameter is the longest diameter of the inlet, it is not fully available for the entrance of the head through the inlet because the presenting part impinges upon the sacral promontory and is thus pushed forward into a smaller diameter. This is the reason that the presenting part often enters the pelvis through the oblique diameters (usually the right).

Oblique diameter (12.75 cm.). The oblique diameter extends from the sacroiliac synchondrosis obliquely across to the opposite iliopectineal eminence. The oblique diameter is called right or left according to the synchondrosis from which it starts.

Plane of greatest dimensions. The plane of greatest dimensions is the largest plane of the pelvis. Anteriorly it passes through the middle of the symphysis pubis, posteriorly through the sacrum between the second and third fused vertebrae, and laterally through the top of the acetabulum. Its anteroposterior diameter averages 12.75 cm., and the transverse diameter averages 12.5 cm.

Plane of least dimensions. The plane of least dimensions is the smallest plane of the pelvic canal, and it passes through the lower

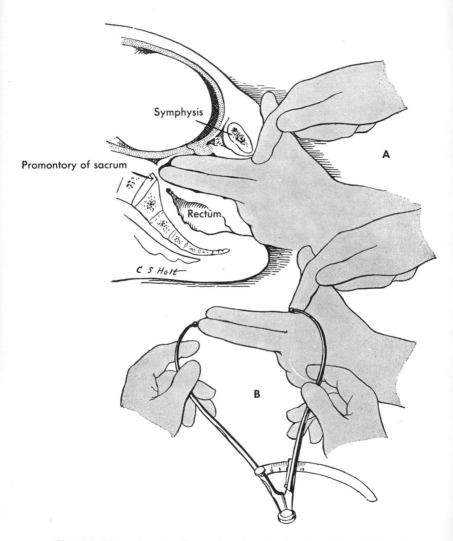

Fig. 9-2. Measuring the diagonal conjugate diameter. (From Falls and McLaughlin: Obstetric and gynecologic nursing, St. Louis, The C. V. Mosby Co.)

margin of the symphysis, the ischial spines, and the tip of the sacrum. Its anteroposterior diameter, from the lower border of the symphysis to the tip of the sacrum, averages 11.5 cm. (to the coccyx tip, 9.5 cm.); the transverse diameter between the ischial spines is the shortest transverse distance in the normal pelvis (10.5 cm.). The posterior sagittal diameter of this midpelvic plane is that portion of the anteroposterior diameter that extends from the ischial spines to the sacrum (about 4.5 cm.). In some respects this is the most important obstetric plane, particularly because shortening of its diameters frequently is associated with obstructed labors.

Plane of pelvic outlet. The plane of the pelvic outlet is really two triangular planes with the same base, which is a line drawn between the two tuberosites of the ischia; the apex of the posterior triangle is at the tip of the sacrum, and the apex of the anterior triangle is at the lower border (arcuate ligament) of the symphysis pubis.

1. The *anteroposterior diameter,* from the middle of the arcuate ligament to the tip of the sacrum, averages 10.5 cm. (to the tip of the coccyx, 9.5 cm.). NOTE: During labor the movable coccyx may be pushed backward by the presenting part; hence, the actual diameter is lengthened to 10.5 cm.

2. The *transverse diameter,* between the inner margins of the ischial tuberosites, averages 11 cm.

3. The *posterior sagittal diameter* extends from the lower end of the sacrum to a right-angled intersection with an imaginary line passing between the ischial tuberosites, and it measures about 7.5 cm.

Pelvic inclination. Pelvic inclination is expressed by the angle that the plane of the inlet forms with the horizon while the woman stands erect, normally 45 to 55 degrees. Unless it departs greatly from the normal, it has little obstetric significance.

Of great significance, however, is the angle between the posterior surface of the symphysis pubis and the obstetric conjugate (usually 90 to 100 degrees), for the obstetric conjugate may be shortened or lengthened by the inclination of the symphysis; therefore, this angle must be considered when one estimates the obstetric conjugate after measuring the diagonal conjugate.

Pelvic axis. The pelvic axis is represented by a line drawn through the centers of all its planes and consequently has the configuration of a gentle right-angle turn (Fig. 12-1).

Pelvic joints

1. In the nonpregnant state the pelvic joints are immovable; however, they do move slightly during pregnancy. At the symphysis this motion can be felt by a finger in the vagina when the woman walks.

2. During pregnancy the normally immobile sacroiliac synchondrosis becomes slightly movable, probably as the result of hormonal activity. Radiologic studies have shown that the interosseous space at the symphysis pubis increases in width during pregnancy. The notion that elasticity of the pelvic joints would lead to an increase in the obstetric conjugate diameter if the patient were placed in extreme hyperextension has been shown to be erroneous.

Variations in pelves

Individual variations. No two pelves are exactly alike, but the differences lie within a narrow range; the measurements just given are averages.

Racial variations. Racial variations have not been scientifically studied for all races. In this country, the pelvis of a black person is likely to be smaller than that of a white person of comparable stature, but obstetrically speaking, this is usually compensated for by the smaller black infant's head.

Sex variations. The female pelvis, designed for purposes of childbearing, differs distinctly from that of the male. The female pelvis is relatively lighter, lower, and less conical; the inlet and the outlet are both larger; the diameters of the inlet of the female pelvis average a centimeter larger and the diameters of the outlet are 2 to 3 cm. larger.

Conversion of fetal pelvis to adult pelvis. The conversion of the fetal pelvis to the adult pelvis is dependent on the fact that the infant's pelvis is more or less "malleable," being composed of bone and cartilage, and the individual bones—ilium, ischium, and pubis—are areas not completely developed and ossified until the individual is more than 20 years of age, and therefore it is subject to change by certain mechanical forces that are applicable when the individual walks.

The pelvis is, as it were, caught between two forces acting in opposite directions when the erect posture is assumed: (1) The weight of the body is transmitted to the pelvis (sacrum) through the spinal column. (2) The resistance to this thrust is transmitted from below through the femurs. Thus the comparatively soft pelvis is compressed by two forces that change its shape, resulting in the peculiar contour of the adult pelvis, which might, paradoxically, be termed "the normally deformed pelvis." Through these same forces a soft rachitic pelvis becomes the rachitic flat pelvis.

The various steps in the change are as follows:

1. The superimposed weight transmitted through the spinal column forces the sacrum toward the symphysis.

2. The sacrum rotates slightly and its tip is displaced upward and backward.

3. The strong sacrosciatic ligaments limit this movement so that the not yet ossified sacrum is bent upon itself vertically.

4. Simultaneously the soft sacral vertebrae are forced forward, thus reducing the transverse sacral concavity.

5. As the sacrum is forced by the body weight downward and forward, it drags the posterior superior spines of the ilium outward; the ilium bends, which accounts for the greater transverse diameter of the pelvis.

These mechanical forces, which act the same in both sexes, evidently cannot be the only factor since they do not account for the differences between the pelves of the two sexes. There must be another as yet unknown influence, perhaps a congenital sexual tendency, to explain the contrast. Quadrupeds have no such "normal deformity," which accounts, in part, for the greater difficulty of labor in the biped woman. A clear concept of the shape and measurements of the female bony pelvis at its various levels is an urgent necessity if one is to understand the mechanism of labor and the possibilities of birth through the pelvic canal.

Classification of major pelvic forms. Caldwell and Moloy (1933) classified pelves from the approach of the architectural structure. The portion of the pelvic cavity anterior to the longest transverse diameter was called the forepelvis and the posterior portion, the posterior or hindpelvis. They divided pelves into four main groups: gynecoid (true female), android (male type), platypelloid (flat), and anthropoid (apelike) (Fig. 9-3).

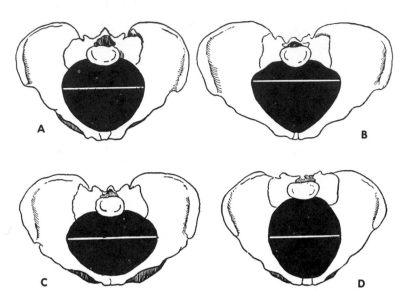

Fig. 9-3. Four main groups of pelves. **A,** Gynecoid pelvis. **B,** Android pelvis. **C,** Platypelloid pelvis. **D,** Anthropoid pelvis. (From Beck: Obstetrical practice, Baltimore, The Williams & Wilkins Co.)

Gynecoid pelvis (true female). The gynecoid or true female pelvis is the most common type (normal) and is approximately round (or slightly oval). The transverse diameter is a little longer than the anteroposterior diameter and is considerably anterior to the sacral promontory, making the hindpelvis roomy, broad, and deep. The sacrosciatic notch is broad, showing that there is ample room in both the anterior and posterior pelvis, and the pubic arch is wide. Normal birth is the rule.

Android pelvis (male type). The inlet of the android or male-type pelvis is heart shaped because the sacral promontory is pushed forward nearer the widest transverse diameter; thus it is nearer the promontory, making the posterior pelvis shallow. The pubic arch is narrow, and the sacrosciatic notch is narrow, with the outlet diameter shortened. This type of pelvis is a frequent cause of difficult labor.

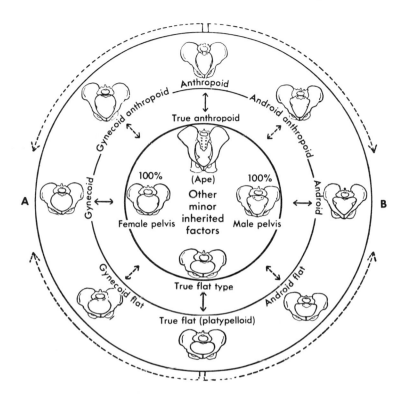

Fig. 9-4. Diagrammatic illustration of the Caldwell-Moloy theory of the development of pelvic form. The vertical axis shows an evolutionary transition from anthropoid to platypelloid type. The transverse axis (**A** to **B**) shows transitions caused by hormonal (sexual) factors. In the outer circle are shown the resulting pure and mixed forms actually observed in adult women. (From Caldwell, Moloy, and D'Esopo: Amer. J. Obstet. Gynec. **28:**482, 1934.)

Platypelloid pelvis (flat). In the platypelloid or flat pelvis the anteroposterior diameter is shortened, and the widest transverse diameter is relatively lengthened and lies approximately equidistant from the promontory and symphysis. Both the forepelvis and hindpelvis are shortened. The sacrosciatic notch appears narrowed, and the subpubic angle is usually relatively wide. The fetal head enters the pelvic brim transversely in pronounced asynclitism.

Anthropoid pelvis (apelike). The anteroposterior pelvic diameter is long and the transverse diameter is short, giving the inlet the shape of a sagittal ellipse. Because the widest transverse diameter is so far from the promontory, the posterior pelvis is deep and the sacrosciatic notch is wide. The head enters the pelvis either obliquely or in the anteroposterior diameter (because of the relatively or actually short transverse diameter of the inlet). The occiput frequently lies posteriorly, and not infrequently the infant may be born with the occiput persistently posterior.

•　　•　　•

X-ray films (anteroposterior, lateral, and stereoscopic) are necessary to determine accurately the different pelvic types in this classification. Not all pelves fall definitely into one of these four parent types. The characteristics of one type may be coexistent with another, for example, gynecoid-anthropoid, android-flat (platypelloid), etc. (Fig. 9-4).

PELVIMETRY

Outlet measurements. The most important external measurement is the distance between the ischial tuberosities—the biischial or intertuberous diameter. This is obtained with the patient in lithotomy position, using the Thoms pelvimeter or some other device to delineate the posterior ends of the tuberosities (Fig. 9-5). If the distance is 8 cm. or more, it is considered normal (adequate).

The posterior sagittal diameter of the outlet (from the line between the tuberosities to the tip of the sacrum) may be measured with the Thoms device externally or by locating the sacral tip with a forefinger in the rectum and noting the distance from the extended fingertip to the anal margin. It is usually 7 to 8 cm. in length.

A rough clinical rule devised by Thoms suggests that a pelvic outlet is adequate to permit passage of a term infant if the sum of the intertuberous and posterior sagittal diameters exceeds 15 cm. (*Thoms' rule*).

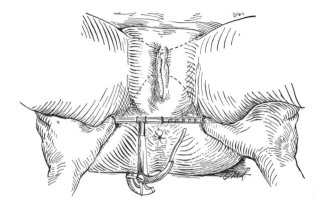

Fig. 9-5. Outlet pelvimetry, using the Thoms pelvimeter for measuring the transverse diameter of the outlet. To measure the posterior sagittal diameter of the outlet, the movable arm is placed at the tip of the sacrum. (From Titus: The management of obstetric difficulties, St. Louis, The C. V. Mosby Co.)

Internal measurements. The diagonal conjugate is the most important of all the inlet measurements. This measurement of the distance from the lower border of the symphysis pubis to the promontory of the sacrum can be obtained easily and with reasonable accuracy simply by a digital examination (Fig. 9-2). If this measurement is 11.5 cm or more, one may usually assume that the inlet is adequate, although occasionally a transverse contraction of the inlet may exist with an anteroposterior value of this magnitude.

Technique

1. Insert the first two fingers gently into the vagina until the middle finger presses against the sacral promontory.

2. Raise the hand until the radial aspect of the forefinger is against the lower border of the symphysis pubis.

3. The point of contact with the symphysis is marked, and the distance from the mark to the tip of the middle finger is measured with the pelvimeter or on a wall-mounted metal scale to obtain the diagonal conjugate.

4. While the fingers are still in the vagina, the pelvic cavity should be palpated for any abnormalities, and an estimate of its capacity should be made.

X-ray pelvimetry. Although x-ray pelvimetry once was used almost routinely for primigravidas by some obstetricians, this practice no longer can be justified because of the obvious genetic hazard of roentgen rays. The dose of radiation to the maternal gonads usually is at least 2 roentgens.

The usual indications for obtaining roentgenograms of the pelvis are as follows:

1. Clinically contracted inlet or outlet; apparent narrowing of interspinous distance

2. Fetal problems—unengaged vertex in primigravida, breech presentation, other malpresentation, or apparently large fetus (over 4,000 grams)

3. History of previous dystocia, birth injury, or stillbirth allegedly related to mechanical problems

4. Unusual maternal stature, build, or gait, stigmas of rickets, or history of inflammatory or other pelvic disease

5. Failure of expected progress in labor despite adequate contractions

Numerous schemes to correct divergent distortion of the image on the film have been devised. Most radiologists use one of the so-called "position" methods, which depend on placing opaque marking devices where they will cast shadows that bear definite relationships to pelvic diameters. Perhaps the best-known example is the procedure of Thoms, in which a perforated grid is placed in the plane of the pelvic inlet (after the patient is removed from the table) and a notched centimeter metallic ruler is placed longitudinally against the sacrum while taking the lateral view. The grid contains *distorted* centimeter scales used to measure transverse pelvic diameters at various levels in the pelvic cavity.

In the other general method of x-ray pelvimetry a *stereoscopic parallax* is employed in correcting for distortion (Fig. 9-6). Although the films produced in this way require somewhat more time for interpretation, they have the advantage of providing stereoscopic views of the pelvis both from the front and from the side. Stereoscopic views are no longer popular because of the additional exposure to x rays, though some radiologists still use the stereoscopic anteroposterior view (Fig. 9-7) combined with a

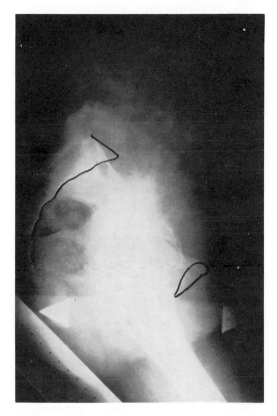

Fig. 9-6. Typical lateral roentgenogram, showing isometric scale between the buttocks and triangular markers for determining parallax by stereoscopic technique. (Modified from McLennan: West. J. Surg. **58:**48, 1950.)

single lateral exposure containing an isometric scale marker. Hodges has described the combination of a lateral film with isometric scale and a frontal film without scale; information from the two views is merged by a procedure known as 90-degree triangulation.* The Colcher-Sussman technique utilizes a frontal film obtained after positioning the patient so that the transverse

---

* Hodges: New developments in radiology, Postgrad. Med. **32:**A59, 1962.

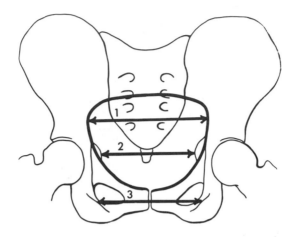

Fig. 9-7. Diameters usually measured on anteroposterior film. **1,** Greatest transverse of inlet; **2,** interspinous; **3,** intertuberous of outlet. (From McLennan: West. J. Surg. **58:**48, 1950.)

diameters of the inlet, midpelvis, and outlet lie in the same plane, along with an isometric scale. A lateral film with isometric scale is included for anteroposterior measurements.

Pelvimetry films must, of course, be measured and described by someone with radiologic experience, but the information thus provided must be weighed and interpreted by someone skilled in obstetric matters. The wise radiologist does not make sweeping predictions or recommendations from films alone. Radiologic pelvimetry is a valuable aid in the management of certain labors, but only in a very small percentage of instances can it be the prime factor in the decision as to the method of delivery.

See Chapter 25 for a discussion of the consequences of pelvic contraction.

PELVIC SOFT PARTS

It is quite as urgent to know the anatomy of the pelvic floor and the part it plays in the mechanism of labor as to understand the role of the bony pelvis in childbirth (Fig. 9-8).

Pelvic floor. The pelvic floor, which must be overcome by the

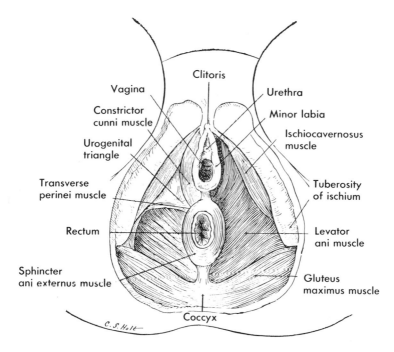

Fig. 9-8. Muscles of the pelvic floor viewed from below. The superficial muscles on the left are removed to expose the deep muscles. (From Falls and McLaughlin: Obstetric and gynecologic nursing, St. Louis, The C. V. Mosby Co.)

powers of expulsion before birth can occur, is composed of two diaphragms—pelvic and urogenital.

Pelvic diaphragm. The pelvic diaphragm consists chiefly of the levator ani and coccygeus muscles with their fasciae, forming a strong, troughlike structure, which almost closes the pelvic outlet, leaving a hiatus between the inner edges of the levators for the passage of the rectum, vagina, and urethra. The levator ani of each side arise from the posterior surface of the pubis and the arcus tendineus, which extends from the pubis to each spine of the ischium, and are inserted chiefly in the central raphe, between the rectum and the vagina, to the sides of the lower vagina and the rectum and behind the anus (hence their name, levator ani). The space behind the levators is occupied by the coccygeus, which on each side arises from the ischial spine and inserts into the lateral margin of the lower sacral and upper coccygeal vertebrae.

Urogenital diaphragm. The urogenital diaphragm closes the hiatus between the openings, adding strength to the pelvic floor. It consists of the following:

1. The perineal fasciae (deep, middle, and superficial)
2. The superficial muscles (constrictor cunni and ischiocavernosus) and the transversus perinei muscles (superficial and deep).

These muscles add little strength to the pelvic floor. The fasciae, however, lend considerable aid to the muscles of the pelvic floor.

• • •

The *action of the levator ani* tends to draw the lower vagina, rectum, and anus forward. Inasmuch as strong action of the levators pulls the posterior wall of the rectum against the anterior wall, they are sometimes called the "sphincters of the rectum." During labor the pelvic floor offers considerable resistance that must be overcome by the expulsive forces. Sometimes the levators are overdeveloped, leading to dystocia, for example, in women who indulge in horseback riding and other active athletic pursuits.

The troughlike structure of the pelvic floor is a factor in the normal internal rotation of the head. Its resistance also causes the extension of the fetal head at birth. It is easy to understand why rapid or careless delivery so often results in lacerations.

The pelvic floor may well be considered the "inferior abdominal wall" that must be overcome by the uterine contractions, anterior abdominal muscles, and diaphragm before birth can take place.

The birth of the baby is always a battle between the forces of expulsion and the resistance of the pelvic floor.

10

Clinical course of labor

PHYSIOLOGY OF LABOR

Cause of onset of labor. Labor is the process by which the mature or nearly mature products of conception (fetus and placenta) are expelled from the maternal body. The term delivery refers only to the actual birth of the infant at the end of the second stage of labor.

The precise cause of the onset of labor is not known. Probably it results from the interaction of a number of factors. Some of the more popular theories include localized progesterone action, progesterone deprivation, oxytocin release, and fetal endocrine activity, alone or in concert with a maternal endocrine response.

Localized progesterone action. Csapo has suggested that progesterone secreted in the placenta exerts a local quieting action on the subjacent uterine muscle. As the uterus increases in size, the area of uninhibited myometrium becomes relatively larger and eventually escapes progesterone control, thus permitting contractions that are strong enough to produce pain and cervical dilation. Local progesterone action is able to protect the placental bed until the third stage of labor.

Progesterone deprivation. The balance between the stimulating action of estrogen and the relaxing action of progesterone (prevention of transmission of contractile impulses) is upset when progesterone production dwindles with placental aging. Theories predicated on a progesterone effect suffer from the observations that progesterone administration does not prevent labor, no consistent fall in plasma progesterone has been shown to precede labor, and labor may be induced successfully despite normal plasma-progesterone values.

Oxytocin release. Theories designating oxytocin from the maternal posterior pituitary gland as the initiating agent have suggested both accentuated release of this material and decreased oxytocinase inhibition as being causative. However, removal of the pituitary does not prevent labor (perhaps oxytocin is secreted by the hypothalamus and merely stored in the pituitary) and oxytocinase blood levels peak at term (perhaps this is overcome by the development of a unique myometrial sensitivity).

Fetal endocrine activity. The newest and to date most reasonable suggestion is that labor is initiated and controlled by an elaborate interlocking system that incorporates, at least in most instances, humoral messages of fetal origin. These are most likely hormonal and hypophyseal. For example, labor is delayed beyond term in 40% of human anencephalic fetuses, which normally are deprived of both hypophyseal and adrenocortical hormones. Additionally, it is known that gestation can be prolonged in the sheep by destroying the fetal pituitary.

Uterine contractions ("pains")

1. In all languages the word **pain** is used to designate the contractions of labor.

2. When the painless contractions that occur at short intervals throughout pregnancy are replaced by painful contractions resulting in cervical dilation, labor has begun; the "pains" gradually increase in severity, frequency, and duration.

3. The cause of the pain:

(a) Early in labor it is caused by the pressure on the nerve endings compressed between the uterine muscle bundles or by anoxia of muscle cells.

(b) Later it is caused by distention of the pelvic soft tissue by the descending fetus.

4. The purpose of the contractions is fourfold.

(a) Effacement of the cervix

(b) Dilatation of the lower uterine segment and cervix

(c) Expulsion of the fetus

(d) Extrusion of the placenta

The uterine contractions of labor are involuntary. Only the final efforts at expulsion by the abdominal muscles and diaphragm are voluntary. Women with paraplegia have normal but painless uterine contractions. Uterine action is under intrinsic nervous control, and, like the heart, the uterus has *pacemakers* that initiate contractions and control their rhythm. But unlike the heart, and even though pacemaker activity is most frequently centered in the area of the uterotubal junction, any group of excited myometrial cells anywhere in the uterus may serve in the pacemaker role and initiate electrical propagation throughout the myometrium. Muscle contraction results from an interaction between actomyosin (protein) and adenosine triphosphate, and it is affected by the quantity of potassium ions in the muscle cell.

5. Interval between contractions:

(a) Early in labor the contractions occur every 15 to 30 minutes and are usually felt in the back (sacral region).

(b) The interval between contractions gradually shortens to 2 or 3 minutes.

6. Duration of each contraction: The contractions increase in length as labor proceeds and last from 30 to 90 seconds (average, 1 minute).

7. Force of each contraction: The force transmitted to a hydrostatic bag in the uterus varies from 25 to 50 mm. Hg, but intramuscular pressure varies from 25 to 150 mm. Hg in various areas.

8. Effect of uterine contractions:

(a) The pregnant uterus between contractions lies on the spine.

(b) During contractions it rises from the spine, possibly because of contraction of the round ligaments, and forces the abdominal wall forward.

(c) The longitudinal diameter lengthens.

(d) The transverse diameter becomes shorter and decreases the capacity of the uterine cavity. The infant and the "bag of waters" are forced against the lower part of the uterine body and cervix, resulting in dilation of these structures and eventually expulsion of the infant.

Formation of upper and lower uterine segments

1. Before labor begins the uterus is composed of the uterine body and the cervix.

2. However, uterine contractions soon cause the uterine body to differentiate itself into:

(a) The *upper segment*—active, thick, muscular, contractile, and retractile.

(b) The *lower segment*—a thin-walled, passive, muscular tube.

3. The *physiologic retraction ring* separates the two segments.

4. The upper segment increases in thickness as labor progresses, whereas the lower segment becomes thinner and is retracted (pulled up) by the shortening of the muscle fibers of the upper active segment. The musculature of the lower segment relaxes to permit more and more of the intrauterine contents to distend its walls. This stretching is increased when labor is obstructed.

5. At such times, the retraction ring (now pathologic) ascends, sometimes nearly to the umbilicus, which is a warning of impending rupture, and labor should be terminated.

Contraction and retraction

Contraction. When the muscle fibers of the upper segment contract, they become thicker and shorter. The uterine cavity becomes smaller, forcing the baby and the amniotic sac in the direction of least resistance toward the lower segment and the cervix. The stretched fibers of the lower segment do not contract to their previous length at the termination of each contraction. They remain fixed at the longer length and maintain their tension.

Records of uterine contractions obtained with the tokodynamometer (Reynolds) show greater intensity in the upper corpus than in the lower corpus (midzone) and greater intensity in the midzone than in the lower uterine segment. Likewise, the duration of the contraction is greater, zone by zone, from above downward. Such gradients do not exist in false labor; therefore no progress is made.

Retraction. The fibers of the upper segment interlace with the circular fibers of the cervix, so that when the contracting fibers of the upper segment shorten they pull the lower segment up against the presenting part, thus aiding in dilatation. As labor progresses the upper segment grows thicker and shorter; late in the expulsive stage it covers not more than half of the baby, illustrating the degree and significance of both contraction and retraction.

When the cervix is completely dilated, the same process retracts (pulls) the lower segment up over the presenting part.

Intra-abdominal pressure. After full dilatation of the cervix, expulsion of the fetus is aided greatly by contraction of the abdominal muscles. Pressure of the fetal head on the perineum produces a reflex that causes the woman to "bear down" vigorously. When regional anesthesia or spinal cord injury has blocked the action of the abdominal muscles, the fetus only rarely is expelled by uterine action alone.

COURSE OF LABOR
Preparatory phase

Before actual labor begins, there are certain physiologic preparatory events, which might well be called the preparatory stage of labor: "lightening," "settling," or "dropping" and effacement of the cervix.

"Lightening," "settling," or "dropping." Two or more weeks before labor the fetal head in most primigravidas settles into the brim of the pelvis and becomes fixed in the brim or may even become completely engaged, with the vertex entering the pelvis to the level of the ischial spines. "Lightening" in multiparas usually does not occur until early labor.

1. The upper abdomen becomes flatter because the fundus uteri is lower.

2. Consequently, the lower abdomen is more prominent.

3. Pressure against the diaphragm is relieved because the baby is lower.

4. Previous difficulty in breathing is relieved.

5. Urination, attributable to pressure by the presenting part, is more frequent.

Preliminary contractions often accompany "settling"—false labor pains. Sometimes the cervix is almost completely effaced and the head engaged before any true labor contractions occur, especially in primigravidas.

Effacement of cervix. Effacement of the cervix is a process of shortening or obliterating the cervical canal, blending it with the lower uterine segment. Thus the external cervical os remains as a circular opening into a spheroidal cavity lined by fetal membranes and filled with amniotic fluid and the presenting part (head). Effacement is aided by an unfolding of the extensive pattern of cervical clefts (Fluhmann) and their mucus content.

Progress of labor

The *first stage* of labor is the period of effacement and dilatation of the cervix uteri. It lasts from the beginning of labor to the complete elimination of the barrier of the cervix.

The *second stage* or stage of expulsion extends from the complete dilatation of the cervix to the birth of the fetus.

The *third stage* or stage of placental extrusion lasts from the birth of the fetus to the birth of the placenta.

Labor also may be summarized graphically for the primigravida (Fig. 10-1) by relating the passage of time to the cervical dilatation, as a sigmoid curve (method of E. A. Friedman). Usually

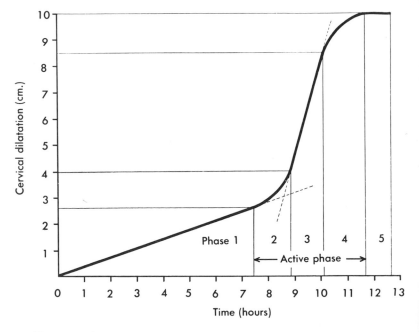

Fig. 10-1. Graphic representation of labor in a primigravida. Phase **1,** latent; **2,** period of acceleration; **3,** steady; **4,** deceleration; **5,** second stage of labor. (Redrawn from Friedman.)

there is a latent period between the onset of contractions and the beginning of *active* cervical dilatation. Next comes a period of acceleration (between 2 and 4 cm. dilatation), followed by the most rapid change in cervical patency. Deceleration sets in toward the end of the first stage of labor. This general concept of the "norm" is useful in evaluating the progress of labor of the individual patient, whose performance may, of course, differ appreciably from the standard sequence of events.

A similar graph for the multiparous patient shows a shorter latent phase (about 5 hours), a shorter active phase (2 hours), and a total labor time of about 8 hours.

First stage. The stage of labor consists of two phases: effacement and dilatation of the cervix uteri. At the onset of labor "the plug of mucus" that has corked the cervical canal soon escapes, mixed with a little blood, hence its name "show."

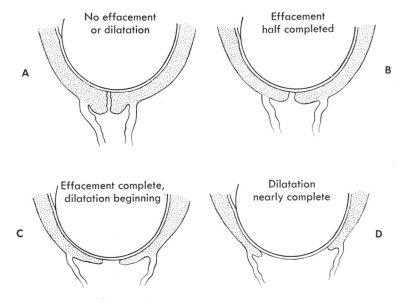

Fig. 10-2. Effacement and dilatation of the cervix.

Effacement

1. The process of effacement (Fig. 10-2) has been variously designated. The cervix is "thinned out," "obliterated," "taken up," or "shortened," but "effaced" is the generally accepted term.

2. Effacement begins before labor, in the last weeks of gestation; in first pregnancies it may be almost complete before full term.

3. First the cervical walls became gradually thinner, decreasing in thickness from more than a centimeter to a few millimeters.

4. At the same time the thinned walls are "taken up" into the thinned lower segment—retraction.

5. Effacement is really the last step in the formation of the lower segment.

6. The factors that bring about effacement are the following:

(a) Preliminary softening begins because of anatomic changes.

(b) Contractions force the uterine contents in the direction of least resistance.

(c) Retraction occurs when the upper segment pulls against the presenting part.

(d) The hydrostatic dilator, composed of the bag of waters, exerts its force equally in all directions so that it acts in the direction of least resistance, thus pushing a small segment of the bag into the internal os more and more as labor progresses. Because of the plausibility of this explanation, we may have placed too much emphasis upon the relative importance of the hydrostatic dilator, since it often happens that effacement and dilation are actually hastened when the membranes are ruptured accidentally or artifically to induce labor.

(e) There is another factor that enters into consideration—stabilization of the uterus by the round and uterosacral ligaments. These, being projections of uterine muscle, contract with each general myometrial contraction. The round ligaments pull the fundus forward, and the uterosacral ligaments pull backward on the lower segment, thus assuring that the force of each contraction will be exerted in the direction of the pelvic axis.

7. Effacement occurs from above downward; first, the hydrostatic bag of waters or the fetal head enters the internal os and then, aided by the factors mentioned, gradually thins out the cervix from the internal os to the external os until its walls have been reduced to a thickness of only a few millimeters.

Dilatation of cervix uteri. Both dilatation and effacement are accomplished solely by the involuntary contractions of the uterus. In a primigravida effacement usually is almost complete before any appreciable dilatation is achieved, whereas in a multipara the two processes are more likely to advance concomitantly. When the more or less circular opening into the lower segment of the uterus is about 10 cm. in diameter, dilatation is said to be "complete" or "full." At this stage of dilatation a fetal head of average size can slip through the cervical barrier, and usually the residual ring of cervical tissue moves superiorly toward the fetal neck. It can then no longer be easily palpated vaginally because the fetal head is well below it and occupies most of the available vaginal space.

The membranes may spontaneously rupture at any moment in this process. Exceptionally, they do not rupture during labor and the baby is born with the membranes over the head—the "caul." Not infrequently rupture occurs prior to labor. Labor usually sets in soon after such premature rupture but may be delayed for days or in exceptional cases even weeks.

After the membranes rupture there often is a temporary cessation of contractions. Soon, however, the contractions recur with increasing force and frequency.

Second stage or expulsion of fetus

1. The second stage of labor begins upon completion of cervical dilatation. A variable degree of fetal descent has occurred during the dilatation process and the remainder is accomplished during this stage.

2. Now the patient wishes to "bear down," the diaphragm is fixed, and she cannot resist contracting the abdominal walls and pushing. She indeed labors; her face is suffused and the face and neck vessels are distended—she inhales deeply, holds her breath as long as she can, pushes mightily, and then suddenly exhales with an explosive grunt as the muscles of the abdomen and the diaphragm relax.

3. The patient is relieved for a short interval.

4. The process is then repeated at varying intervals and with ever-increasing force and strain.

5. Vaginal examination will reveal a completely dilated cervix retracted over the presenting part.

6. Descent of the infant is progressing through the pelvis.

(a) Descent is caused by the force of uterine contractions, reinforced by the voluntary efforts of the abdominal wall and diaphragm.

(b) The force is applied to the breech.

(c) The force is transmitted directly to the fetal spinal column and thence to the fetal head.

(d) The curve of the fetal spine tends to straighten, which adds power to push the head downward.

7. The head, after retraction of the lower segment, occupies the pelvic cavity.

8. Soon the head impinges upon the pelvic floor. The pressure upon the rectum gives the desire to defecate.

9. After a varying period of such effort, the pelvic floor begins to bulge with each contraction.

10. The anus opens.

11. Soon the fetal scalp becomes visible at the vaginal orifice.

12. The perineum bulges and the vulva dilates more and more with each contraction.

13. The head usually recedes nearly or completely out of sight between contractions, until it "crowns."

14. The pelvic floor is thus gradually stretched, and the perineum becomes thinned out, so much that with each contraction it appears about to rupture.

15. The anus is now distinctly dilated, and the anterior wall of the rectum protrudes.

16. The head is born by extension, the occiput hugging the undersurface of the symphysis pubis, with the sinciput, brow, and face following each other, sliding off the perineum.

17. As soon as the head is born, it drops down over the perineum.

18. The neck, which has been twisted as the head rotated internally, now unwinds, turning the head to one side, according to the yet unrotated position of the shoulders (restitution of the head).

19. Then, when the shoulders rotate internally, they turn the head farther to the side (external rotation of the head).

20. Birth of the shoulders and body.

(a) The anterior shoulder impinges on the undersurface of the symphysis pubis, which acts a fulcrum, and the posterior shoulder is then born over the perineum by lateral flexion.

(b) The anterior shoulder soon follows under the symphysis pubis.

(c) Rarely the anterior shoulder is born first.

(d) The body quickly follows by lateral flexion at the waist.

Third stage of labor or birth of placenta

1. After the baby's birth the uterine contractions usually cease for a short interval.

2. The contractions, however, soon recur. The sudden shrinkage in uterine size after delivery of the infant is accompanied by a decrease in the area of the placental site. The placenta becomes about twice as thick as it was at the onset of labor, and the uteroplacental union soon is disrupted through the layer of endometrial (decidual) spongiosa.

3. After a few minutes the placenta separates completely, as noted by a modest gush of blood.

4. It then is forced into the lower uterine segment, where it may be observed as a slight bulging above the symphysis pubis.

5. Further contractions push it into the vagina, and this is indicated by a distinct lengthening of the cord outside the vulva.

6. Finally, it is totally expelled.

7. The whole process lasts for 5 to 30 minutes; occasionally the placenta is extruded almost immediately after the birth of the fetus.

8. Because it is below the contraction in the upper segment, it will often lie in the lower segment or vagina until manually expressed by the obstetrician.

9. Labor is ended. The uterus lies as a hard mass above the symphysis, extending almost or completely to the umbilicus.

Birth injuries. Small tears or areas of minor mucosal separation are common after natural delivery, but they, as well as more extensive lacerations, may usually be avoided by careful technique and prophylactic episiotomy. The cervix and vagina should be thoroughly inspected and lacerations should be repaired at once. This will be considered in greater detail in Chapters 12 and 27.

Length of labor

1. There is great individual variation in the length of labor. A recent study has shown the *mean* duration of labor in white primigravidas to be about 13 hours, the median, 10.6 hours, and the mode, 7 hours. For multiparas, the figures were 8, 6, and 4 hours. Labor usually is 5 or 6 hours longer in primigravidas than in multiparas. Occasionally labor is of very short duration even in a primigravida. For statistical purposes, labors lasting over 30 hours usually are classed as "prolonged." The median duration of the second stage is around 50 minutes in primigravidas and only 20 minutes in multiparas. Primigravidas will deliver within the space of 20 contractions after the head has reached the pelvis floor. Multiparas require only 10 or even fewer contractions to effect delivery from the perineal level.

2. There is very little lengthening of labor in older primigravidas, that is, after 35 years of age, but perinatal mortality is increased two to three times in this group.

3. There is some evidence that the greatest incidence of deliveries is between 5 and 8 A.M. However, analyses of large series of labors indicate that there is only a fraction of 1% difference between the incidence of day and night deliveries.

11

The mechanism of labor in vertex presentations

In the lower orders of primates, with their cylindric pelves and relatively smaller fetal heads, the passage of the fetus through the pelvis is usually simple.

In a woman, however, the pelvis has been altered because of her erect posture and the pelvic canal has different diameters at varying levels; therefore, the large, tightfitting head, always seeking the easiest way out, adjusts and readjusts itself to the changing diameters of the pelvis. This process is the *mechanism of labor*. It is complex and not completely explained. We know what happens but not exactly why it occurs.

Inasmuch as vertex presentations occur in more than 95% of all patients, a thorough knowledge of the mechanism must be mastered. Also it will serve as a model, because all cephalic and breech presentations must repeat the same mechanism, modified only by the spatial arrangements peculiar to each presentation.

L.O.T. POSITION AT INLET
Diagnosis
Abdominal palpation
First maneuver. In the first maneuver a soft, irregular mass is felt in the fundus uteri (Fig. 8-6).

Second maneuver. In the second maneuver the long, resistant back is found on the left, and the nodular small parts are found on the right.

Third maneuver. The third maneuver determines that the hard, round head is at the pelvic inlet.

1. If not fixed or engaged, it is freely movable.

2. If not movable, fixation has occurred.

3. If the head is engaged, the anterior shoulder may be felt.

Fourth maneuver. The fourth maneuver determines that the cephalic prominence is on the mother's right.

Vaginal palpation

1. Vaginal palpation is not of much value until the head is at least fixed or engaged.

2. The sagittal suture lies transversely across the pelvis.

3. The posterior, small, triangular fontanel lies to the left.

Auscultation. The point of maximum intensity of the fetal heart is usually found on the line from the umbilicus to the left anterior superior iliac spine.

Steps of mechanism

Flexion. Flexion is caused by the force of uterine contraction resisted by the pelvic brim and also by the fact that the long arm of the "head lever" is anterior to the articulation of the head and spine.

Fixation. Fixation occurs when the head has entered the pelvic brim and cannot be moved from side to side, although it is not engaged; that is, it is not yet at the ischial spines.

Engagement. Engagement occurs when the large diameter of the fetal head is in the pelvic brim, shown by the fact that the vertex is level with a line between the ischial spines.

Descent. Descent begins when the barrier of the cervix is removed by complete effacement and dilatation. Descent continues once it has begun.

Internal rotation. When the head reaches the pelvic floor, it rotates from left to right until the sagittal suture lies anteroposteriorly. A head of average term size cannot be born until it rotates into the anteroposterior diameter of the pelvic outlet.

What happens is known, but why it occurs is still subject to differences of opinion. Probably the shape of the bony pelvis is a cause, particularly the shape of the midpelvis. The chief factor is the peculiar troughlike sling of the pelvic floor, composed of the two levator ani muscles and their fasciae. When the occiput (lowest part of the head) lies in the transverse or right oblique diameter and strikes the left side of the "perineal gutter," the resistance of the levators forces the occiput to slide down the inclined plane into the trough. To accomplish this, it must rotate from left to right into the anteroposterior diameter.

In about two thirds of all patients, internal rotation is complete by the time the head reaches the pelvic floor, and in about 30% rotation is completed shortly thereafter. Delay in rotation is far more common in primigravidas. The role of the levator trough has been demonstrated in experiments involving pushing dead infants through female cadaver pelves.

Even more difficult to understand is the fact that when the occiput is posterior, it also usually rotates to the symphysis pubis and not through the shorter arc to the sacrum. About 4% of fetal heads do not rotate anteriorly.

Birth by extension

1. When the flexed head reaches the pelvic floor, it meets its last barrier—the perineum—which it greatly distends.

2. The nape of the neck hugs the symphysis pubis, with the head occupying the pubic arch (Fig. 11-1).

3. The back of the head (occiput) lies between the labia in the vulvar opening—the only way out.

4. The contractions press the head against the pelvic floor, which, by its resistance, forces the head in the direction of least resistance, upward and outward through the vulvar opening, the head extending over the perineum. The occiput is born first, then the bregma, forehead, eyes, nose, mouth, and chin (Fig. 11-2).

Restitution. The neck has been twisted by internal rotation. It untwists as soon as the head is free, restoring the natural relation between the head and body—restitution. The face turns toward the mother's right thigh (Fig. 11-3).

External rotation

1. Turning of the face accompanies the internal rotation of the shoulders until the head is transverse—external rotation.

2. The shoulders must be born by the same mechanism as the head, rotating, however, in the opposite direction because they engage in the left oblique diameter, which accounts for the turning of the face to the right (Fig. 11-4).

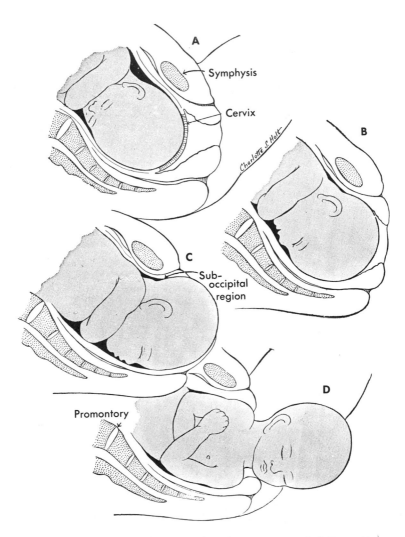

Fig. 11-1. Mechanism of labor in left occiput transverse (L.O.T.) position. (From Falls and McLaughlin: Obstetric and gynecologic nursing, St. Louis, The C. V. Mosby Co.)

Birth of the shoulders and body (expulsion)

1. As internal rotation of the shoulders is completed, the anterior shoulder comes to the symphysis pubis (Figs. 11-5 to 11-7).

2. The posterior shoulder distends the perineum and is usually born first.

3. Immediately the anterior shoulder slips under the symphysis.

4. The body then is quickly expelled.

● ● ●

If one learns thoroughly all the steps of the mechanism of the L.O.T. presentation, he has the foundation for a complete

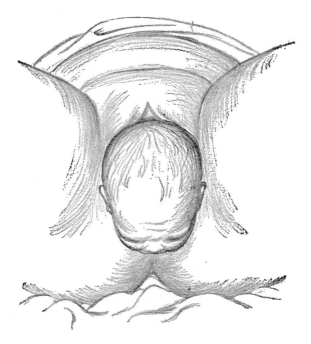

Fig. 11-2. Head dropping back after passing vulva. (From Beck: Obstetrical practice, Baltimore, The Williams & Wilkins Co.)

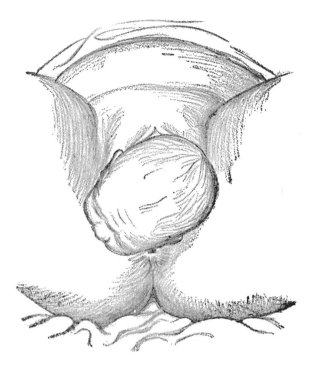

Fig. 11-3. Restitution in L.O.T. position. During internal rotation the neck is twisted. It untwists when the head is born, which turns the face toward the right thigh. (From Beck: Obstetrical Practice, Baltimore, The Williams & Wilkins Co.)

understanding of the mechanism of labor in all presentations, because the same forces of expulsion and resistance obtain. However, certain peculiarities of some presentations need to be considered.

The classic description just given implies that the fetal head routinely enters the pelvis in the transverse position with the sagittal suture equidistant from the sacral promontory posteriorly and the symphysis pubis anteriorly. Very often, however, during the course of engagement and descent, the fetal head will be

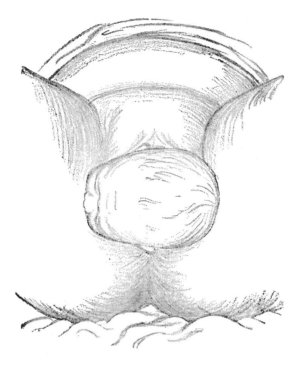

Fig. 11-4. External rotation. As the shoulders rotate internally, the head turns with them so that the head directly faces the right thigh. (From Beck: Obstetrical practice, Baltimore, The Williams & Wilkins Co.)

cocked slightly toward the anterior or posterior shoulder. In this event the sagittal suture will lie anterior or posterior to the transverse midline of the maternal pelvis and one of the parietal bones will be more dependent and more fully palpable from below than the other. If the more dependent parietal bone is anterior to the sagittal suture, the condition is called *anterior asynclitism.* If the more dependent parietal bone is posterior to the sagittal suture, *posterior asynclitism* exists. Modest degrees of transient or alternate asynclitism occur normally and facilitate

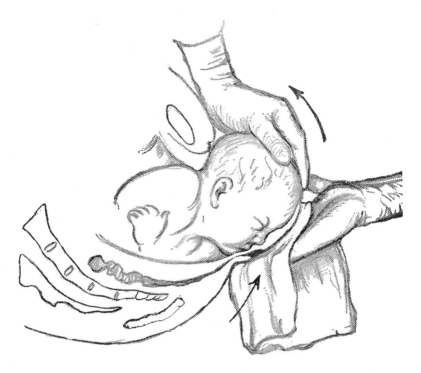

Fig. 11-5. Delivery of the head between pains by the Ritgen method. Note how both hands aid extension; the fingers of the right hand behind the anus push upward, and the left hand pulls the head upward. (From Beck: Obstetrical practice, Baltimore, The Williams & Wilkins Co.)

accommodation of the fetal head to the maternal pelvis. This accommodation is also facilitated on occasion by a spontaneous and gradual *molding* or reshaping of the fetal head. This occurs by an overlapping of the normally ununited bones of the fetal cranium and is often associated with the development of edematous swelling of the fetal scalp at its most dependent point immediately over the cervical os (caput succedaneum).

In understanding the mechanism of labor, one must bear in mind that the various movements mentioned do not occur in-

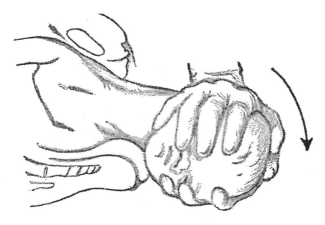

Fig. 11-6. Delivery of the anterior shoulder. Forcible traction must not be used for fear of injury to the brachial plexus and consequent Erb's paralysis of the baby. (From Beck: Obstetrical practice, Baltimore, The Williams & Wilkins Co.)

dependently of one another but rather that several maneuvers may manifest themselves simultaneously.

R.O.T. POSITION

The steps of the mechanism in the R.O.T. position follow identically those in the L.O.T. position except that they are in the opposite direction.

OCCIPUT POSTERIOR POSITIONS

The diagnostic procedures are the same as in the L.O.T. position. The fetal back is posterior instead of anterior, lying in either the right or left flank. The fetal small parts are easily felt on the opposite side at the front. The small fontanel is found opposite the sacroiliac articulation; the large fontanel is found near the iliopectineal eminence (Fig. 11-8). True occiput posterior positions are uncommon.

The fetal heart is best heard in the mother's right or left flank, depending on the fetal position. If the head is partly extended, not infrequently the heart sounds are best transmitted through

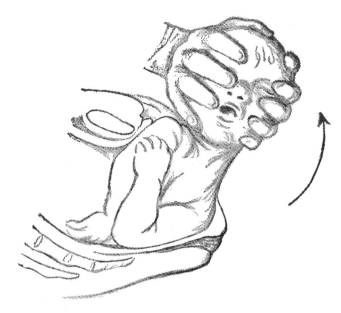

Fig. 11-7. Delivery of the shoulders should occur chiefly by bearing-down efforts by the patient or by pressure from above by the physician or an assistant. (From Beck: Obstetrical practice, Baltimore, The Williams & Wilkins Co.)

the fetal thorax and heard near the midline of the mother's abdomen.

About 8% of vertex presentations observed late in labor are of the occipitoposterior variety—5% are R.O.P. and 3% are L.O.P. Inadequate space in the forepelvis fosters lack of anterior rotation. Other factors are abnormally short bispinous diameter, prominent ischial spines, and convergent pelvic sidewalls. Extension of the head tends to occur when the occiput enters the lower pelvis and meets the resistance of a prominent sacrococcygeal shelf. Incomplete flexion is a major factor in the lack of normal progress that characterizes many occiput posterior labors.

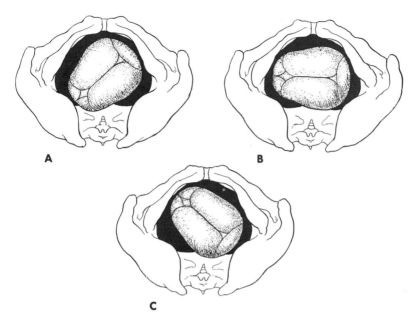

Fig. 11-8. Fetal head landmarks in occiput left positions as palpated through the vagina. **A,** Small fontanel anterior and to left, L.O.A. **B,** Transverse position, L.O.T. **C,** Posterior and to left, L.O.P.

Steps in mechanism

1. Internal rotation is usually toward the symphysis pubis, despite the fact that the head must rotate through an arc of 135 degrees instead of merely 90 or 45 degrees.

2. There are sometimes difficulties in the rotation. The head must be well flexed to be favorable for rotation.

(a) The head *may* rotate backward into the hollow of the sacrum.

(b) The anterior rotation may stop when the sagittal suture lies transversely—deep transverse arrest.

(c) Rotation may entirely fail—persistent occiput posterior position.

(d) Without complete rotation forward or backward, the fetus cannot be born spontaneously.

3. *Labor is prolonged* because the rotation takes longer, but nearly all fetuses rotate eventually.

4. When *posterior rotation* of the occiput occurs, birth may occur by one of two mechanisms:

(a) *With a well-flexed head.* By extension the brow, eyes, nose, mouth, and chin slip under the symphysis pubis.

(b) *With a poorly flexed head.* The root of the nose impinges against the symphysis pubis; then by flexion the brow, bregma, and occiput appear in order over the perineum; the face then passes under the symphysis pubis.

5. There is great danger of deep tears in all cases of posterior internal rotation because of the gross distention of the pelvic floor.

6. Rotation anteriorly frequently does not occur in the presence of caudal or spinal anesthesia, and operative rotation then becomes necessary.

For further discussion of the mechanism in posterior positions see Chapter 24.

12

The management of normal labor

PREPARATORY CARE

The patient is advised to enter the hospital at the onset of labor in order that certain preliminary preparations may be made.

Admission examination. At the admission examination the physician performs a brief general examination, looks for evidences of respiratory infection, and inquires about recent exposure to contagious diseases, as well as recent episodes of diarrhea. When there is any possibility that the patient may transmit an infectious disorder to others, particularly to the newborn infant, she must be properly isolated. Attention then is turned to the obstetric situation, and the following are determined:

1. Blood pressure (to be taken frequently during labor)
2. Fetal presentation, position, and estimated weight
3. Fetal heart sounds (rate varies from 120 to 140 per minute)
4. Duration, interval, and strength of uterine contractions
5. Vaginal findings

(a) Station of presenting part (distance above or below ischial spines (Fig. 12-1)

(b) Degree of effacement of cervix

(c) Dilatation of cervix in centimeters

(d) Presence or absence of bulging membranes

6. Presence of protein or sugar in the urine

The question of whether the patient really is in labor usually is settled by determining that contractions appear at regular intervals. A bloody "show" often is present, and progressive cervical effacement and dilatation will be demonstrated. False

167

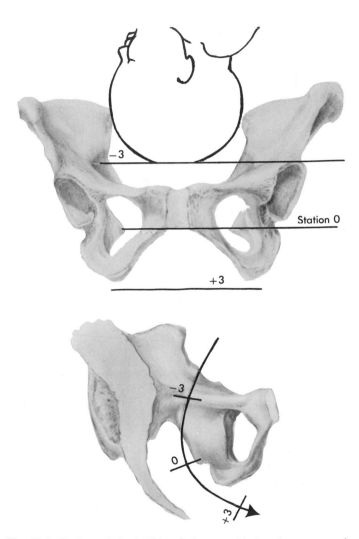

Fig. 12-1. Stations of the fetal head above and below the zero or reference line between the ischial spines.

contractions tend to vary in interval, duration, and intensity and do not efface or dilate the cervix.

The onset of labor and premature membrane rupture occur most often during the usual hours of sleep, with a peak incidence between 2 and 4 A.M. A recent study indicates that about 65% of labors begin between 9 P.M. and 9 A.M. Membranes rupture prior to labor in about 20% of patients. In the majority this premature rupture of membranes occurs at term and, after a variable lag period, is followed by the spontaneous onset of labor.

Because of the great potential for the development of chorioamnionitis and fetal pneumonia with prolonged rupture of the membranes, it is generally advantageous to ensure that delivery is accomplished within 24 to 48 hours after membrane rupture if the fetus is mature. This can ordinarily be accomplished by inducing labor with an intravenous infusion of dilute oxytocin. However, if the fetus weighs less than 2,000 gm., the risk of prematurity and respiratory distress after induced delivery may be greater than the peril of intraamniotic infection while awaiting fetal maturation. Maternal antibiotic therapy has not been shown to protect the fetus under these circumstances. A delicate balance is often drawn in this situation and the obstetrician's clinical judgment and intuition are often put to a severe test. Use of the assessments for fetal maturity described in Chapter 7 may be of considerable aid in making the appropriate decision as to when to conclude the pregnancy. Prolapse of the cord is uncommon in premature rupture of the membranes unless the presentation is abnormal.

Vulvar and rectal preparation. As soon as the physician is convinced that the patient is truly in labor, he directs the nurse to shave and cleanse the pubic area, vulva, and inner thighs and to administer an enema. Shaving the pudendum probably is an unnecessary ritual for those women in whom uncomplicated, spontaneous deliveries are expected. If episiotomy is to be done, the surgical repair may be somewhat simpler in the absence of perineal hair. Allegedly perineal hygiene post partum is simplified by shaving the area, but this is not invariably true.

Detecting rupture of membranes. When the patient is uncertain and the physician cannot decide by examination if the membranes are ruptured, it may be desirable to determine the pH of the vaginal fluid. Normal vaginal secretions are acid, but amniotic fluid is alkaline. Nitrazine paper is widely used for this test. Demonstration of fat globules or fetal epithelium in the vaginal fluid may be helpful. For this purpose a standard Papanicolaou smear may be adequate, but various special staining techniques have been developed for rapid use at the bedside.

One should be aware that a variable amount of amniotic fluid not infrequently collects between the dependent portions of the amnion and the chorion. Rupture of the chorion alone in this situation will provide a clinical picture indistinguishable from the more typical, simultaneous rupture of both membranes. This is most commonly the explanation for the discovery of an intact membrane in circumstances in which history and examination both conclusively pointed to previous membrane rupture. It is an element for concern and debate only in instances of premature membrane rupture in preterm pregnancies inasmuch as the presence of an intact amnion should essentially relieve any fear of intraamniotic infection.

CARE DURING LABOR

Patience is a prime requisite because labor requires time for its spontaneous conclusion and must not be hurried unless there is a definite reason for operative interference.

Labor may be a painful experience; therefore, suffering must be reduced as much as possible and eliminated when wise and possible. However, unwise administration of analgesics may lead to unnecessary operative deliveries, with attendant dangers to the mother and the child.

Although labor should be conducted conservatively and with patience, the physician should not hesitate to undertake any operation promptly and with courage when the welfare of the mother or child demands interference, using the method that will be the least dangerous. The true conservative is not he who hesitates or fears to operate but he who knows how, why, and when to be radical.

MANAGEMENT OF FIRST STAGE OF LABOR

1. Provided that analgesia has not been instituted, the patient may sit up or walk around her room if she desires.

2. Solid food usually is withheld during labor to avoid vomiting and aspiration at the time of delivery. Fluids may be taken during early labor, and when labor is prolonged, it is desirable to give glucose solution intravenously.

3. The degree of fullness of the bladder must be observed frequently. Voiding may be difficult during labor and it may be necessary to empty the bladder with a catheter. In general, though, cathetcrization should be avoided because the procedure may introduce pathogenic bacteria into the urinary tract.

4. Vaginal examinations are made at variable intervals, depending on the apparent progress as judged by the frequency and duration of uterine contractions. When delivery is conducted in a hospital, there is provided, as a rule, a special "progress of labor" record on which are recorded periodically the dilatation of the cervix, station of the presenting part, fetal position and heart rate, maternal blood pressure, and other significant items.

5. The intensity and frequency of uterine contractions are improved by having the patient lie on her side rather than on her back. Placental perfusion and fetal oxygenation are also optimized.

6. If abnormalities are present, it is wiser not to worry the patient by informing her. However, many women appreciate and respond positively to compassionate objectivity and are calmer and more helpful when they are kept abreast of developments. Regardless, the husband or other responsible relative should be apprised of the situation.

7. The physician must be in constant attendance after the os is nearly dilated in primigravidas or after 5 cm. dilatation in multiparas.

8. *Warning:* The patient must be cautioned against voluntary bearing-down efforts during the first stage. They do not aid dilatation and they exhaust the patient.

ASSESSMENT OF FETAL STATUS

Various methods are currently under investigation for continuous or intermittent monitoring of the physiologic status of the intrauterine fetus during labor. These methods include the simultaneous recording of the fetal heart rate (FHR) and intra-amniotic pressure (IAP), plus sampling of capillary blood from the fetal scalp for determination of pH, O_2 saturation, blood gas partial pressure etc.

FHR monitoring may be conducted indirectly (Fig. 12-2) by phonocardiographic or Doppler auscultation through the maternal abdominal wall or directly by electrodes attached to the presenting fetal part. IAP is monitored by a tokodynamometer attached to the abdominal wall or directly by a intraamniotic

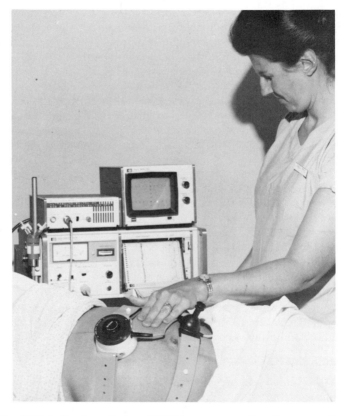

Fig. 12-2. Indirect monitoring of fetal heart rate and uterine contractions by Doppler auscultation and tokodynamometry.

transcervical catheter attached to an external pressure transducer. Direct monitoring requires ruptured membranes.

Although most uterine contractions are not associated with a significant variation in FHR, a fall and recovery in FHR that directly mirrors the rise and fall of the IAP is currently believed to be acceptable and to represent response to normal compression of the fetal head. However, a fall in FHR starting during late contraction, with recovery occurring slowly or incompletely between contractions, is believed to signify deficient villous perfusion with fetal jeopardy. This appears to be particularly true if the prefall FHR is above normal (for example, 170 to 180 per minute) and appears to remain true even if the FHR does not fall below 120 per minute. Thus FHR determinations made only occasionally and auscultatively between contractions may not detect fetal distress exemplified in this manner. Constant recording is required. Falls in FHR with patterns and relationship to IAP different from those noted above are also believed to represent fetal circulatory embarrassment, most likely from cord compression.

Slowness of the FHR, regardless of the method of observation, calls for attentive concern but is not automatically a cause for alarm or instant action directed to fetal delivery. Its temporal relationship to the uterine contraction, its rapidity and completeness of recovery, and its prefall value are important elements in its evaluation.

Tachycardia apparently is not serious, but if persistent for over 2 hours or associated with abnormal FHR decelerations, it may suggest severe fetal compromise.

The FHR baseline is consistently variable within a 3% to 10% fluctuation. A smoothing out or loss of this normal fluctuation of heart rate is considered to be an ominous sign although this can be benignly induced by maternal administration of certain drugs such as diazepam (Valium) and atropine.

Positioning the patient on her side, elevating her legs, administering oxygen, diminishing the oxytocin drip rate, correcting maternal hypotension, etc., are recommended, with the hope of eliminating these abnormal patterns and avoiding ill-advised intervention.

Correlations of 99% have been noted between normal FHR

patterns and a high Apgar score at birth. However, accuracy in predicting neonatal depression when FHR patterns are abnormal is low, being variously judged as between 20% and 60%.

Fetal hypoxia results in acidosis and may be detected by the demonstration of an abnormal pH in capillary blood obtained from the fetal scalp. Acidosis usually develops slowly and repeated sampling is required for adequate monitoring. Fetal blood pH should be above 7.30. Values below 7.20 are ominous particularly if the mother is ventilating normally and the low pH is accompanied by an abnormal FHR pattern. Many investigators suggest immediate cesarean section if the scalp blood pH is below 7.10.

It is fair to say that not all investigators find the above relationships to be clear cut, and considerable additional investigation will be required before techniques that will regularly and precisely reflect the physiologic status of the intrauterine fetus are perfected.

MANAGEMENT OF SECOND STAGE OF LABOR
Passage through pelvis
1. Rupture of the membranes often marks the beginning of the second stage of labor (full cervical dilatation).

2. After a short lull the contractions are renewed with increasing vigor and decreasing intervals.

3. The patient soon feels like bearing down. These voluntary efforts grow increasingly irresistible and involuntary.

4. *Examination of the patient* includes the following:

(a) Condition of the cervix (retracted?).

(b) Station of the head above or below the ischial spines.

(c) Location of the fetal landmarks, such as sutures and fontanels; in breech presentations, location of the sacrum.

(d) Position of the cord. If the membranes break when the presenting part is above the brim, with a sudden gush of much water, the cord may prolapse. One will probably need to examine vaginally to detect this as overt prolapse of the cord beyond the vulva is uncommon.

(e) Monitoring of the fetal status, as previously noted, is as equally applicable to the second as to the first stage of labor and should be regularly performed, even if this is only by the discontinuous method of auscultative FHR determination.

Delivery

1. As a rule, multiparas should be taken to the delivery room when the cervix is dilated to 7 or 8 cm., but primigravidas need not be moved until dilatation is complete.

2. After the patient has been cleansed and draped for delivery, catheterization may be performed by the physician (gowned for delivery) if it seems indicated. This ritual is not, however, essential. Indeed, it may be impossible to pass a catheter without displacing the fetal head, and occasionally the urethra may be damaged by the catheter. Additionally, a symptomatic or asymptomatic bacteriuria may be initiated.

3. The patient should be instructed in the technique of using her abdominal muscles to assist the uterine expulsive effort. While flexing her thighs and holding a deep breath, she should exert downward pressure identical to that used for defecation.

4. Intermittent administration of nitrous oxide, or other safe, short-acting, gaseous agent, may provide helpful analgesia at the onset of each contraction.

5. The head (or breech) distends the pelvic floor, and the introitus gapes with each contraction. The head recedes between contractions and advances a little farther each time until it "crowns." Finally, the biparietal diameter separates the vulva widely.

6. The perineum and anus should be frequently wiped downward and backward with cotton balls soaked in antiseptic solution to prevent feces from contaminating the field.

7. Until the head "crowns" the chief function of the obstetritian is not to hurry the delivery but to prevent too rapid progress and to preserve flexion of the head. Both are accomplished by pressing upon the head near the occiput, backward toward the table, which preserves the flexion, and slightly upward, which keeps the head from advancing too rapidly.

8. Severe leg cramps, presumably caused by pressure of the fetal head on the pelvic nerves, are common during the second stage. They are relieved by changing the position of the legs and by massage.

9. Many methods have been recommended for *preservation of the perineum,* and most of them are adequate. The method

chosen is not so important as mastery of the technique selected, provided it fulfills the prime essentials of tear prevention.

(a) Prevent too rapid birth.

(b) Preserve flexion until the head may be delivered safely by gradual extension over the perineum.

(c) Tears may be prevented by using *Ritgen's maneuver* to deliver the fetal head. It consists of covering the anus with a sterile towel and exerting upward or forward pressure on the area beneath the fetal chin while maintaining pressure against the occiput with the other hand. This may aid in controlling the egress of the head or may effect delivery between uterine contractions. (Fig. 11-5).

10. *Episiotomy* (perineal incision):

(a) Episiotomy is an incision designed to substitute a clean cut for a ragged tear.

(b) Not all patients need it, but most primigravidas do. Many multiparas have a relaxed perineum, and some primigravidas have tissues so elastic that an episiotomy is not required if the infant is small.

(c) Early (prophylatic) episiotomy may be unwise; the best time to perform episiotomy is when the head "crowns" slightly.

(d) In forceps deliveries it is best to defer episiotomy until after the blades have been applied, because blood loss is lessened by immediate tamponade of the perineum by the fetal head.

Types of episiotomy include the median, lateral, midlateral and the Schuchardt incision (Fig. 12-3).

(a) The *median* episiotomy is made along the perineal raphe, to within about ½ inch of the anus. This is the best for general use since it is easily and most accurately repaired; with careful delivery it seldom extends. Deliberate section of the anal sphincter (episioproctotomy) is not advised, although some physicians prefer to do this if tearing into the rectum is anticipated.

(b) The *lateral* episiotomy is almost at right angles to the vagina. It is not recommended.

(c) The *midlateral* episiotomy extends from the midline outward and downward to the outer margin of the sphincter ani. It is preferred by many to the central incision, but greater care is required in its repair to avoid impaling the rectum with the sutures. There is also more bleeding from the hemorrhoidal

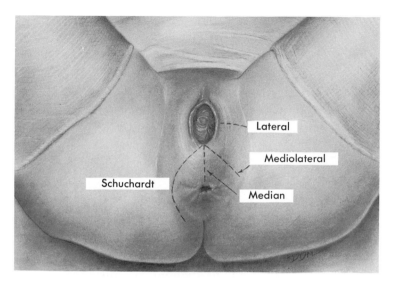

Fig. 12-3. Types of episiotomy incisions.

and other vessels, and postpartum discomfort is often greater than with the median incision.

(d) The *Schuchardt incision* is a very deep sulcus incision extending in an outward curved line to or behind the anus. It has been advocated in place of episiotomy for the aftercoming head of breech presentations, versions, and very large forecoming heads but is rarely used in modern obstetrics.

11. The problem of the *cord around the neck* is common and occurs in 25% or 30% of deliveries.

(a) Immediately feel or look for the loop of cord around the neck.

(b) Loosen the loop and gently slip it over the head.

(c) When this is not easily accomplished or the baby seems endangered, occlude the cord with two clamps and cut between them.

12. *Delivery of the shoulders:*

(a) Do not yield to the urge to hasten delivery as soon as the head is born.

(b) There is usually a lull in the contractions at this time.

(c) Wait until the head rotates externally, which is an indication that the shoulders have rotated internally. There is no hurry as long as fetal color is good. Bulb aspiration of the nose and pharynx may be conducted at this time.

(d) When sure that the shoulders lie directly anteroposterior and contractions have recurred, one may assist delivery.

(1) Pull the head gently downward and backward until the anterior shoulder is behind and against the symphysis pubis.

(2) Now lift the head gently until the posterior shoulder delivers over the perineum. (Gentle assistance may be given to the delivery of the posterior arm if necessary.)

(3) The anterior shoulder now can be delivered easily under the pubic arch.

(4) Some obstetricians deliver the anterior shoulder first or both at the same time by first pulling the anterior shoulder under the arch and delivering both shoulders simultaneously; however, this method puts more stretch upon the perineum than delivery of one shoulder at a time.

(e) *Caution:*

(1) When pulling the head downward and backward, be careful not to pull too far or too strongly backward because the brachial plexus may be injured or even ruptured and Erb's paralysis may occur.

(2) The same injury may occur if the fingers are used for strong traction in the axillae.

13. *Delivery of the body* usually follows quickly and spontaneously. If the infant is unusually large and assistance is necessary, always pull by grasping the shoulders externally and not by pulling on the head or in the axillae.

14. The issuance of greenish (meconium-stained) amniotic fluid, whether viscid or thin, may signify fetal hypoxia and resuscitative efforts (Chapter 14) may be required.

Immediate care of infant

1. As soon as the infant is born, place it crosswise on the mother's abdomen.

2. The head should hang low over the mother's side, so that the mucus may drain.

3. If delivery occurs on a table without stirrups, usually there is ample room for the infant at the foot of the table.

4. The excess mucus may be sucked out with a tracheal catheter or aspiration bulb.

5. The cord should be tied with a sterile tape ligature, or clamped with a plastic cord clamp, and cut. (The question of whether sustained benefit accrues to the infant by waiting for cessation of pulsations before clamping the cord has not been resolved despite numerous studies.)

6. If the infant does not breathe promptly, institute resuscitation procedures (Chapter 14).

7. After birth the infant should be wrapped in a warm covering or placed in a heated bassinet to prevent heat dissipation and hypothermia.

8. *For prevention of ophthalmia neonatorum* (gonorrheal) drop 1% solution of silver nitrate in each eye. This is a legal requirement in most states. The sale and use of penicillin ointment for this purpose has been halted by the Food and Drug Administration because the potential hazard to infants and attendants of penicillin sensitization is believed to outweigh its usefulness.

9. If birth occurs in a hospital, the infant must be labeled for identification before being taken from the delivery room.

MANAGEMENT OF THIRD STAGE OF LABOR

Location of placenta

1. May be situated on the anterior or posterior wall
2. Occasionally laterally
3. Rarely in the fundus
4. Sometimes may touch or cover the internal os—placenta previa

Mechanism of separation

1. *Uterine contractions* reduce the area of placental site.

2. The spongy, weak portion of the decidua basalis cannot long resist this sheering and separates, leaving the placenta free in the uterine cavity (a foreign body). The uterus becomes smaller and changes in shape from discoid to globular. At the same time, more of the umbilical cord appears externally, and there is a gush of blood from the vagina.

3. A small portion of the spongy layer of decidua basalis remains attached to the uterine muscle.

4. When separation is complete, the contractions expel the placenta into the lower segment, the vagina, and out.

5. The membranes gradually peel off because of the contractions and the weight of the descending placenta.

Manner of extrusion. The manner of extrusion is by one of two methods (Fig. 12-4):

1. *Schultze*—like an inverted umbrella (80%)

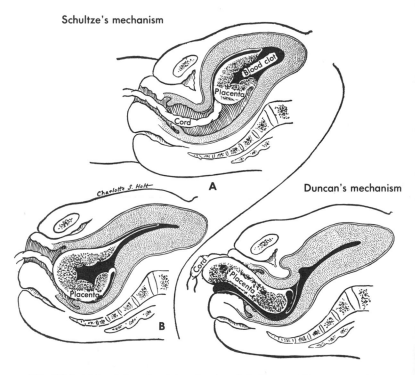

Fig. 12-4. Birth of the placenta, showing Schultze and Duncan mechanisms of separation. (From Falls and McLaughlin: Obstetric and gynecologic nursing, St. Louis, The C. V. Mosby Co.)

2. *Duncan*—rolled up and born edgewise (20%)

Management of placental delivery

1. As soon as the infant is born, the hand of the obstetrician or an assistant should gently grasp the fundus uteri.

2. This is only for observing the action of the uterus. *It must not be massaged* at this time.

3. If contractions need stimulation, after a few minutes the uterus may be mildly irritated.

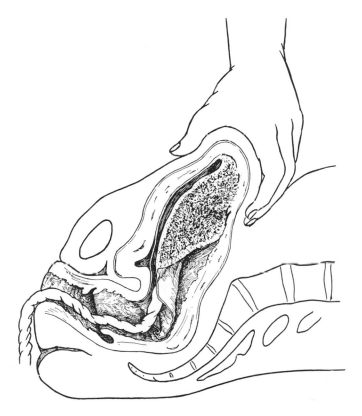

Fig. 12-5. Credé's method of expressing the placenta. (Redrawn from Bumm.)

4. The placenta will usually be born spontaneously if the physician waits long enough, but there is no logic in waiting after it is known that separation has occurred and that the placenta is in the lower segment of the uterus.

5. Then it should be expressed:

(a) By simply pushing down on the fundus, with moderate pressure in the axis of the pelvis, *being careful not to force the cervix down to the introitus.*

(b) By *Credé's technique* (Fig. 12-5):

(1) Place the fingers and palm as far down over the posterior surface of the uterus as possible.

(2) Place the thumb on the anterior surface in the center.

(3) Compress the uterine body firmly with downward pressure in the pelvic axis.

(4) *Warnings:*

(a') Do not persist in using Credé's method of expression if it is not quickly effective.

(b') Do not pull on the cord. Inversion of the uterus may result.

6. Immediate delivery is demanded only when bleeding is alarming.

7. Retained or adherent placenta may require manual removal (Chapter 26).

Management of membranes

1. The membranes usually slide out easily.

2. However, they frequently peel off slowly, remaining adherent after the placenta is delivered.

3. Therefore, the physician should not let the weight of the placenta tear off pieces of membranes that will be retained in the uterus.

4. If the membranes begin to tear, grasp them with a clamp and tease them out slowly.

5. The membranes should be carefully examined to make sure they are intact.

6. If despite your efforts a piece of membrane remains, it may be ignored, but a retained piece of placenta must be removed because of the danger of subsequent hemorrhage.

Management of blood loss

1. Some loss of blood during the third stage of labor is inevi-

table. When one considers perineal lacerations and tearing of vessels occasioned by placental separation, the opening of the large uterine sinuses, and the failure of the uterus to close them by firm contractions, it is not strange that hemorrhage is the great danger of the third stage of labor and the immediate puerperium. Therefore, meticulous care during this stage is imperative. The average normal blood loss should be less than 400 ml.; if care is exercised, it can be kept between 100 and 300 ml.

2. *To prevent too much blood loss* the following procedures should be observed:

(a) Immediately after expulsion of the placenta be sure that the uterus is well contracted, "like a croquet ball," and kept so by manual massage as required.

(b) Oxytocin, 1 ml., may be given intramuscularly after the birth of the baby, followed by 0.2 mg. ergonovine intramuscularly after delivery of the placenta. Some obstetricians prefer to give ergonovine intravenously at the time the anterior fetal shoulder is being delivered in order to produce immediate placental delivery without preliminary oxytocin. It should be pointed out that these oxytocic agents are not absolutely essential in all patients, but their use has become routine in virtually all hospitals.

Also noteworthy is that ergot preparations not infrequently induce blood pressure elevation and are probably best not used in hypertensive or toxemic patients.

(c) Examine the maternal surface of the placenta to make sure that no piece is missing; also examine the fetal surface to see that no vessels are torn off at the edge of the placenta, which occurs when a *placenta succenturiata* is left in the uterus.

EPISIOTOMY REPAIR

Generally episiotomy repair is deferred until completion of the third stage of labor. However, if placental separation has not occurred within a few minutes after delivery of the infant and the obstetrician is not intending to electively separate and remove the placenta manually, he may proceed with the perineal repair. An assistant should keep one hand on the uterine fundus to detect evidences of relaxation or of placental separation. If necessary, the repair is interrupted to permit placental explusion. Disruption of the repair may occur, however, if manual extraction of the placenta is required later.

Chromic catgut, size 2-0 or 3-0, is recommended. Suturing is started at the apex of the vaginal incision and a continuous suture is used for closure of the vaginal mucosa. Several interrupted sutures ordinarily are required to approximate the fascial and muscle structures, and the subcutaneous fascia may be

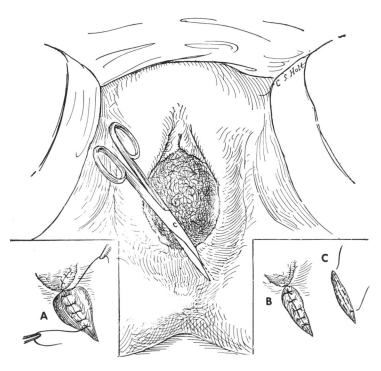

Fig. 12-6. Repair of midlateral episiotomy. (From Falls and McLaughlin: Obstetric and gynecologic nursing, St. Louis, The C. V. Mosby Co.)

closed with the remainder of the vaginal suture (Fig. 12-6). The latter should be sufficiently long to be carried forward as a subcuticular stitch to complete the skin closure. Some physicians prefer not to close the skin layer with sutures, believing this provokes edema and postoperative pain. They merely coapt the skin edges briefly with Allis clamps and then apply ice packs to the perineum to minimize transudation of fluid.

If the episiotomy has extended to involve the anal sphincter muscle and rectal wall, these structures must be approximated first. Various techniques have been described, and all seem satisfactory, provided accurate anatomic restoration of the parts is effected.

VAGINAL AND PERINEAL LACERATIONS

1. *First-degree* lacerations involve only mucosa and skin.
2. *Second-degree* lacerations are deeper and involve muscular structures in the perineum but not the sphincter ani. Such tears usually extend up along the posterior vagina on one or both sides. They may occur even if episiotomy has been done.
3. *Third-degree* or *complete* lacerations involve the mucosa, skin, perineal body, and anal sphincter. In some instances the anterior rectal wall is lacerated.

The vagina also may be torn at higher levels, particularly in the region of the urethra. All lacerations should be repaired immediately. The technique is essentially that already described for repair of the episiotomy.

CONTROL OF PAIN IN LABOR

As maternal mortality rates decline, the role of anesthesia in producing maternal death becomes more prominent. About 10% of maternal deaths now are attributable in some way to the anesthetic used. Aspiration of vomitus and excessively high levels of spinal anesthesia are the chief problems.

Obstetric anesthesia presents several general problems that must be considered in arriving at a choice of technique.

1. In normal labor anesthesia is not absolutely necessary, although the mother may, of course, experience considerable pain at intervals for varying periods of time.
2. The fetus is peculiarly susceptible to sedative and anes-

thetic drugs given to the mother, and fetal respiration is easily embarrassed.

3. Anesthesia merely for the actual delivery often is considered inadequate. Relief of pain during many hours of labor may be demanded in addition.

4. Certain anesthetic agents will stop uterine contractions and in the immediate postpartum period may lead to excessive hemorrhage from an atonic uterus.

5. Obstetric anesthesia may be required promptly, without adequate preparation of the patient. Vomiting and aspiration of gastric contents may occur, and this can be fatal.

6. *No completely safe and satisfactory form of obstetric anesthesia is currently available.* Although a small percentage of patients may be carried through labor with positive conditioning (that is, "natural childbirth") or hypnosis, the more usual approach is to use some combination of analgesic, sedative, and amnesic drugs. Such drugs may be supplemented later in labor by various local, regional, or general anesthetics.

Scopolamine and barbiturates. Most of the barbituric acid derivatives have been used for analgesia and amnesia although their major effect is sedation. Pentobarbital and secobarbital may be used early in labor, do not materially lessen uterine contractions, and may be used with scopolamine or any of a number of other drugs. When labor is well established (cervical dilatation is evident) 100 to 200 mg. of pentobarbital may be administered orally. If scopolamine is to be used, 0.4 mg. may be given intramuscularly and repeated every 2 to 4 hours as desired thereafter for its amnesic effect. With the use of scopolamine, constant supervisory attendance is mandatory as various degrees of excitement, physical and vocal activity, hallucinations, and even delirium occur with this medication. The mother must be watched carefully to guard against self-injury and the attendant must be broadminded and skilled to some extent in evasive action. This medication has very largely fallen into disfavor.

Meperidine (Demerol) and scopolamine. Demerol, a synthetic substitute for morphine, is not only analgesic but also seems to relax the cervix. It may be given intramuscularly or intravenously in doses ranging from 50 to 100 mg. at intervals of about 4 hours. In some patients it produces euphoria. Demerol may be combined with scopolamine (0.4 mg.) to produce amnesia. Supposedly, as has been stated for so many drugs, it is not a respiratory depressant. Yet, as with essentially all drugs, fetal apnea is not an uncommon occurrence when the drug is administered in fully analgesic dosages or within a short time prior to delivery.

Fads in obstetric analgesia come and go with considerable rapidity, and it would serve no useful purpose to list the hundreds of pharmaceutic regimens that have been used in childbirth. Currently it is popular to use potentiating and tranquilizer drugs, such as promethazine (Phenergan) and diazepam (Valium), with sedatives, analgesics, and, rarely, amnesics.

Gas and volatile anesthetics

Nitrous oxide. Nitrous oxide may be used in 80% concentration with 20% oxygen for intermittent analgesia during contractions in the second stage of labor. It may be used continuously to induce deeper anesthesia for episiotomy and delivery, as well as for episiorrhaphy.

Trichloroethylene (Trilene). Trichloroethylene may be self-administered through a properly regulated portable inhaler, adjustable to give concentrations of vapor from 0.1% to 1.35%. Analgesia is obtained in about 15 seconds. This agent is a useful supplement in the second stage of labor. It cannot be used in a gas machine with soda lime, or when a subsequent anesthetic requiring such a machine is to be employed, since it then changes to dichloracetylene, a neurotoxic substance.

Cyclopropane. Cyclopropane is a good anesthetic for rapid induction and relaxation and is effective with high concentrations of oxygen. A concentration of only 20% to 25% cyclopropane is needed for surgical anesthesia, but respiratory failure may occur if the concentration is much higher. The range between effectiveness and safety is narrow. Additionally, the explosion hazard is great. Twenty to 30% of fetuses exposed to cyclopropane require resuscitation, and serious maternal cardiac irregularities may be produced, especially if cyclopropane is employed with drugs having vasopressor activity.

Ether. Ether is a relatively safe anesthetic when given by the open-drop method, but it may provoke vomiting, excessive uterine relaxation, and bleeding. This agent should always be available for emergency use when other varieties of anesthesia are not available (usually because of lack of trained personnel).

Halothane. Halothane is a rapid acting, nonexplosive and easily tolerated volatile anesthetic that may be combined with nitrous oxide and oxygen. It produces substantial uterine relax-

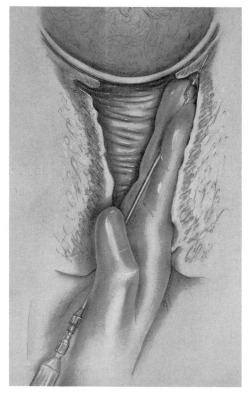

Fig. 12-7. Technique of paracervical block anesthesia during labor. (From Baken, Freeman, and Barno: Surg. Gynec. Obstet. **114:**375, 1962.)

ation, increasing the potential for postpartum hemorrhage, and occasionally results in liver damage. It crosses the placenta readily.

Regional anesthesia

Paracervical anesthesia. Paracervical anesthesia (Fig. 12-7) is given when the cervix is 4 to 5 cm. dilated to relieve pain until the presenting part reaches the introitus. Through a long needle with a special guide, such as the "Iowa trumpet," the physician injects 5 ml. of 1% lidocaine (Xylocaine), or similar agent, in the region of the uterovaginal fold of mucosa, just posterior and lateral to the cervical rim on each side (approximately 4 o'clock and 8 o'clock positions). Indwelling plastic catheters may be inserted if the continuous technique is to be employed.

Labor may be retarded briefly, and a transient fetal bradycardia is not infrequent. FHR of less than 100 per minute has been noted in 3% to 30% of patients in different studies and may be associated with fetal hypoxia and acidosis if prolonged. The dosage should be kept to a minimum. It is not recommended in cases of placental insufficiency, preexisting fetal distress or prematurity.

Paracervical anesthesia effectively provides relief from the discomfort of uterine contractions during labor but must be supplemented if perineal anesthesia is desired for delivery.

Local infiltration. For episiotomy, local anesthetic agents may be injected into the perineum and adjacent tissues prior to incision.

Pudendal block. If time permits, the physician may block the pudendal nerves near the ischial spines (Fig. 12-8), using any local anesthetic agent. Five to 10 ml. of anesthetic solution should be injected into the area of the internal pudendal nerve as it passes immediately inferior and posterior to each ischial spine. This will relieve the discomfort of delivery, including that of low forceps extraction, and is particularly useful for repair of an episiotomy or perineal lacerations. Infiltration may be accomplished either by the transperineal or transvaginal route. Drug sensitivity and regional infection are about the only contraindications.

Spinal anesthesia. Low-dosage hyperbaric solutions designed

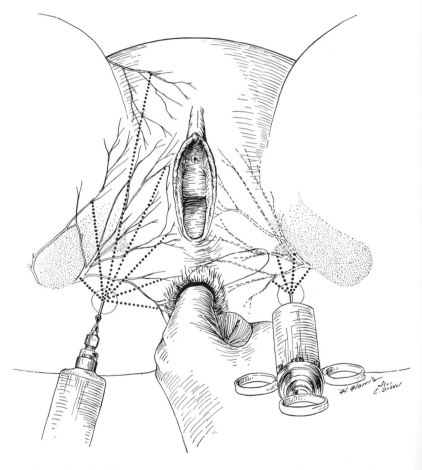

Fig. 12-8. Pudendal block technique. Superficial and deep innervations on both sides injected through only two skin wheals. Dotted lines show paths of needle infiltrating both pudendal and ilioinguinal nerves.

to give "saddleblock" anesthesia to the level of the navel are very popular because the obstetrician can act as the anesthetist and administer a single injection of anesthetic solution just prior to or early in the second stage of labor. Uterine contractions are unaffected and relaxation and anesthesia of the pelvic tissues are achieved with 5 to 10 minutes; failures are infrequent. Although dibucaine (Nupercaine) has been widely used because of its relatively long action, tetracaine (Pontocaine) appears to be a safer agent, the recommended dose being 5 mg. (weighted with 10% glucose). During an interval between contractions, a low lumbar injection is made with the patient in the sitting position, but a supine posture is resumed in about 30 seconds. Since this procedure produces effective anesthesia for only 1 to 2 hours, it is used merely as a terminal form of pain relief after drug-induced analgesia. Maternal hypotension may occur and should be combated with the usual remedies (elevation of the lower extremities and the administration of mild pressor agents). Postpartum headache occurs in 5% to 10% of women delivered under spinal anesthesia.

Caudal anesthesia. Although the single-dose method of caudal anesthesia has been used on occasion over a period of many years, it did not become popular until the continuous technique was introduced in 1942. The anesthetic solution is introduced into the caudal canal via the caudal hiatus through a small catheter previously inserted through the lumen of a 16-gauge needle. After the catheter has been placed, the needle is withdrawn, and the catheter is attached to a closed system containing the anesthetic solution.

If there are no untoward reactions from a small test dose and subarachnoid injection was not inadvertently performed (as confirmed by the lack of an anesthetic level occurring after the test dose), an amount sufficient to produce anesthesia to the umbilicus is given. Additional amounts of solution are injected every 45 to 60 minutes, and in this way complete relief from the pain of labor may be afforded for many hours. Since the patient has no desire and little ability to exert voluntary bearing-down efforts, the second stage of labor usually must be terminated by forceps extraction. Caudal anesthesia should not be attempted by the inexperienced anesthetist and should be used only in those hospitals where physicians with special experience are on duty continuously to observe patients in labor.

The principal causes of trouble are extensive sympathetic blockade, inadvertent subarachnoid injection (spinal anesthesia), and excessive absorption of anesthetic into the bloodstream. In the main these problems can be prevented or promptly corrected by an experienced anesthesiologist. Though there are few absolute contraindications to the use of caudal anesthesia, such as infection in the caudal area or disease of the spinal cord, each patient must be considered individually and jointly by the obstetrician and anesthetist.

Caudal anesthesia is suitable for management of labor in abnormal presentations but will not relax the uterus for operative manipulation. Therefore, supplementary inhalation anesthesia may be required in this situation. Under ideal conditions, caudal anesthesia offers the greatest number of advantages to the mother, her infant, and her doctor.

Lumbar epidural anesthesia. Continuous lumbar epidural anesthesia may also be utilized in essentially the same manner as continuous caudal anesthesia. The advantages and disadvantages are essentially the same for the parturient and the obstetrician as with caudal anesthesia, and the choice of the route employed largely depends on the technical preference of the anesthesiologist.

In essentially all circumstances, but especially when regional block anesthesia is employed, some degree of lateral positioning of the patient is desirable during labor. This will reduce the uteroplacental hypoperfusion typically associated with aortocaval compression by the pregnant uterus when the parturient is in the supine position.

Natural childbirth. The term "natural childbirth" is used to describe a system of treating and educating the pregnant woman, with a view to eliminating her fears of pregnancy and helping her to accept and bear the discomfort of labor and delivery. During pregnancy the patient practices relaxation, muscle control, and various patterns of breathing and receives elementary instruction in the anatomy and physiology of reproduction. Emphasis is placed on using minimal amounts of sedative and anesthetic drugs for labor and delivery, although these are not denied if the patient requests them. Spontaneous delivery is encouraged, as well as breast feeding and a "rooming-in" arrangement for the mother and baby during the immediate puerperium.

Hypnosis. Hypnosis may be a useful procedure in carefully selected patients, provided that the obstetrician attempting to use it has had adequate instruction in the technique and is fully aware of its limitations and contraindications. Because prenatal training of the patient is involved, this is not a practical device for widespread use.

13

The puerperium

The puerperium is the stage of recovery extending from delivery until approximately 6 weeks thereafter and characterized by distinctive tissue catabolism.

CLINICAL FEATURES

Uterus. The uterus on the first postpartum day should be palpable as a firm, rounded mass, with the upper margin just below the umbilicus. If it tends to relax, it should be massaged until firmness is restored. Oxytocic drugs may be required to maintain adequate contraction. Although the common practice is to give such agents routinely by mouth for a few days after delivery, there is no evidence that this is essential. After about 10 days the uterus has shrunk considerably and no longer is readily palpable through the abdominal wall (Fig. 13-1).

Care of perineum. The perineum should be covered by a clean pad held in place by a T-binder. The external genitalia should be cleansed regularly with soap and water or an antiseptic solution. A heat lamp may be used several times daily if needed to relieve pain in the episiotomy wound or from hemorrhoids. Anesthetic ointments are popular, but their value is open to question. Warm sitz baths, several times per day, are appreciated by most parturients, as the baths significantly reduce perineal edema and discomfort and are believed by many to improve bladder function. They do not aggravate puerperal morbidity.

Temperature. The temperature should be taken several times daily while the patient is hospitalized. Any significant elevation above normal should be considered a sign of puerperal infection until proved otherwise.

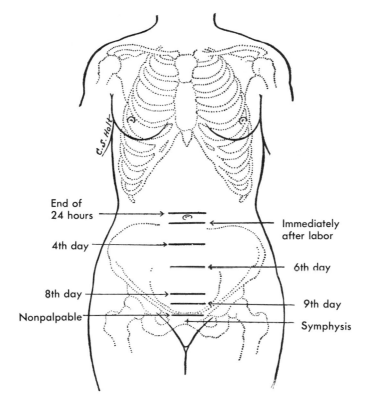

Fig. 13-1. Height of the fundus uteri at different stages of the puerperium. (From Falls and McLaughlin: Obstetric and gynecologic nursing, St. Louis, The C. V. Mosby Co.)

Puerperal morbidity is defined as fever exceeding 38° C. (100.4° F) on any 2 days of the puerperium, excluding the first 24 hours after delivery.

Some patients exhibit a brief (12 hours or less) temperature elevation if breast engorgement on the third or fourth day is extremely great. In general, however, so-called "milk-fever" is not a routine phenomenon.

Postpartum chills. Shaking chills of short duration and unknown etiology are noted by approximately 20% to 25% of par-, turients during the first 5 to 60 minutes after delivery. Treatment is unnecessary and no residual effect is obvious. Type of delivery and/or anesthesia may be incriminated, as the incidence is greater with regional anesthesia and operative delivery than it is with local anesthesia and spontaneous delivery. On the other hand, the event also correlates moderately well with the appearance of fetal blood cells in the maternal plasma and may represent a fetomaternal transfusion reaction. Chills at later periods in the puerperium are of more obvious etiology and usually denote septicemia.

Bathing. Showers and tub baths are permissible, beginning the day after delivery. Frequent sitz baths should be encouraged if perineal discomfort or bladder dysfunction is significant.

Pulse. Bradycardia is common after delivery (rates of 50 to 70 per minute). The precise explanation for this is not known.

Afterpains. The uterus in a primipara tends to remain in tonic contraction and usually is not painful. The multiparous uterus has less ability to maintain constant contraction and relaxes and contracts at intervals. Such activity provokes afterpains. These are most noticeable during the first 2 days and during breast feeding and may require anodynes for relief.

Lochia. Lochia is the postpartum vaginal discharge that at first is bloodstained *(lochia rubra)*. In a few days it pales to become the *lochia serosa,* and after 10 days it is usually yellowish white from leukocytes *(lochia alba)*. Foul-smelling lochia denotes putrefactive bacteria. Most lochial discharges contain anaerobic streptococci and often colon bacilli and staphylococci. Persisting bloody lochia usually indicates retention of small pieces of placental tissue with associated subinvolution of the placental site.

Bladder. Diuresis occurs between the second and fifth postpartum days. This increase in output of the kidneys, coupled with a difficulty in initiating normal voiding, may lead to serious overdistention of the bladder. If prompt and adequate voiding cannot be achieved, catheterization or suprapubic aspiration must be performed. Urinary antibiotics should be employed if catheterization is necessary. A midstream urine culture should be obtained within a week or so after discontinuation of the antibiotic to ensure that an asymptomatic bacteriuria has not been established. This is particularly true if continuous catheter drainage has been necessary. Numerous routines for the poorly functioning bladder have been devised, but the perfect solution to this common problem is not at hand.

Sugar in the urine is common after delivery because of lactose from the mammary glands. Acetonuria is common after prolonged labor, because of muscular activity and starvation.

Diet and fluids. Regular diet as well as fully elective oral fluids may be initiated as soon as the previously administered analgesics and anesthetics have been fully metabolized and the potential for nausea and vomiting has been eliminated.

Bowel function. Puerperal constipation is common, engendered by a prepartum enema, liquid diet during labor, bed rest, painful perineal incision, or hemorrhoids. Whether to administer another enema a few days postpartum or give one of a great variety of recommended cathartics is a matter of individual judgment. Often a gas-forming rectal suppository will provide the stimulus for a spontaneous bowel movement.

Breasts and nipples. Breasts should have adequate support but not a tight binder. Milk appears 48 to 72 hours after delivery, and breasts may become greatly engorged for a day or two at the onset of lactation. If there is adequate reason for not nursing, an attempt may be made to suppress lactation with estrogen or androgen administered immediately after delivery, but success is not invariably achieved. Lactation will cease within a few days if suckling is discontinued or if it is never started, and the necessity or desirability of hormonal suppression has not been established.

Oxytocin, released from the posterior pituitary as a response to suckling, has a galactokinetic effect and initiates the so-called milk ejection or milk letdown associated with nursing. Synthetic oxytocin is occasionally used (intranasal, sublingual, or intramuscular application) to relieve breast engorgement or to promote the flow of milk at the beginning of a period of nursing, but its use is not an established obstetric practice.

Breast feeding is convenient, inexpensive, and emotionally satisfying for most women. Breast milk is digestible, sterile, and nutritionally ideal, except possibly for a deficiency in fat-soluble vitamins (A, D, E, and K) and fluoride. The mechanism for control of the nutritional composition of breast milk is wholly unknown. The only disadvantages of breast feeding are restrictions on the mother's activities, the possibility of puerperal mastitis, and the passage of a large number of maternally ingested drugs to the infant in pharmacologic dosages.

Full milk production is reached in 10 to 14 days, with yields of 120 to 180 ml. of milk per feeding. During the early days of lactation the milk ejection reflex may be deficient, the breasts become greatly engorged, and the infant is unable to cope with the unyielding areolae. Manual expression of milk, aided by oxytocin, will improve this situation. The infant may be nursed at both breasts at each feeding to avoid overfilling and reduction in milk secretion.

Nipples should be kept clean and free from dried milk crustations. Bleeding fissures and tenderness of nipples can usually be corrected within 24 to 48 hours without discontinuing nursing by simply protecting the nipple on each occasion with a nipple shield. Other treatment is usually not required, but antibiotic ointments may be used if they are thoroughly washed away before nursing.

Ambulation and length of time in hospital. Normal puerperal patients may be out of bed as soon after delivery as their postanalgesic and postanesthetic condition allows. The number of days spent in the hospital varies from area to area and is dictated by local custom rather than by scientific reasoning. Commonly multiparas go home from 2 to 4 days after delivery. Primiparas tend to remain a day to two longer, depending on adequacy of lactation, perineal pain, and the personal convictions of the patient's obstetrician. From the standpoint of avoiding infection with bacteria that are resistant to antibiotics, early departure from the hospital may be advisable, but the danger of infection must be weighed against the possible advantages of more prolonged hospital care.

Special medications. Rh_0 (D) immune globulin should be administered within 72 hours after delivery to all Rh_0 (D)—negative and D^u-negative, unsensitized women who have borne an Rh_0 (D)-positive or D^u-positive infant.

Immunizations withheld during pregnancy for fear of fetal infection may be administered during postpartum hospitalization. For example, immunization should be offered to all women who demonstrated a low rubella antibody titer in the prenatal period.

Follow-up examinations. Although the examination 6 weeks after delivery has become a ritual in obstetric practice, some patients will require attention earlier and others may be seen later without harmful effect. Every effort should be made to encourage patients to present themselves at least within 3 months of delivery. The breasts, abdomen, perineum, cervix, and pelvic cavity should be examined meticulously. Contraception should be discussed and initiated (see Chapter 32).

Resumption of menses. In the absence of lactation, menstruation usually reappears 7 to 9 weeks after delivery. Although lactation may be associated with amenorrhea, this is not invariably the case, and about one third of lactating primiparas will have menstruated 3 months post partum. But by this time about 90% of nonlactating primiparas will have had a menstrual flow.

The first episode of bleeding after delivery may be heavier and persist longer than previous menses and will be preceded by ovulation in approximately 25% of patients, a point of importance when scheduling reinitiation of contraception.

Advice on dismissal. Postpartum patients, especially primiparas, need advice on numerous minor matters, and an opportunity for discussion of these items should be provided on the day of dismissal.

1. Full ambulation, both in and out of the house, is encouraged. Flights of stairs may be climbed as necessary. Physical endurance is usually quite limited for the first 1 or 2 weeks. This lack of endurance and perineal discomfort are the common restricting factors. Oral analgesics should be regularly prescribed for the latter.

2. Tub baths may be taken if showers are unavailable or distasteful to the patient.

3. Sexual intercourse and vaginal douching should be avoided until the lochial discharge has ceased and the episiotomy scar is no longer tender. A diminution of libido as well as an increase in frictional dyspareunia caused by disruption of the thin, estrogen-deprived vaginal mucosa is not uncommon during the

puerperium in both nursing and nonnursing patients. However, sexual pleasure and excitement may evolve from nursing and may be sufficiently guilt-provoking for some women to induce them to reinitiate coitus earlier than would otherwise be the case.

4. The lactating mother should consume at least 1 quart of milk a day and probably should continue any vitamin supplement she may have been using prenatally. Any localized redness or tenderness of either breast, especially if coupled with fever and axillary tenderness, should be immediately brought to the physician's attention.

5. Any sharp increase in uterine bleeding during the first 4 to 6 weeks should be reported at once in order that a decision may be made as to its likely cause and that the indicated therapeutic measures may be started before blood loss becomes unnecessarily great.

6. Some provision should be made for assistance with major household duties during at least the first 2 to 3 weeks after delivery.

7. Contraception should be discussed and a schedule derived for its resumption. In some institutions, oral contraceptives are initiated before the patient leaves the hospital (for nonnursing mothers) and intrauterine devices are inserted immediately after delivery. Such zeal is not required routinely but is obviously strategic in given circumstances.

8. *Postpartum exercises* of various sorts may improve the tone of abdominal muscles, but they exert no obvious effect on the generative organs. Assumption of the knee-chest posture to prevent uterine retroversion is a useless procedure.

ANATOMIC AND PHYSIOLOGIC CHANGES

Involution of uterus. The uterus decreases rapidly in weight from about 1,000 grams at delivery to 500 grams a week later and to 50 grams a week thereafter. This stupendous rate of tissue absorption, eliminating a growth of 9 months within 2 weeks, is accomplished by a poorly understood autolytic process that breaks down uterine muscle protein, and especially the tremendously increased volume of connective tissue collagen and elastin, into simpler compounds that are absorbed and eliminated in the urine.

The mechanism for the initiation and control of this process is unknown.

Endometrial regeneration occurs in about 10 days except at the placental site. In this area lie many thrombosed vascular sinuses that undergo typical organizational changes. The placental site eventually is undermined and exfoliated by growth of new endometrial tissues, so that no permanent scar remains.

The cervix is soft and flabby after delivery, and minor depressions in its margin represent lacerations. Within a week it will scarcely admit a finger; new muscle cells have been added to its substance, and minor lacerations are healed. The external os rarely assumes its nulliparous appearance because lacerations at the lateral angles never heal without leaving visible depressed scars.

Vagina. The vagina never returns entirely to its nulliparous state. The hymen is replaced by tags of mucosa called *carunculae myrtiformes,* and the introitus is larger than it was before delivery. Rugae reappear during the third week. Supportive tissues of the pelvic floor regain a varying degree but seldom all of their former tone within 2 to 6 months after vaginal delivery. For most women repetitive delivery leads to increasingly poor pelvic floor tone and for some to symptomatic tissue relaxation.

Vascular system. For several hours after delivery, presumably because of the return of uterine blood to the general circulation, the cardiac work load is substantially increased, a point of importance in caring for patients with cardiac disease. Plasma and red blood cell volume return to normal within 2 weeks. A modest leukocytosis is present for several days after delivery.

Abdominal wall. Involution in the abdominal wall requires at least 6 weeks. Silvery striations in the skin often persist indefinitely, but the linea nigra gradually fades. There is great individual variation in the degree to which rectus muscle tone returns, and some women exhibit midline separation of the rectus muscles *(diastasis recti).*

Breasts. During the first 2 days only colostrum can be expressed from the nipples, but by the third or fourth day milk appears in response to prolactin from the pituitary. Breast milk is an emulsion of fat droplets, protein, lactose, salts, and water. The quantity produced varies enormously and presumably is related to diet, mental state, fluid intake, and other factors, notably certain drugs.

Suckling provokes a reflex stimulation of the uterus and appears to hasten involution.

If breast nursing is not undertaken, some degree of engorgement appears within 1 to 2 days. The increased pressure diminishes secretory activity, and usually within another 36 hours the breasts are soft and painless. Secretion disappears completely in a week.

Urinary tract. Overdistention and incomplete emptying are common after delivery, particularly in women who have had regional anesthesia. Residual urine with bacteria often leads to cystitis. Ureteral dilatation disappears within 2 weeks and ureteral function usually is normal thereafter.

14

The newborn child

CARE OF NEWBORN CHILD

Before anything specific is done to the infant, an assessment of his general condition must be made and a decision reached as to whether any specific type of resuscitative measure is indicated. The physician looks for color, body tone, respiratory effort, and immediate urination. The Apgar scoring system (1953) (see Table 4) is a useful objective aid; it involves determination of heart rate, respiratory effort, muscle tone, reflex irritability, and color 60 seconds after birth. Scores of each item range from 0 to 2, and thus a score in the range of 7 to 10 indicates that the infant is in good or excellent condition. A perfect score of 10 is rarely given because slight peripheral cyanosis is present in most newborn infants. Eighty to 90% of infants will have scores of 7 or above.

Depressed infants are scored as follows: Agpar 0 to 3, severe; 4 to 6, moderate; 7 to 8, slight. Infants with scores of 6 or above usually require no unusual treatment.

The most important observation is the heart rate. An infant with a rapidly falling heart rate requires immediate resuscitation.

Resuscitation. Generally speaking, 9 out of 10 infants are in excellent condition at birth and need only simple suctioning of pharyngeal mucus. For the infant who requires help, however, prompt intervention with the proper equipment may be lifesaving. Every delivery room should be equipped with oxygen and suction devices, infant laryngoscope, small endotracheal tubes, and a suitable work table.

Treatment. Normally the infant should make inspiratory move-

Table 4. Apgar score of newborn infant

Sign	Score		
	0	**1**	**2**
Color	Blue, pale	Body pink, extremities blue	Completely pink
Heart rate (pulse)	Absent	Below 100	Over 100
Respiratory effort	Absent	Irregular	Good, crying
Muscle tone	Limp	Some flexion of extremities	Active motion
Reflex irritability (catheter in nostril)	None	Grimace	Cough, sneeze

ments a few seconds after delivery. Mucus should be sucked from the pharynx and nares with a rubber bulb syringe, and simple cutaneous stimulation may be applied. These measures usually suffice to initiate respiration, but more radical measures may be needed; if so, place the infant on a table and start the following procedures:

1. If the trachea or bronchi contain amniotic fluid or mucus, a soft rubber catheter may be introduced into the larynx and the foreign material sucked out.

2. If these measures do not suffice, and positive-pressure equipment is not at hand, mouth-to-mouth breathing may be employed, always being careful not to cover the nose so that air may escape if the physician blows too hard.

3. If oxygen equipment for producing intermittent positive pressure is available, this should be used in preference to mouth-to-mouth insufflation. Mixtures containing carbon dioxide should not be used.

4. An infant asphyxiated during the birth process requires immediate tubation, using an infant laryngoscope and endotracheal tube of appropriate size. Attach a bag with oxygen inflow through a T-tube connection and gauge the inflation by

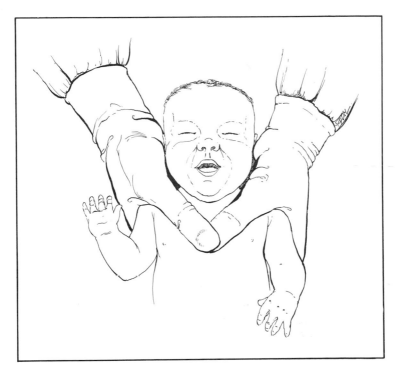

Fig. 14-1. Method of applying external cardiac massage to newborn infant (sternal compression).

observing the chest and listening to the entry of air with a stethoscope.

5. If the heart is inaudible at birth, use external cardiac massage after immediate intubation and pulmonary inflation. With the hands around each shoulder and thumbs superimposed over midsternum, depress the sternum about 100 times per minute, between lung inflations (Fig. 14-1).

6. Nalline (0.2 mg.) or Lorfan (0.05 mg.) may be used intravenously to counteract narcosis from morphine or Demerol. Do not use these drugs if the mother has had barbiturates, because the infant will become more depressed. Respiratory stimulants

are not useful, but in the event of cardiac arrest, intracardiac epinephrine (1 : 2,000) may be injected through the fourth interspace to the left of the sternum.

Oxygen should be continued as long as there is cyanosis. Aspirate the stomach if delivery was by cesarean section or if the abdomen appears greatly distended. Glucose and bicarbonate solution are given as indicated by serum pH and bicarbonate values. Because resuscitated infants often develop infections, cultures of blood and spinal fluid, chest x-ray examination, and antibiotic therapy must be considered.

Efforts at resuscitation should be kept up as long as the heart beats. Successful results occasionally are obtained after 30 to 60 minutes. Whatever method of resuscitation is employed, gentleness must always be observed and an attempt should be made to prevent hypothermia, since it is detrimental to infant survival.

Care of umbilical cord. The umbilical cord should be tied with a sterile tape ligature or occluded with a plastic cord clamp, a centimeter or two from the skin margin. A second clamp is then applied further from the skin margin and the cord is cut between the clamps. A longer stump of umbilical cord should be left attached to the infant if a need to catheterize the umbilical vein for blood sampling or transfusion is anticipated.

If the infant is premature, anoxic, or presumed to have erythroblastosis, there is nothing to be gained by waiting for cord pulsations to cease before clamping or tying the cord. Although approximately 80 ml. of placental blood may be shifted to the infant by delayed clamping, this has not been proved to be of value to the infant and only delays the initiation of resuscitative care. Indeed, experiments in fetal lambs suggest that hemodynamic changes that occur after interruption of the umbilical circulation are among the stimuli that initiate respiration.

Later, the stump of the cord becomes dry and dark. A line of demarcation appears just beyond the abdominal skin surface and the stump usually sloughs off during the second week. The granulating wound heals to form the umbilicus.

Care of eyes. As soon as the head is born, each eye should be wiped gently (away from the nose) with a separate pledget of cotton or gauze. Later a drop of 1% silver nitrate should be instilled in each eye to prevent gonorrheal ophthalmia and then washed out with saline solution. This is a requirement of law in most states. Silver nitrate produces a mild chemical conjunctivitis in essentially all infants properly treated, but this is usually transient.

The use of penicillin ophthalmic ointment for this purpose has been discontinued by a decision of the Food and Drug Administration. The potential for the sensitization in the infant was held to be greater than the demonstrated benefit of the medication. Additionally, allergic skin reactions have developed in personnel handling the ointment.

Care of skin. Nothing special need be done to the skin in the delivery unit other than wiping away excess vernix caseosa and blood. In the newborn nursery it is common practice to cleanse the skin daily with mild soap and water.

Icterus neonatorum. About one third of all newborn infants show some degree of jaundice between the second and the fifth day of life, with the serum bilirubin reaching levels of 4 to 5 mg. per 100 ml. It has been suggested that this transient phenomenon is caused by immaturity of the bilirubin conjugation mechanism necessary for bilirubin excretion.

Fluids and nursing. The baby may be put to the breast in the delivery room or at any time thereafter as long as there are no abnormalities. The first breast milk, colostrum, has little food value, but suckling is desirable to stimulate the normal flow of milk. The typical interval between breast feedings is 4 hours. The duration of each feeding will depend on the ease and the quantity of the milk flow and the strength of the suckling. It is unnecessary for infants to suckle for long periods; 5 to 10 minutes at each breast is usually sufficient.

Rooming-in. Rooming-in refers to keeping the infant in a crib at the mother's bedside and permitting the mother to take care of her child. Usually an adjacent small nursery is provided so that the infant may be removed from the mother's room at night. In addition to the alleged educational benefit for the primiparous mother, this is an excellent method for prevention of epidemic infections in large nurseries.

SPECIAL PHYSICAL FEATURES OF NEWBORN CHILD

Skin. Usually covered by *vernix caseosa,* a white, creamy mixture of exfoliated cells, sebaceous material, and lanugo. The latter is downy hair scattered over the face, back, and extremities.

Petechiae and erythematous patches are common on the scalp, face, and neck. The trauma of delivery may create abrasions, contusions, and impressions from obstetrical forceps.

Head. The head is large in proportion to the body, but, unlike the adult, the infant's face is much smaller than its cranium. (See Chapter 4 for details of skull bones and sutures.)

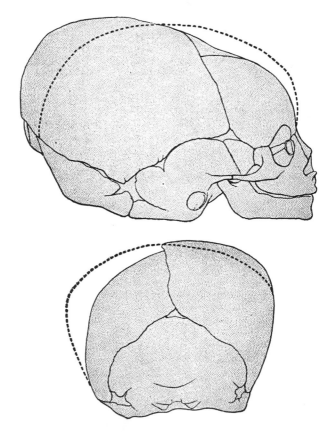

Fig. 14-2. Molding of the head during labor. Lateral and frontal views show how the head bones overlap. (Redrawn from Bumm.)

Immediately after birth the head of the newborn infant may present one or more of the following temporary phenomena, particularly if the labor has been protracted or if there has been some degree of cephalopelvic disproportion.

Molding (Fig. 14-2). The head is composed of separate bones so that it may accomodate itself to the shape and the size of the pelvis. By movements of the various bones at the sutures, diameters are shortened where necessary, with compensatory lengthening in other diameters. It is these movements of the cranial bones that put the tentorium and falx under stress, occasionally causing tears and cerebral hemorrhage, even in normal deliveries. Pressure upon the occipital bone by the symphysis pubis in delivery of the aftercoming head accounts for the large number of infants with intracranial bleeding in breech deliveries.

Caput succedaneum. The caput succedaneum is a blood-stained serous swelling of that part of the scalp that lies over the os uteri. It forms only after rupture of the membranes. In left positions it is found on the right parietal bone and vice versa in right positions because it forms on the lowest part of the presenting head. By its location the presentation can be determined after delivery.

Cephalhematoma (Fig. 14-3). Cephalhematoma is a hemorrhage under the periosteum of the skull, not in the scalp. It usually makes its appearance several days after delivery.

Neck. The neck is short and the head appears to rest directly on the shoulders, which are relatively narrow.

Thorax. Breast tissue is palpable in both males and females. Respirations are shallow and rapid (38 to 44 per minute), and abdominal breathing is common. The heart rate is 120 to 140 per minute; there may be sinus arrhythmia and transient, functional murmurs.

External genitalia. In the male there is an adherent foreskin completely covering the glans penis, and testes usually are within the scrotum. The female has prominent labia minora and often a mucoid secretion at the introitus. One should determine that the anus is patent and the anal sphincter competent.

Temperature. Cooling of the body surface at birth reduces the temperature somewhat, but normal values usually are observed after the infant has been in a warmed bassinet for a short time.

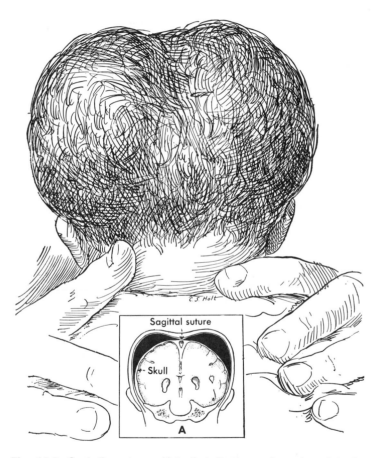

Fig. 14-3. Cephalhematoma. Note that the hemorrhage is not in the scalp (since it is in the caput succedaneum) but is under the skull periosteum. (From Falls and McLaughlin: Obstetric and gynecologic nursing, St. Louis, The C. V. Mosby Co.)

Such a device, kept constantly warm, should be in every delivery room for immediate care of the infant. The temperature-regulating mechanism in a newborn infant is quite unstable during the first few days of life.

Intestinal content. The brownish green meconium of the intestine of a newborn infant is initially sterile, but bacteria soon enter the intestinal canal. After ingestion of milk, the feces become light yellow, and eventually formed cylindric fecal material is expelled once or twice daily.

Urine. The bladder contains urine at birth, so if the baby does not soon urinate, the cause should be investigated. It may be caused by simple phimosis or a serious congenital defect of the kidneys or ureters.

Primary weight loss. Primary weight loss, from lack of milk and loss of fluids, is usual until the mother's milk "comes in." The loss may be reduced by giving an ounce of a 5% solution of glucose every 3 or 4 hours. The loss is generally regained in 8 or 10 days.

Circulatory changes. Circulatory changes are discussed in Chapter 4.

15

Multiple pregnancy

Litter size is roughly inversely proportional to the adult size of the mammal concerned. Animals with unicornuate uteri tend to produce a single fetus, as do animals with only two breasts. Species with the longest span of life and the greatest duration of gestation produce the fewest offspring. The birth of human sextuplets has been reported by reliable sources several times, and quintuplet births are rather well known. It is unusual, however, for all the infants to survive.

TWIN BIRTHS

Etiology. Twinning may result from the simultaneous fertilization of two ova (fraternal or dizygotic twins) or from the abnormal development of a single ovum (identical or monozygotic twins). Double-ovum twins are not twins in the strict biologic sense— merely two individuals resulting from the maturation and fertilization of two ova at once. Presumably the ova may come from a single ovarian follicle, from two different follicles in the same ovary, or one from each ovary. Single-ovum twinning may be due largely to environmental conditions that affect the embryo's rate of growth shortly after fertilization. Triplets may come from one, two, or three ova. The famous Dionne quintuplets presumably were derived from a single ovum.

Identical twins are always of the same sex; fraternal twins may be of the same or of different sex. Only about 25% to 30% of twins develop from one ovum. Multiple pregnancies from multiple ova are most common in Negroes and least common in Orientals. The rate of single-ovum twinning is almost the same in all races and is not familial. Dizygotic twinning is clearly a familial phenomenon, but only females carry the trait for multiple ovulation and, hence, multiple pregnancy.

Induction of ovulation with gonadotropins or clomiphene in instances of anovulatory infertility not infrequently results in multiple pregnancy, which is the direct result of multiple ovulation.

Incidence. Twins occur in Caucasians in the United States about once in 99 deliveries or in 1.01% of births, but in 1.34% (1:74) of Negro births and 0.64% (1:155) of Oriental births.

The twinning rate by age of mother increases up to the age of 40 and decreases thereafter. The greater the mother's parity, the more likely she is to bear twins, but this difference according to parity is dependent on the incidence of dizygotic twinning, because the monozygotic rate remains constant.

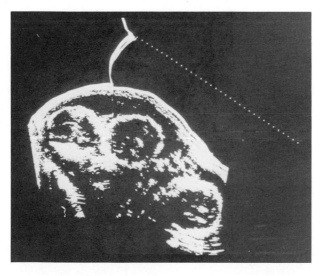

Fig. 15-1. Sonogram of a triplet gestation at term. (Courtesy Dr. Louis Bartolucci, San Francisco.)

Diagnosis. There is usually some exaggeration of the minor discomforts of pregnancy, such as pelvic pressure, backache, varicosities, hemorrhoids, and difficulty in breathing. The relatively large size of the uterus in relation to presumed duration of gestation may be the initial diagnostic clue, or fetal activity may seem excessive. The diagnosis may be made as follows:

(a) Various parts of two fetuses may be felt.

(b) Two asynchronous fetal hearts may be heard with either auditory or Doppler auscultation.

(c) Dual fetal electrocardiographic tracings may be obtained.

(d) X-ray or B-scan ultrasonographic examination (Fig. 15-1) will give positive evidence in most doubtful cases.

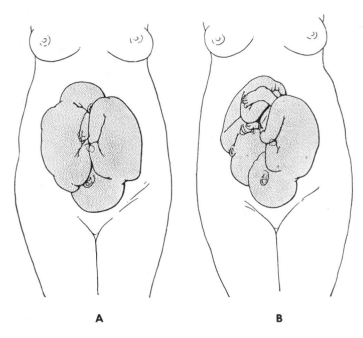

A   B

Fig. 15-2. A, Twin pregnancies, showing presentation of head and breech. **B,** Both heads in twin pregnancy presenting. (Redrawn from Bumm.)

A correct diagnosis of twinning is made clinically in only about 70% of patients.

Both fetuses present by the vertex in about one half the patients; in one third there is a combination of vertex and breech presentations, in one tenth there are two breech presentations; and in another one tenth there are single or double transverse presentations (Fig. 15-2).

Placenta and membranes. Fraternal twins have two amnions, two chorions, and two placentas, although they may fuse and appear to be one (Fig. 15-3).

Identical twins usually have two amnions, one chorion, and one placenta. Occasionally, however, monoamniotic twins (with one chorion) will develop as a result of a late splitting of the germ disk after formation of the amnion. Moreover, a single ovum may divide so early in its development that the placental relations are like those of a two-egg pregnancy with two amnions and two chorions. The possible identicality of dual amniotic, dual chorionic twins of the same sex cannot be established until hematologic, dermatoglyphic, or tissue grafting tests are applied.

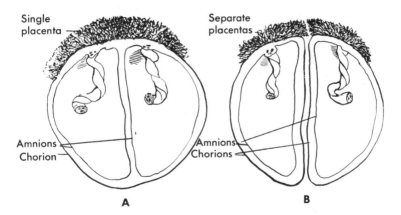

Fig. 15-3. Diagram showing membranes and placenta formation in **A,** identical single-ovum twins, and **B,** fraternal double-ova twins. Note that there are two amnions and two chorions in double-ova twins. (From Titus: The management of obstetric difficulties, St. Louis, The C. V. Mosby Co.)

Placental relationships are best studied by histologic section of the partitioning membrane at the point where it joins the fetal surface of the placenta. Microscopic examination of the apposed membranes will show either (1) amnion on each surface and two layers of chorion in the center, often with trophoblastic remnants of the chorion laeve, or (2) merely two apposed amnions. Grossly the dichorial membranes often are opaque, and the amnion is an extremely thin sheet readily separable from the underlying chorion. The chorionic layer cannot be stripped from the surface of the placenta because of numerous ramifications of the villi from its inferior surface.

In monochorionic placentas there are usually anastomoses between placental vessels of the two fetuses. They are established early in intrauterine life and may be artery to artery, vein to vein, or artery to vein. Arteriovenous anastomoses can produce the *transfusion syndrome,* a cause of prematurity and stillbirth in monochorionic twins. An artery-to-vein anastomosis transfers arterial blood from one twin to the venous system of the other, and the recipient becomes hypervolemic and hypertensive. The heart, liver, and kidneys enlarge, and extra urine creates hydramnios. The donor twin becomes malnourished and oligohydramnios develops. On occasion this may occur rapidly, and the sudden development of hydramnios in a single sac is cause for alarm, especially if the cardiac rhythm of either of the twins becomes abnormal. This is presumptive evidence of an acute transfusion syndrome. A distinct difference in the appearance of monochorionic twins upon delivery is also presumptive evidence of such an event.

A similar, though earlier and slower occurrence, can also be used to explain the development of *acardius amorphus,* a heartless and shapeless blob of tissue representing the malformed and atrophied loser in a quiet struggle between twins for blood and nutrition. *Fetus papyraceus* or *compressus,* a dead but small and normally formed twin, may develop in the same manner.

About 7% of twin placentas have velamentous insertion of the cord combined with vasa previa. These unprotected blood vessels may easily be torn, particularly during rupture of the membranes, and exsanguination of one or both twins may occur unless delivery is accomplished speedily.

Clinical course

1. Hydramnios occurs in 5% to 7% of multiple pregnancies. This may lead to premature labor and thus to an increase in fetal mortality.

2. Preeclamptic and eclamptic toxemia occurs in about 20% of multiple pregnancies. The incidence is approximately 33% in primigravidas.

3. Circulatory and respiratory disturbances are more noticeable—dyspnea, varicose veins of the vulva and lower extremities, and edema of the legs. Maternity corsets and elastic stockings may be useful.

4. Maternal anemia is more frequent and more severe.

5. Because of the tendency toward premature labor, certain precautions should be observed, such as avoidance of coitus and orgasm in the last 3 months, additional rest, and minimal travel. Barter has advocated strict bed rest at home, beginning no later than the twenty-eighth week. The patient remains recumbent except for bathroom privileges. Such home care for the expectant mother may be less expensive than the cost of hospitalization for premature infants.

6. Antepartum preparation for blood transfusion in labor or in the puerperium is highly desirable because of the increased incidence of postpartum hemorrhage.

7. Induction of labor rarely is necessary, but artificial rupture of the membranes usually will suffice for this purpose in patients with severe toxemia or pronounced respiratory distress.

8. Fetal death in utero is common because of cord compression from entanglement, competition for nutrition, and developmental anomalies. Fetal loss in labor is increased by operative delivery from abnormal positions, prolapse of cord, and premature separation of the placenta before delivery of the second twin.

9. Additional hazards are peculiar to monoamniotic twins and approximately 40% of these fetuses are stillborn. More than two thirds of these twins have knotted cords or other cord complications, and about 10% have congenital malformations. The diagnosis can be made only at delivery by observing knotted cords in the vagina or absence of amniotic sac around the second twin.

Management of twin labors

1. Because of the distended uterus, false labor is common and premature and dysfunctional labor are frequently noted.

2. Labor typically is shorter than with single gestations.

3. Deflexed fetal attitudes and compound presentations are often seen as a result of excess amniotic fluid and small fetal size.

4. The frequency of premature rupture of the membranes is greatly increased, and the incidence of prolapse of the cord is trebled.

5. Only minimal analgesia should be used in order to avoid undesirable effects of drugs in premature infants. Anesthesia to relax the uterus for internal podalic version may be needed for delivery of the second twin if spontaneous delivery is delayed.

6. Usually the labor of the first infant is normal.

7. The physician should be certain to cut the first cord between clamps to prevent loss of blood from the other infant. *Do not give ergonovine or oxytocin!*

8. Reexamine immediately after the first birth to be sure of the presentation of the second fetus.

9. There is often a temporary cessation of contractions after the first birth, but labor usually resumes in a few minutes, and the second infant should be delivered in a half hour or less.

10. If labor is delayed, rupture the second amniotic sac to promote contractions. Version and extraction should be done on the second twin if it does not promptly engage in the longitudinal position. If engagement occurs, spontaneous delivery often will result, or forceps or breech extraction may be effected.

11. Monitor the fetal heart. If fetal distress occurs or there is any evidence of placental separation, deliver promptly by the most conservative method.

12. Finally, remember that the overdistended uterus is particularly likely to bleed; therefore, unusual watchfulness must be practiced to prevent postpartum hemorrhage. Oxytocics should be given routinely after the delivery of the final fetus.

13. Cesarean section is only occasionally necessary for multiple pregnancy. It should be employed for severe malpresentations, when pregnancy must be quickly terminated because of prolapsed cord, severe preeclampsia, or bleeding, and possibly is advisable if the mother has been delivered previously by this method.

14. *Interlocking* of twins refers to the situation in which the chin of a fetus presenting by breech locks into the chin-neck

area of its mate presenting by the vertex. As the breech descends into the pelvis, the locking effect becomes exaggerated. If the two heads cannot be separated by manual manipulation, the only solution is cesarean section or decapitation. This is an exceptionally unusual event and may be expected only once in 800 twin gestations.

Newborn twin. On the average a twin infant is about 700 grams lighter than a singleton infant at birth. Presumably this difference occurs because the duration of pregnancy is shorter, averaging 37 weeks, and the placental bed is somewhat diminished. Congenital malformations are more common in twins than in single children (about 7%). Most malformations appear in both members of a pair of identical twins. The perinatal mortality for twins is more than twice that for single births, and there are twice as many neonatal deaths as there are stillbirths (because of prematurity). On the other hand, a twin or triplet weighing over 2,500 grams at birth has a better prognosis than a single infant of the same weight.

OTHER MULTIPLE BIRTHS

The incidence of multiple pregnancies in which more than two fetuses develop may be calculated roughly from the Hellin-Zeleny hypothesis. According to this concept, if the frequency of twins is 1 in N pregnancies, that of triplets is 1 in N^2, quadruplets 1 in N^3, and quintuplets 1 in N^4 pregnancies. This hypothesis is an approximation rather than a mathematical law, and actual frequencies in census data may be appreciably lower or higher than the predicted values when the sample size is modest. If one assumes that the rate of twinning is about 1 : 100 deliveries, then triplets might be anticipated once in 10,000 deliveries. Vital statistics for the United States in 1964 showed a triplet rate of 0.98 per 10,000 deliveries for all ages and all races. The rate for whites was only 0.86, but the nonwhite (primarily black) rate was 1.62.

Information about the placentas of multiple pregnancies other than twins is scanty. All combinations of zygosity have been reported. Most quintuplets have developed from two to five ova.

16

Abortion and premature labor

Abortion indicates the termination of pregnancy before the fetus is viable (less than 500 grams) and usually before the twentieth week of gestation. The limit of 20 weeks is more legalistic than medical, as birth beyond the twentieth week must be officially reported. However, few infants delivered prior to the twenty-fourth week are likely to survive.

The term "miscarriage," formerly used to designate expulsions from the third month to viability, is now considered unnecessary, confusing, and unscientific.

Premature labor occurs after the fetus is viable but before it is mature. If unchecked, premature labor results in the delivery of an infant weighing less than 2,500 grams.

ABORTION

Abortion is the term now used by most authorities for all interruptions before viability. Abortions are either *spontaneous* or *induced,* and induced abortions may be either *legal (therapeutic)* or *criminal.*

Incidence. The incidence of abortion is variously estimated from 10% to 40%, averaging 20% of all pregnancies. Roughly 10% to 12% of all *identified* pregnancies are terminated by spontaneous abortion, and it is likely that many other pregnancies expire very early without ever being recognized or counted. Nearly 75% occur in the second and third months and less than 10% in the fourth month.

Etiology of spontaneous abortion. The immediate cause of abortions in the early months is usually the death of the embryo or fetus. Though the basic etiology is not determinable in the majority of instances, some of the conditions that may cause spontaneous abortions are as follows:

1. Errors of development inconsistent with life (25% to 50% of abortuses have revealed anatomic or chromosomal abnormalities)

2. Abnormal intrauterine environment

3. Placental abnormalities, for example, large infarcts, premature separation, and placenta previa

4. Maternal factors, such as acute infections, psychic and physical trauma, abnormalities of the reproductive organs, cervical incompetence, and possibly certain poorly understood endocrine dyscrasias

5. Teratogenic factors such as drugs, radiation, viral infections, etc. may result in sufficient malformation to produce abortion.

Stages. Because of the different characteristics of the implantation site at the various stages of placentation, the mechanism, pathologic condition, and clinical course of abortion will be largely dependent on the stage of placentation at which it occurs. For greater clarity, Litzenberg proposed the following classification:

1. *Early* or *decidual stage abortion* occurs during the first 6 weeks or decidual stage of placentation. The conceptus for the first 6 weeks is wholly within the decidua; therefore, it has a very loose attachment (Fig. 16-1).

2. *Intermediate* or *attachment stage abortion* occurs during the second 6 weeks while the anchoring villi are becoming more and more firmly attached.

3. *Late* or *placental stage abortion* occurs after 12 weeks when the placenta is completely formed (Fig. 16-2).

The loose attachment during the *decidual stage* explains why the conceptus is so frequently expelled intact, with all its decidua, or at least the decidua capsularis, attached. Occasionally, the capsularis is torn and the shaggy chorionic vesicle or the embryo is expelled alone. The decidua and any remaining products of conception are subsequently extruded in one mass or in pieces, usually with uterine bleeding.

During the *attachment stage* maternal arterial input into the intervillous space is established and more bleeding is encountered with abortion occurring at this time. Because of the firmer attachment, parts of the developing placenta may be left within the uterus even though the entire conceptus appears to be expelled. Not infrequently the fetus is extruded, and the entire placenta and decidua remain attached.

After the third month, when the placenta is fully formed, abortion resembles the clinical course of a normal labor with

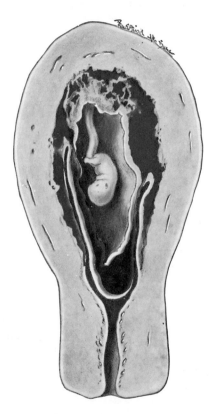

Fig. 16-1. Early abortion, decidual stage. (Redrawn from Bumm, from Litzenberg in Curtis: Obstetrics and gynecology, Philadelphia, W. B. Saunders Co.)

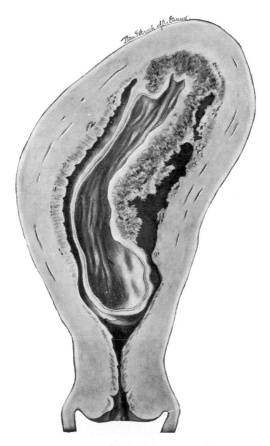

Fig. 16-2. Abortion in the early placental stage, showing beginning separation of the placenta; upper portion still attached. (After Bumm, from Litzenberg in Curtis: Obstetrics and gynecology, Philadelphia, W. B. Saunders Co.)

cervical dilatation, passage of the fetus, and, subsequently, delivery of the placenta, usually intact. Placental disruption at time of separation with intrauterine retention of placental fragments is, nonetheless, more common than at term.

Tissue pathology

1. Because the death of the fetus in early abortion usually antedates the abortion by a considerable time, there are regressive changes in the fetus, such as necrosis and even entire absorption.

2. There is maceration of the fetus, necrosis, and decomposition. If the membranes rupture, thus admitting bacteria, putrefaction converts the fetus and placenta into a stinking mass with a very foul discharge.

3. After fetal death and amniotic fluid absorption, the fetus may become so severely dessicated and compressed by mummification that it resembles parchment—*fetus compressus* or *papyraceus*.

4. Very rarely all the soft tissues disappear by degeneration and resorption until only the skeleton remains—*skeletization*.

5. *Lithopedion* formation may occur. The deposit of salts in the fetus is found more often in abdominal pregnancies and missed abortions than in ordinary abortion.

6. *Atypical abortion specimens:*

(a) When masses of chorion remain attached, they may become encapsulated with blood and fibrin—*placental polyps.*

(b) When the conceptus is not immediately expelled, it may become encased in a large blood clot—*blood* or *carneous mole.*

7. *Pathologic classification of abortuses:* Abortuses showing developmental abnormality have in the past been classified in terms of their gross appearance, for example, empty chorionic vesicle, chorion containing empty amnion, chorion and amnion containing nodular embryo, and so forth.

Symptoms and diagnosis. *Bleeding* and *pain* from uterine contractions are the outstanding symptoms of abortion, varying according to the stage in which abortion occurs.

In the *early* or *decidual stage abortion* the pain and bleeding are considerable but usually are not excessive.

In *intermediate abortion* pain and bleeding are greater than in the early type because of the increased size of the ovum, firmer attachment, and the tendency toward retention of parts of the decidua or placenta.

In *late abortion* there is usually less bleeding and more pain because there is a fetus to be expelled and there is a complete placenta that tends to remain attached until after the birth of the fetus.

Ordinary clinical varieties of abortion

1. *Threatened abortion* is defined as bleeding of intrauterine origin with or without uterine contractions.

2. *Inevitable abortion* is diagnosed when continuous and progressive dilatation of the cervix is noted. Bleeding and uterine contractions are invariably present and the membranes may have ruptured.

3. *Complete abortion* is noted when the products of conception are expelled in toto.

4. *Incomplete abortion* is the expulsion of some but not all of the products of conception. Hemorrhage persists until the uterus is empty.

5. *Missed abortion* is classified as the intrauterine retention of a fetus for 8 or more weeks after its demise.

6. *Habitual abortion* is the occurrence of three or more spontaneous, consecutive abortions.

Generally the diagnosis of abortion is easy when the patient is known to be pregnant. When pregnancy is doubtful, it may be quite difficult. This can usually be determined by the presence or absence of the usual signs of pregnancy or by the methods noted in Chapter 6.

Treatment

Threatened abortion

The diagnosis of pregnancy should be established by the methods noted in Chapter 6, and the possibility that the bleeding is originating from the cervix, vagina, or vulva should be excluded. If the bleeding is uterine in origin and threatened abortion seems the most likely diagnosis, bed rest, mild sedation, smooth muscle relaxants, or one of the orally active progestogens may be prescribed individually or simultaneously. However, the value of these modalities has not been established.

Coitus and orgasm should probably be avoided until symptoms have ceased.

Symptoms usually abate or progress unchecked, although occasionally protracted mild bleeding and cramping may occur. It is well to keep in mind that prognostically the pregnancy is still intact until such time as cervical dilatation, membrane rupture, or extrusion of a piece of the conceptus (fetus or placenta, *not* decidua) occurs. Patients may bleed for weeks and still go to term. If the uterus decreases in size, however, the fetus is probably dead.

It may be of help to remember that at least 25% to 50% of abortuses demonstrate structural or chromosomal abnormalities. If one were to accept these as maximal percentages, it is nonetheless impossible, prognostically and therapeutically, to ascertain prior to expulsion which fetus is normal and which is not. Although this might engender a nihilistic attitude toward treatment, even assuming that treatment is effective, one should remember that the incidence of anomalies in fetuses born at term after threatened abortion, regardless of the type of treatment, is no greater than in those born without this history.

Inevitable abortion. When an abortion becomes inevitable, time, effort, blood, and the health of the patient will be conserved by terminating the pregnancy promptly. The method to be employed depends on the amount of hemorrhage and the degree of dilatation of the cervix.

1. If the os will admit one or two fingers, the contents of the uterus may be digitally removed, intact or piecemeal. Remaining pieces may be removed with the ring sponge holder.

2. When the os is insufficiently dilated, it may be enlarged by the finger or metal dilators. The stretching must be deliberate and slow to avoid tearing, and anesthesia is required.

3. Since there is danger of perforating the uterus with instruments, curettage of the uterus must be done with judgment, skill, deliberation, and gentleness. The cavity should be explored afterward digitally or with a sound to make certain the myometrium is intact. Sharp or suction curettage may be used.

4. In certain instances, instrumental means may be avoided and the abortion may be completed by the use of oxytocin administered intramuscularly or by intravenous infusion. Relatively large doses or high concentrations are often required, as noted

below. This may also be useful after complete expulsion to minimize blood loss.

Incomplete abortion. In incomplete abortion the same methods are employed as when emptying the uterus in inevitable abortion.

If the fetus has been expelled and there is evidence of placental fragmentation, currettage is almost invariably required to staunch the continuing blood flow. If there is no evidence of placental fragmentation, it is usually possible to achieve passage of the intact placenta by alternating the administration of 10 units of oxytocin intramuscularly and 0.2 mg. of ergonovine intramuscularly ever 30 minutes for a total of 3½ hours (four doses of each). If this is successful, curettage is not required.

Complete abortion. When the uterus is empty, there is no need for further interference, and as a rule if the decidua vera in early abortion is not cast off, it is unnecessary, in the absence of considerable hemorrhage, to remove it because it usually comes away spontaneously. However, by careful inspection the physician must always make sure that the uterus is entirely empty. Therefore, patients and attendants must be instructed to save everything that has come from the uterus for the physician's examination.

Missed abortion

Definition. Missed abortion is the failure of the uterus to expel its contents within 8 weeks after the death of the embryo or fetus. Mall and Streeter established the fact that the fetus is ordinarily retained for 6 weeks after its death, except in the early stages of pregnancy. In missed abortion it may be retained for months or years.

Etiology. The cause of missed abortion is unknown.

Termination. The fetus is usually ultimately expelled. Mummification, areas of calcification, lithopedion formation, or skeletization may be seen and complete absorption of the embryo may occur in very early abortions.

Symptoms

1. Early signs of abortion subside, with the patient thinking she had a threatened abortion.

2. Weeks or months later she notices that her abdomen is not increasing but decreasing in size.

3. The physician finds a hard uterus, not hard like a myoma or yet with the characteristic elastic softening of a normal pregnancy, but rather between the two in consistency.

4. The breasts regress in size.

5. Often there is variable vaginal bleeding.

Diagnosis

1. Most failures to diagnose missed abortion are attributable to a lack of consideration of the diagnosis rather than to a lack of technical diagnostic skill.

2. Missed abortion should be suspected when:

(a) A woman skips one or two menses.

(b) Then she threatens to abort but does not.

(c) The uterus ceases to grow or decreases in size between two examinations a month apart.

(d) The symptoms of pregnancy abate or regress.

(e) Pregnancy tests become negative. This, however, is not an invariable occurrence.

Treatment. Waiting for the ultimate expulsion may be psychologically distressing for the patient and her family. Intervention in the form of intra-amniotic instillation of hypertonic saline to induce uterine emptying is probably the treatment of choice. The same result may be obtained by repetitive intravenous infusion of oxytocin or by cervical dilatation with sharp or suction curettage.

Disseminated intravascular coagulation, with resultant incoagulability of the blood, may occur after lengthy retention of a dead fetus in the uterus, particularly after the fourth month of gestation. This is typically a slow process and, if the presence of a dead fetus is recognized and temporization to achieve spontaneous resolution is desired, the development of life-endangering disseminated intravascular coagulation can usually be prevented. This may be accomplished by following the plasma fibrinogen level at regular intervals and extracting the fetus promptly should this level significantly decline. As with the other obstetrical causes for intravascular activation of the coagulation system (amniotic fluid embolism, abruptio placentae, infected abortion) the consumption coagulopathy will usually spontaneously remit with correction of the primary disease. In the event that blood incoagulability develops, it should be managed as noted in Chapter 18.

If fibrinogen levels are noted to be severely depressed in a patient with an intrauterine fetal death, but bleeding is not occurring, heparin therapy for 2 to 3 days prior to elective evacuation of the uterus may be used to correct the coagulopathy and prevent hemorrhage.

Abortion in second trimester

Abortion in the second trimester occurs in about 2% of pregnancies and the causes are numerous. The common etiologic factors are premature separation of the placenta, incompetent cervix, cord complications, trauma, pelvic operative procedures, toxemia, chronic maternal disease (diabetes, nephritis, hypertension, etc.), and uterine malformations. However, in over 40% of instances, it has been impossible to assign a specific cause.

Loss of a pregnancy in the middle trimester tends to occur in women with poor previous obstetric performances. Perhaps at least one fourth of these late abortions are preventable. Another reason for grouping these patients on the basis of the time of occurrence of abortion is to emphasize the fact that the middle portion of pregnancy is not as free from fetal loss as it is commonly assumed to be.

Habitual abortion

Habitual abortion is defined as a condition in which a woman has had *three or more spontaneous and consecutive abortions.* The etiologic factors are largely those already noted for spontaneous abortion. Treatment is directed toward correction of nutritional deficiencies, thyroid dysfunction, uterine anomalies, and psychic disturbances.

Late abortions sometimes appear to be related to *incompetency of the internal os of the cervix.* This may be demonstrated radiographically, and various surgical procedures have been devised to strengthen this portion of the uterine canal.

To qualify as having an incompetent cervix, the patient must experience painless, partial dilatation of the cervix in the second trimester, followed by membrane rupture and rather prompt delivery of an immature fetus. These events tend to repeat themselves in subsequent pregnancies. If the situation is detected during pregnancy, the cervix may be reinforced or the os occluded by any of several vaginal operative procedures. The

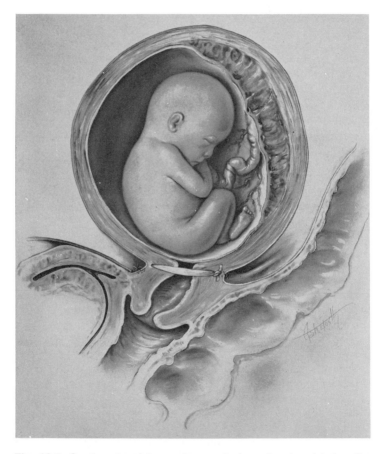

Fig. 16-3. Cerclage band for an incompetent cervix, placed below the fetus in utero by means of transabdominal operation. (From Benson and Durfee: Obstet. Gynec. **25:**145, 1965.)

most popular are those described by Shirodkar, McDonald, and Wurm. Benson and Durfee advise placement of a cervical band through a laparotomy incision if the vaginal portion of the cervix is very short or deformed by previous operative maneuvers (Fig. 16-3). Other operative techniques have been advised for use between pregnancies.

Habitual abortion currently is the subject of a vast literature, and enormously extensive clinical investigations often are recommended. The prognosis in terms of successful pregnancy is 70% to 80% regardless of the treatment method employed.

Infected abortion

Infection commonly occurs after criminal abortion. It usually is caused by the colon bacillus or by an anaerobic streptococcus. If the infection appears to be confined to the uterus, the residue of gestational material should be evacuated. Very large doses of antibiotics should be used at once to control or prevent peritonitis and septicemia.

Chronic pelvic infection originating in an abortion may proceed to the formation of a pelvic abscess that can be drained through the posterior vaginal fornix. In other instances abdominal removal of the reproductive organs may be required, and this should not be postponed until the patient is extremely ill.

Bacterial endotoxic shock is a rare but often lethal complication of infected abortion. Hypotension is related to hypersensitivity to endotoxins, usually of gram-negative bacilli, most commonly the colon bacillus. The mechanism may be that of disseminated intravascular coagulation, peripheral or sphincteric vasoconstriction, generalized loss of vascular tone, or a combination of these and others currently unknown. Prompt and concentrated therapy is required, including correction of hypovolemia under central venous pressure (CVP) monitoring, correction of the usual metabolic lactoacidosis with sodium bicarbonate, antibiotics in massive doses, and large amounts of adrenal glucocorticoid. The choice of a vasoactive agent for the direct treatment of the hypotension is empirical. In general, patients with warm, dry skin and low or normal central venous pressure are candidates for vasoconstrictor agents (for example, metaraminol), whereas those with cold, clammy skin and high or high-normal CVP are better candidates for vasodilator agents (for example, isoproterenol), both given by continuous intravenous infusion. In the event of hemorrage associated with incoagulability of the blood, disseminated intravascular coagulation should be suspected and the condition managed as noted in Chapter 18. The uterus should be promptly evacuated by sharp or suction curettage. If this cannot be accomplished easily through the vagina or if the infection appears to have spread beyond the uterus, hysterectomy, with or without the excision of additional tissue, should be considered. The mortality, even with well-designed and vigorous therapy, is 20% to 30%.

The demonstration of gram-positive encapsulated rods in the cervix or uterine cavity of a hypotensive patient with an infected abortion is essentially diagnostic of *Clostridium welchii* (gas gangrene) infection. Hemolysis and renal failure resulting from septicemia and the exotoxin produced by this organism are very frequently fatal. Treatment with massive doses of antibiotics, polyvalent antitoxin, and immediate hysterectomy without consideration of curettage and without awaiting the results of microbial culture is recommended.

Acute renal failure may appear in patients after abortion, either as a result of infection and shock or the destructive action of some drug taken to produce the abortion. Urinary output must be watched with care, and if oliguria or anuria appears, appropriate medical consultation should be sought at once. Some of these patients may be helped by treatment with peritoneal dialysis or an artificial kidney (hemodialysis). Despite heroic treatment, the mortality in this situation is 25% to 30%.

Therapeutic abortion

Therapeutic abortion is an operative procedure and is described in Chapter 31.

PREMATURE LABOR

Definition. Premature labor is spontaneous labor occurring after fetal viability and before fetal maturity. However, it is customary to consider fetuses weighing 1,000 to 2,499 grams (29 to 36 weeks of gestation) as *premature* and fetuses weighing 500 to 999 grams (20 to 28 weeks of gestation) as *immature*.

Although few in the latter group survive birth, some do, and thus labor at that stage must be included in the above definition.

Premature birth is by far the most common cause of neonatal mortality. Five to 10% of labors are premature, but in less than half of them can any definite cause be shown.

Etiology. The more common causes of premature labor are chronic vascular disease, toxemia, placenta previa, abruptio placentae, hydramnios, multiple pregnancy, fetal anomalies, uterine anomalies, uterine fibromyomas, incompetent internal cervical os, and maternal urinary tract infection.

The course of premature labor differs very little from that of normal labor, but it may be somewhat slower because of weak contractions. Lacerations are less frequent. Sometimes the fetus is expelled in its intact sac (caul). Malpositions are more frequent.

Treatment. When seen early, premature labor may sometimes be stopped by complete rest in bed and sedatives. The use of intravenous and oral ethyl alcohol has also been suggested. The rationale is that alcohol inhibits the release of antidiuretic hormone from the posterior pituitary and may also inhibit the release of oxytocin from the same organ. Results to date are inconclusive. Smooth muscle relaxing agents have also been tried with equivocal results. The urine should be regularly examined and bacteriuria treated with the appropriate antibiotic.

Heavy sedation or narcosis is very undesirable and will severely limit the potential for fetal survival should delivery inadvertently occur.

If *premature rupture of the membranes* has occurred and labor has not ensued, it is often difficult to decide whether to initiate labor and effect delivery of the fetus prematurely or to seek additional intrauterine maturation at the risk of amnionitis and fetal septicemia. Use of the methods for assessing intrauterine fetal maturation as outlined in Chapter 7 may be helpful in this decision. Prophylactic use of antibiotics is not recommended. It is desirable, however, to give antibiotics during actual labor to prevent dissemination of infection if amnionitis or endometritis is known to be present. It is claimed that the premature rupture of the membranes is not caused by an inherent weakness since membranes will withstand pressures that exceed those resulting from the uterine contractions of labor.

Douching, intercourse, and orgasm must be avoided.

If the pregnancy has advanced to 36 weeks or if the infant clearly weighs over 5 pounds, labor may be stimulated with oxytocin intravenously.

Regional or local anesthesia is advised for premature labor, and episiotomy may be helpful in avoiding undesirable trauma to the small infant. Competent pediatric care should be arranged in advance of delivery.

The most important point of all is to make every effort to determine the cause, so that prophylactic measures may be employed to prevent recurrence.

17

Ectopic pregnancy

An *ectopic pregnancy* is any pregnancy situated outside of the uterine (endometrial) cavity. Most ectopic pregnancies (over 95%) are tubal gestations, but others occur in such places as the ovary, cervix, rudimentary uterine horn, and abdominal cavity (Fig. 17-1).

The incidence is approximately 1 in every 150 to 200 infants delivered, and it is commoner in women with a history of infertility, especially the "one-child sterility" group. The frequency is greater in lower socioeconomic groups, probably because of their predisposition to inflammatory disease of the uterine tubes. An increase in the frequency of ectopic pregnancy may be related to the use of antibiotics to treat gonococcal salpingitis. Authorities believe that such treatment may prevent complete tubal occlusion, though adhesions between tubal folds or impaired peristalsis may persist.

ETIOLOGY

The following conditions may lead to ectopic pregnancy:

1. Endosalpingitis, leading to agglutination of mucosal folds and formation of blind pockets
2. Tubal anomalies (diverticula, accessory ostia, hypoplasia)
3. Peritubal adhesions after puerperal infection or appendicitis
4. Tumors distorting the tube
5. Previous tubal operations
   a. To restore patency
   b. Tubal ligation or resection
6. External migration of ovum, providing time for development of invasive blastocyst while still within tube (theoretical only)

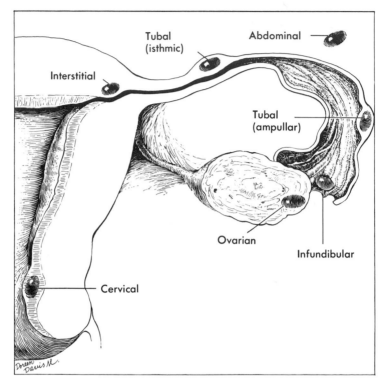

Fig. 17-1. Sites of ectopic pregnancies.

7. Menstrual reflux and late fertilization of ovum could combine to delay progress of blastocyst or even wash it out of tube prior to implantation

8. Ectopic endometrium in tubal mucosa (uncommon); a decidual reaction in the fallopian tube is the usual response to implantation and not an indication of true endometriosis

PATHOLOGIC ANATOMY

The implantation of the ovum in the tube follows exactly the normal processes of nidation as they occur in the uterus,

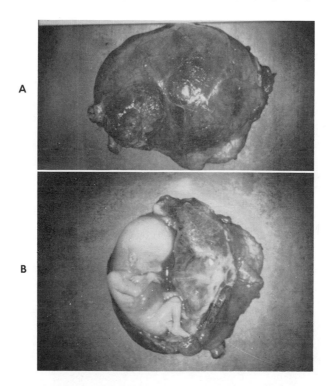

Fig. 17-2. A, Tubal pregnancy of 10 weeks' duration, perforation of tube wall with portion of placenta protruding. **B,** Tube opened, showing 9 cm. fetus, cord, and placenta. Opposite tube was previously removed because of ectopic pregnancy.

but the results are inevitably pathologic from the beginning because the tube is unsuited, anatomically and histologically, for the reception and development of the fertilized ovum. The tube is incapable of forming extensive decidua, although there is a feeble "decidual reaction" in the form of patches, islands, and single cells.

The fertilized ovum may develop in the ampullar, isthmic, or interstitial portions of the tube. The commonest site is the ampulla, whereas interstitial pregnancies comprise only about 1% of all tubal gestations. The ovum promptly burrows through the tubal epithelium, comes to lie in the subjacent connective tissue, and then proceeds promptly into the muscularis because the tube lacks a well-developed decidual layer. The ovum of an intact early tubal pregnancy is separated from the lumen of the tube by a layer of connective and muscular tissue that may contain a few isolated decidual cells. This covering membrane is invaded by trophoblast, undergoes fibrinoid degeneration, and eventually fuses with the mucosa of the opposite side of the tube. The enlarging gestational mass, advancing as a sphere of increasing diameter, then pushes against the intact tubal wall opposite the nidation site to create a bulbous swelling that is grossly obvious (Fig. 17-2).

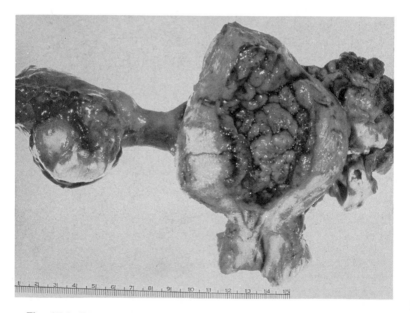

Fig. 17-3. Right tubal pregnancy and conspicuous decidual formation in uterus. (From Titus and Willson: The management of obstetric difficulties, St. Louis, The C. V. Mosby Co.)

TUBAL RUPTURE AND TUBAL ABORTION

The tube wall forms the outer part of the gestational capsule and the tubal mucosa forms the inner portion. Rupture may occur either through the external capsule into the abdominal cavity or *through the internal capsule into the tubal lumen*. Internal rupture is commonly called *tubal abortion*.

When no external rupture is seen, the ectopic pregnancy is often erroneously said to be unruptured, even when there is blood in the abdominal cavity. This is fallacious, for when there is blood in the abdomen there must have been a rupture, either of the external or of the internal capsule. An ovum protruding from the fimbriated end of the tube is usually said to be a tubal abortion, but according to the observations of Litzenberg, it is usually due to implantation of the ovum near the ostium abdominale; hence, it grows in the direction of least resistance out through the end of the tube.

External or extracapsular rupture occurs when a portion of the villous covering of the ovum extrudes through the serosal surface of the tube. The amount of bleeding from the area of disrupted tubal wall depends on the caliber and number of blood vessels penetrated by the advancing trophoblast, as well as on the degree of trauma produced by diagnostic efforts.

UTERINE CHANGES

The uterus becomes slightly enlarged and rather soft, and decidua develops in the endometrium (Fig. 17-3).

When the ovum dies, the decidua degenerates, bleeds (the source of the characteristic vaginal bleeding), and is discharged in small pieces, or as a decidual cast of the uterine cavity. Histologic sections of endometrium may show the Arias-Stella phenomenon, a characteristic change in the glandular epithelium attributed to the action of chorionic gonadotropin. The epithelial cells are large and their nuclei are hyperchromatic and irregularly shaped and tend to occupy the luminal portion of the cell. The cytoplasm often is vacuolated or foamy.

The endometrium begins to regenerate as soon as the ovum dies, often before the ectopic pregnancy terminates. Thus the absence of decidua and presence of proliferative endometrium does not exclude the possibility of ectopic pregnancy, and microscopic examination of curetted endometrium may not be a helpful diagnostic exercise.

TERMINATION OF TUBAL PREGNANCY

A common outcome is *tubal abortion,* as described above. If abortion is incomplete, blood continues to escape through the fimbriated end of the tube and may encapsulate in the cul-de-sac to form a *hematocele.* If the fimbriated end is occluded, blood will slowly distend the tube to form a *hematosalpinx.*

Rupture into the peritoneal cavity, through an area of tubal wall weakened by trophoblastic invasion, usually occurs spontaneously but may be provoked by the trauma of coitus or bimanual examination of the pelvis. If only the fetus escapes and the placenta maintains its tubal attachment, further development of a secondary abdominal pregnancy theoretically is possible.

When the implantation site is directed toward the mesosalpinx, rupture into the broad ligament may occur. This may lead to embryonic death and formation of a *broad ligament hematoma,* or conceivably to further development of the pregnancy in its new site (intraligamentous or broad ligament pregnancy).

SYMPTOMS AND SIGNS

Prior to disruption of a tubal pregnancy through abortion or rupture, the clinical patern is not characteristic. The patient may believe she is normally pregnant because of some delay in the onset of an anticipated menstrual flow, but commonly she does not suspect that pregnancy exists.

Postponed, protracted, or any pattern of anomalous menstruation is suggestive of extrauterine pregnancy, particularly when accompanied by pain, vaginal bleeding, fever, leukocytosis, and a mass to one side of the uterus.

Symptoms vary with the time the patient is seen—before, during, or after rupture.

Before rupture the pain is vague and described as only discomfort, indefinite distress, soreness, or very mild cramps. There is no fever or leukocytosis because there is no peritoneal irritation from blood in the abdomen. All symptoms are elusive and diagnosis is difficult. The mass at the ectopic site is often too small to be palpated.

The period *during rupture* is the critical period because the diagnosis missed before rupture may now be made, and the tragedy of a complete rupture may be avoided by recognizing the now more definite signs and symptoms. The pain is more severe and located on one side. Exacerbations of pain followed by complete relief are particularly significant. The cervix is exceedingly sensitive to movement. Dribbling vaginal bleeding is constant or intermittent. Fever and leukocytosis may be present because there is bleeding into the peritoneal cavity. Now a tense, exquisitely tender mass is usually palpated with ease.

Diagnosis *after rupture* is often easy because of the usual history of agonizing, one-sided pain, and signs of internal hemorrhage followed by shock, with a rapid, feeble pulse, cold sweat, pallid skin, shallow breathing, air hunger, restlessness, and extreme anxiety. On the affected side the abdominal wall may be tender and rigid. Pain radiating to the top of the shoulder and the side of the neck is fairly common and is attributed to diaphragmatic irritation by blood (usually 500 ml. or more in peritoneal cavity). A mass is palpable in about 70% of patients, and much of it may be a hematoma surrounding the gestational site, or adherent ovary, bowel, or omentum (Fig. 17-4). Massive intraperitoneal bleeding in a thin woman or one with an umbilical hernia may create bluish black discoloration of the periumbilical skin, known as Cullen's sign.

Temperature elevations to 38° C. are noted in about one third of patients with bleeding tubal pregnancies and may be related to hemoperitoneum. Leukocyte counts are likely to be normal, though sudden and massive hemorrhage may provoke a leukocytosis of 15,000 or higher. Within the first few hours after acute hemorrhage the hematocrit may be an unreliable index of the amount of blood lost. But progressive hemodilution will depress the hematocrit, so that serial determinations will be helpful in making the correct diagnosis.

At least half of all tubal pregnancies become subacute, chronic, or atypical. Bleeding from the tube is intermittent and never massive, and a more or less indolent hematoma produces moderate pelvic discomfort. The true nature of the problem may be recognized only after operation is undertaken on the basis of some other tentative diagnosis.

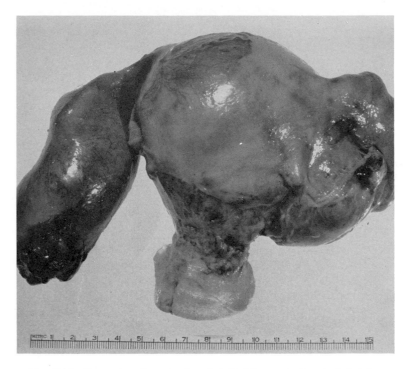

Fig. 17-4. Pregnancy in ampulla of right tube and chronic left tubo-ovarian abscess. (From Titus and Willson: The management of obstetric difficulties, St. Louis, The C. V. Mosby Co.)

DIAGNOSIS

Tests for chorionic gonadotropin are not particularly useful because they are positive in only 35% to 40% of cases. A negative pregnancy test does not exclude a disrupted ectopic pregnancy surrounded by a hematoma.

Anemia may be severe if there has been appreciable intraperitoneal bleeding, and there may be mild leukocytosis. The icterus index is elevated and hematin may be detected in the peripheral blood.

Culdocentesis (aspiration of fluid through the posterior vaginal

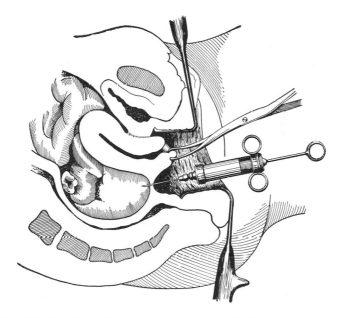

Fig. 17-5. Needle colpotomy to demonstrate blood in the cul-de-sac. (After Greenhill, from Titus and Willson: The management of obstetric difficulties, St. Louis, The C. V. Mosby Co.)

fornix) may demonstrate intraperitoneal blood. Fluid that appears bloody and does not clot is diagnostic. If the aspirate subsequently clots, it is most likely that it was obtained from a blood vessel rather than from the cul-de-sac (Fig. 17-5).

Colpotomy (surgical incision through the posterior vaginal fornix) will disclose free blood if tubal rupture has occurred. In this event, the peritoneum should be closed and laparotomy performed. Otherwise tubes and ovaries may be exposed to rule out the possibility of an unruptured tubal pregnancy or other adnexal disease.

Laparoscopy or *culdoscopy* may be useful in the diagnosis of either an unruptured or a very chronic tubal pregnancy, but these approaches should be used only when the diagnosis is obscure. Large collections of blood in the pelvic area obviously interfere with visualization through lenses.

Hysterosalpingography may demonstrate a tubal pregnancy, but the procedure is dangerous in this situation; the tube may be ruptured and bleeding aggravated.

Dilatation and curettage of the uterus may disclose decidual changes in the endometrium and absence of chorionic villi, thus suggesting pregnancy at another site. But if uterine bleeding has been in progress for a considerable time, the decidual stroma may have sloughed, being replaced by proliferative endometrium not at all suggestive of pregnancy.

Frequently it is extremely difficult to diagnose ectopic pregnancy because no single, invariably reliable feature can be elicited in every instance. Diagnostic success can be improved if one is constantly alert to the possible significance of lower abdominal pain in any woman during her reproductive years and if one is meticulous about obtaining an accurate history.

DIFFERENTIAL DIAGNOSIS

Many pathologic conditions share the signs and symptoms of ectopic pregnancy, the most common being appendicitis, salpingitis, ruptured ovarian follicle or corpus luteum cyst, uterine abortion, torsion of ovarian cyst, and urinary tract infection. The adnexal mass, consisting of gestational site and surrounding hematoma, may on occasion be confused with a neoplasm.

In *intrauterine abortion* the bleeding is usually more profuse, and the pain is caused by characteristic uterine cramps. Villi or fetal parts may be seen in the expelled material.

In *salpingitis* there may be a history of gonorrhea, purulent discharge, gradual onset, no enlargement or softening of the uterus, and less circumscribed mass than in tubal pregnancy.

In *appendicitis* there are no menstrual anomalies, no evidence of pregnancy, and usually no mass, unless an abscess has already formed.

Ovarian cysts (except the small retention cysts) are larger

than a pregnant tube, not very tender, and there are no uterine changes.

A myoma at the uterine cornu may be confusing but can usually be differentiated by the history and the firmness of the tumor.

TREATMENT

It is best to remove the afflicted tube as soon after the diagnosis is made as feasible. Prompt operation before or during rupture will avoid the frank bursting of the tube with its tragic consequences. After rupture and the attendant blood loss, collapse, and shock, there is no certain safety until the bleeding artery is tied. Immediate blood transfusion is the best treatment of shock, *provided always that the bleeding vessels are ligated soon to prevent loss of the transfused blood.* If no blood is immediately available, the shock should be combated with infusion of blood substitutes until blood can be obtained.

If a large amount of blood is found in the abdominal cavity, it may be disposed of in various ways: (1) sucked out and discarded, (2) used as an autotransfusion, or (3) allowed to remain in situ. The first choice is preferable whenever banked blood is quickly available for transfusion.

Removal of the ovary on the affected side may be necessary if it is involved in the gestational mass. Indeed, some authorities have suggested routine removal of the ovary along with tube to prevent future ectopic pregnancies related to external migration of the ovum. Others suggest that fertility might be improved if ovulation always occurred immediately adjacent to a fallopian tube, but most gynecologists preserve the ovary whenever possible. Removal of the outer half of the interstitial portion of the tube (cornual resection) may be advisable to minimize the very rare occurrence of pregnancy in the remaining tubal stump.

In the absence of shock and massive hemorrhage, and depending on age and parity, removal of the opposite tube may be advisable if it is clearly abnormal. Hysterectomy may be desirable in selected instances when the only remaining tube is being removed because of tubal pregnancy. Rupture of an interstitial pregnancy often leaves a massive anatomic defect requiring hysterectomy.

If one is so fortunate as to operate upon a person with an early tubal pregnancy before perforation of the tube wall has occurred, it may be feasible merely to open the tube longitudinally, evacuate the gestational mass, and ligate or coagulate small bleeding vessels (*salpingostomy*). Thus the tube may be preserved, particularly if it is the only one remaining in an infertile patient. Even if the opposite tube is present, the afflicted one may be the better of the two in terms of possible future pregnancies.

Maternal mortality for ectopic pregnancy in the United States is about 1 in 800 cases. Ectopic pregnancy recurs in about 10% of patients. Normal pregnancies are achieved subsequently by more than half of the women who have had an ectopic pregnancy.

RARE TYPES
Interstitial pregnancy

The interstitial portion of the tube is very thin, so that when nidation occurs there it ruptures almost at once into the musculature of the uterine wall. It resists rupture into the abdominal cavity much longer than does the free tube, but it rarely resists a second rupture into the peritoneal cavity beyond the fourth month. Because of the abundant blood supply at the site of implantation, hemorrhage after rupture may be massive and lead to death before the patient can be brought to a hospital. Fortunately, only about 1% of tubal gestations occur in this location.

When a soft mass is found at one uterine cornu with the characteristic history of an ectopic gestation, a diagnosis of interstitial pregnancy is justifiable (Fig. 17-6).

Ovarian pregnancy

Ovarian pregnancy is extremely rare. The condition usually is confused with tubal pregnancy or ovarian cyst, and the proper diagnosis is not made until after laparotomy. The pregnancy usually terminates within the first 2 months, but an occasional ovarian pregnancy has gone to term.

A hematoma in an ovary is much more likely to be associated with one of the more common lesions, such as endometriosis, hemorrhage into a physiologic cyst, or torsion.

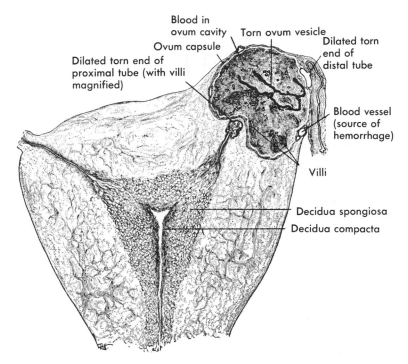

Fig. 17-6. Composite drawing of various serial sections of an interstitial pregnancy brought to the same plane by the artist. (From Litzenberg: Amer. J. Obstet. Gynec. **9:**22, 1925.)

The pathogenesis of ovarian pregnancy is not entirely clear, and the situation is always difficult to reconstruct from sections of the damaged organ. It has been suggested that fertilization and implantation may occur inside a ruptured follicle or in a sulcus on the ovarian surface (perhaps at a focus of endometriosis).

Abdominal pregnancy

Primary abdominal pregnancy was long denied, but a few well-authenticated cases have proved the possibility.

Secondary abdominal pregnancy occurs when a living embryo escapes from its primary location, usually the tube, and implants elsewhere on a peritoneal surface or maintains its trophoblastic attachment to the ruptured tube. Abdominocyesis does not include intraligamentous or advanced tubal pregnancies.

Over 400 patients with abdominal pregnancy have been re-

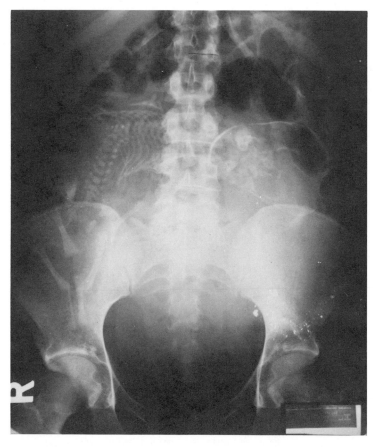

Fig. 17-7. Abdominal radiograph in a patient with advanced tubal gestation (34 weeks). Note deformed fetal skull, angulation of spine, and upper abdominal position of fetus.

ported and some have gone to term. The incidence is about 1 in 3,500 pregnancies in large public hospitals in the southern United States. Usually the correct diagnosis is not made until fetal movements produce nausea, abdominal pain, and diarrhea. The cervix may be displaced upward and forward, so that it is difficult to visualize vaginally. Radiologic examination will show a fetus in transverse or oblique lie, absence of uterine shadow, and perhaps fetal parts overlying maternal vertebrae in the lateral view. Compare Fig. 17-7.

Laparotomy should be performed as soon as the diagnosis is made. The operation may precipitate massive hemorhage, therefore it is essential to have at least 2,000 ml. of compatible blood available in the operating room and additional amounts in a nearby blood bank. Two intravenous infusion systems should be in operation before the procedure is started. If the blood supply to the placenta can be ligated, it is safe to remove the placenta, otherwise it should be left in situ. Occasionally a second operation is required for removal of the placenta. Fetal mortality ranges from 75% to 95% in various reports; nearly all the fetuses have malformations. Maternal mortality is about 5%.

Simulataneous extrauterine and intrauterine pregnancies have carried to term. There are about a dozen reports of survival of the mother and both infants.

Cervical pregnancy

Cervical pregnancy is a rare phenomenon usually accompanied by slight but fairly continuous vaginal bleeding. The cervical walls become very thin and distended but the internal os is closed. The surmounting corpus may be mistaken for a tumor. Such a pregnancy rarely advances beyond the fourth lunar month. Because of the danger of hemorrhage, cervical gestations of 8 weeks or more are best treated by abdominal hysterectomy. Earlier ones may be evacuated vaginally, but suturing of cervical arteries and packing will be required to control bleeding.

18

Abruptio placentae and placenta previa

Placental abruption and placenta previa are the major causes of obstetric bleeding in the third trimester, and bleeding is a major cause of maternal mortality and morbidity. The other causes of bleeding in late pregnancy are nonplacental, and the bleeding is generally slight. Because of the potential danger of the placental disturbances that lead to bleeding, every effort must be made to reach the proper diagnosis without provoking unnecessary hemorrhage and without sacrificing the fetus by premature delivery. Virtually all patients with third trimester bleeding will cease to bleed if kept in bed for a day or two; hospitalization for rest and observation usually is the initial therapy. Rarely is the first episode of bleeding a matter of such magnitude that it requires heroic treatment.

PREMATURE SEPARATION OF NORMALLY SITUATED PLACENTA (ABRUPTIO PLACENTAE, PLACENTAL APOPLEXY, OR ABLATIO PLACENTAE)

Etiology. The etiology of premature separation of the normally situated placenta is unknown. It occurs in about 1% of late pregnancies. Approximately one half the patients with abruptio placentae show signs of preeclamptic toxemia, as well as evidence of necrotic lesions of the decidual vessels, but the agents responsible for the necrosis are unknown. Placental abruption occurs, by definition, after the twentieth week and most commonly in the last 10 weeks of pregnancy. Placental detachment earlier in pregnancy is regarded as an *abortion*.

Predisposing factors include preeclampsia, chronic renal disease, hypertension, trauma, and multiparity. Many precipitating factors have been invoked to explain placental disruption in individual patients, but these may have been coincidental rather than truly causative.

Pathology. Separation of the placenta may be complete, but more often it is incomplete. The amount of bleeding depends on the number of uterine sinuses exposed.

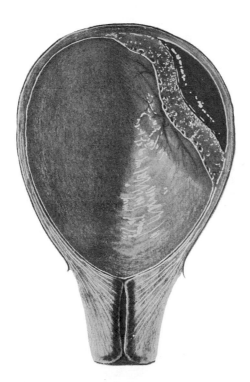

Fig. 18-1. Abruptio placentae with concealed hemorrhage. (From Bland: Practical obstetrics, Philadelphia, F. A. Davis Co.)

As the subplacental hematoma spreads, it may:

1. Be confined to the limits of the placenta (invisible hemorrhage) (Fig. 18-1)

2. Cleave the membranes from the uterine wall, permitting the blood to escape into the vagina (visible hemorrhage) (Fig. 18-2)

3. Rupture into the amniotic cavity (invisible hemorrhage) (Fig. 18-3)

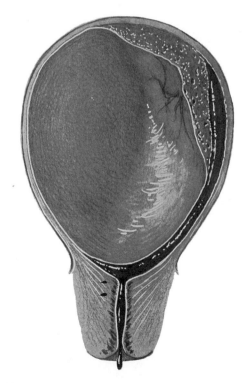

Fig. 18-2. Abruptio placentae with external hemorrhage. (From Bland: Practical obstetrics, Philadelphia, F. A. Davis Co.)

Once the hematoma is established, separation continues until the following occur:

1. Bleeding ceases by coagulation.

2. Blood pressure falls enough to prevent bleeding and further separation.

3. The entire placenta is detached.

4. The blood escapes through the vagina or into the amniotic cavity.

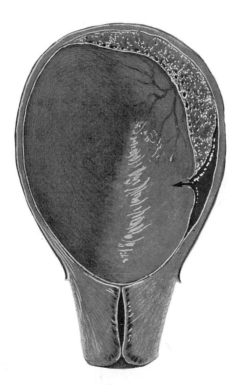

Fig. 18-3. Abruptio placentae with concealed hemorrhage and rupture into the amniotic sac. (From Bland: Practical obstetrics, Philadelphia, F. A. Davis Co.)

In the most severe cases there is extensive hemorrhagic infiltration between the muscle bundles, and this produces a bluish mottling of the uterus, broad ligaments, tubes, and ovaries (*Couvelaire* uterus). The uterus may lose its ability to contract.

Disseminated intravascular coagulation with resultant incoagulability of the blood (p. 256) may occur with some of the more severe grades of abruptio placentae. Similar incoagulability has been noted in occasional patients with amniotic fluid embolism, infected abortion, and prolonged intrauterine retention of a dead fetus.

Acute renal failure has been observed with severe abruption. It has been suggested that myoglobin is released from damaged muscle fibers and produces spasm of renal arterioles. It may, however, result from a prolonged lack of renal perfusion associated with hemorrhagic hypotension or from the obstruction of periglomerular arterioles with fibrin from disseminated intravascular coagulation.

Symptoms. The severity of the symptoms varies from very mild to fulminant. The *maternal* signs and symptoms are as follows:

1. Vaginal bleeding usually, but may be concealed
2. Shock disproportionate to the apparent blood loss
3. Uterine pain and tenderness
4. Anemia
5. Firm consistency (tetany) of the uterus, which may be extremely hard when the hemorrhage is concealed

In most patients with abruptio placentae, the bleeding and pain are moderate, but in concealed abruption they are alarmingly severe. The uterus enlarges if the bleeding is concealed. Contractions are dysrhythmic and very painful. When severe uterine tetany is established, it is not possible to discern any alternating consistency of the myometrium as in normal labor.

Varying degrees of fetal distress may be evident, depending on the degree of fetal hypoxia, and may be assessed by the methods noted in Chapter 12. Fetal death is not uncommon.

One must recognize, however, that less than half the patients with partial separation of the placenta present the classical picture described. In many circumstances, nothing unusual is noted during labor except slight vaginal bleeding, and the diagnosis is made during routine inspection of the placenta after delivery.

Treatment. The urgency of the situation is related to the degree of placental abruption and the clinical status of the patient and fetus. Obstetrical management should be designed to effect delivery within 5 to 6 hours. There is no advantage in delay or watchful expectancy once the diagnosis has been established even if the abruption appears to be mild and the fetus uncompromised. In other situations, the status of the patient or fetus may be so imperiled that more immediate and definitive therapeutic action is required. Regardless, expeditious delivery of the fetus and placenta is the sine qua non of obstetrical management.

1. *Grade 1:* External bleeding is evident, uterine tetany may or not be present, maternal shock and fetal distress are absent. Labor may or may not be in progress. The membranes should be ruptured artifically regardless of the dilatation of the cervix or the station of the presenting part unless precluded by other obstetric considerations. Bleeding commonly declines after this procedure, and uterine contractions are often readily initiated. If contractions are not present and do not readily begin, they should be initiated by the intravenous administration of oxytocin by constant infusion. The latter may also be utilized to augment contractions that are dysrhythmic, weak or infrequent.

2. *Grade 2:* External bleeding may or may not be present, but the uterus is firm and tender. Fetal distress develops and death in utero may occur, but as a rule the classical findings of maternal shock are not evident. Cesarean section may be justified if fetal rescue appears possible and if vaginal delivery cannot be achieved within a few hours by membrane rupture and oxytocin. Grade 2 situations often worsen and become grade 3 problems.

3. *Grade 3:* The cardinal features are maternal shock, tetanic uterus, dead fetus, and possibly a coagulation defect. External bleeding may or may not be present. Rupture the membranes, and after vigorous treatment of the shock and coagulation defect deliver vaginally if possible (usually feasible in multiparas); otherwise deliver by cesarean section. Whole blood and intravenous fluids should be used to restore normovolemia. Treatment of shock should be monitored by observation of central venous pressure and urinary output.

Constant intravenous infusion of oxytocin should be used for several hours post partum. Continued bleeding from a stimulated but atonic uterus may on rare occasion require hysterectomy.

Cesarean section. The use of cesarean section is limited to the following:

1. To those patients with severe abruption seen so early in the course of the separation that the fetus is still living and in whom there is some hope of recovering a living, viable infant by prompt delivery

2. To those few patients with uneffaced, undilated cervices not permitting intrauterine manipulation through the vagina

3. To those who show no progress in labor after rupture of the membranes and use of oxytocin and in whom it appears unlikely that vaginal delivery can be accomplished within 5 or 6 hours.

Surgery should not be performed in the presence of hemorrhagic shock or blood incoagulability or until treatment of these abnormalities has, at least, been initiated.

Fewer and fewer uteri (Couvelaire type) are now being removed to prevent postpartum hemorrhage after cesarean section for premature separation; more than 75% of them can be made to contract vigorously enough to justify their retention.

Prognosis. The prognosis obviously depends on the degree of placental separation and the adequacy of treatment. Maternal mortality from hemorrhage or subsequent renal failure ranges from 0.5% to 5% in different areas of the world. Fetal mortality is 50% to 80%. Many infants that survive the initial intrauterine insult die in the neonatal period because of immaturity or prematurity.

Disseminated intravascular coagulation. *Disseminated intravascular coagulation* (DIC) may develop in association with abruptio placentae and is also occasionally seen with other obstetrical complications such as amniotic fluid embolism, infected abortion, and prolonged intrauterine retention of a dead fetus. The precise mechanism for its development is unknown, but it results in activation of the intrinsic or extrinsic coagulation system, or both. Free thrombin appears in the circulation, disseminated coagulation occurs with conversion of fibrinogen to fibrin, and a consumption coagulopathy results. There is a significant

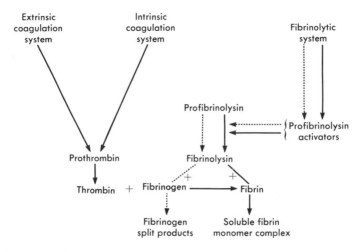

Fig. 18-4. Schematic representation of the hematologic pathways involved in consumption coagulopathy. Solid lines, Pathways associated with *disseminated intravascular coagulation*. Dotted lines, Pathways associated with *primary activation of the fibrinolytic system*. Clinically, these conditions may occur independently or together.

depression in the platelet count and a substantial decline in circulating levels of fibrinogen, factors V, VIII, and XIII, and, to a lesser extent, prothrombin. A blood smear reveals characteristic, bizarre alterations in the structural form of the red cells associated with increased erythrocyte fragility. Some degree of mild, beneficial activation of the fibrinolytic system normally occurs to ensure lysis of the fibrin thromboemboli and to maintain patency of the microcirculation (Fig. 18-4).

Consumption coagulopathy may also occur on the basis of a wholesale *primary activation of the fibrinolytic system*. This rarely occurs alone in obstetric situations but, on occasion, may accompany and further complicate DIC. With primary activation of the fibrinolytic system, fibrinogen undergoes lysis by fibrinolysin before fibrin can be formulated. When accompanying DIC, this further depresses fibrinogen levels, accentuates the consumption coagulopathy, and decreases the potentiality for clot formation at the site of bleeding. Moreover, the resulting fibrinogen split products have a profound anticoagulant effect on the coagulation system and can exacerbate the hemorrhagic diathesis.

Clinically, there is great variability in the severity of these processes and in the condition of the patient. The end result may be a minimal degree of abnormal bleeding that is subclinical and spontaneously remitting. At its worst, however, the abnormal bleeding may be intractable and exsanguinating because of total incoagulability of the blood.

In the clinical conditions noted above, the appearance of DIC, its severity, and its response to therapy should be monitored by serial determinations of the following:

1. Platelet count (reduced) (fibrin monomer is known to coat platelets and to potentially render them less functional; consequently, the bleeding time may be a more reliable index of blood coagulability)

2. Plasma fibrinogen level (reduced)

3. Prothrombin time (prolonged)

4. Partial thromboplastin time (prolonged)

Additionally, the ethanol gelation test or the plasma protamine paracoagulation test should be used, both of which detect soluble fibrin monomer complex resulting from the *normal* lysis of the disseminated fibrin. They will be positive with DIC and negative in the event of primary activation of the fibrinolytic system. The latter should be confirmed by demonstrating a substantial shortening of the euglobulin lysis time, which is a measure of profibrinolysin activators essential in the conversion of profibrinolysin to fibrinolysin.

Treatment should consist of the following:

1. *Eliminate the underlying problem* with as much dispatch as possible.

2. If there is no bleeding, there is no necessity to treat the coagulopathy, as it will usually spontaneously remit with correction of the primary disease.

3. If bleeding is present, prevent hypovolemia by administering lactated Ringer's solution or other suitable infusion fluid. Administer fresh whole blood or packed red cells only as necessary to treat any concomitant hemorrhagic shock. The

platelet count may vary in response to the administration of blood and will be less reliable in monitoring the clinical situation once transfusion is initiated.

4. Heparin primarily inhibits the function of the intrinsic coagulation system and also accelerates the neutralization of thrombin by antithrombin. It should be employed regularly if hemorrhage is occurring as a result of blood incoagulability induced by DIC. Initially, administer 5,000 to 15,000 units of heparin intravenously. Thereafter, administer 10,000 to 30,000 units of heparin per 24 hours by continuous infusion, as guided by changes in the results of the tests above. The partial thromboplastin time is an overall measure of the general activity of the intrinsic coagulation system and will be greatly prolonged and of no further benefit once heparin therapy has begun.

Heparin may be discontinued as soon as the underlying problem has been eliminated, bleeding has ceased, and the laboratory values have reverted to normal. These values should be monitored for a 24-hour period thereafter, however, for detection of any recurrence of the coagulopathy.

5. Epsilon aminocaproic acid is useful in treating primary activation of the fibrinolytic system, as it inhibits the action of profibrinolysin activators. It will not inhibit fibrinolysin itself, however, and consequently a therapeutic lag of some degree must be expected with its use. It should be employed *only* if there is substantial evidence of primary activation of the fibrinolytic system (shortening of the euglobulin lysis time and demonstration of circulating fibrinogen split products). If used in the treatment of DIC, it theoretically will inhibit the lifesaving action of the secondarily activated fibrinolytic system, which prevents capillary occlusion by removing fibrin as it is formed.

PLACENTA PREVIA

When the placenta is attached in the lower uterine segment and encroaches upon the internal cervical os (when fully dilated), placenta previa exists (Fig. 18-5). This occurs in approximately 0.5% of late pregnancies.

Etiology. The cause is unknown. Many plausible theories

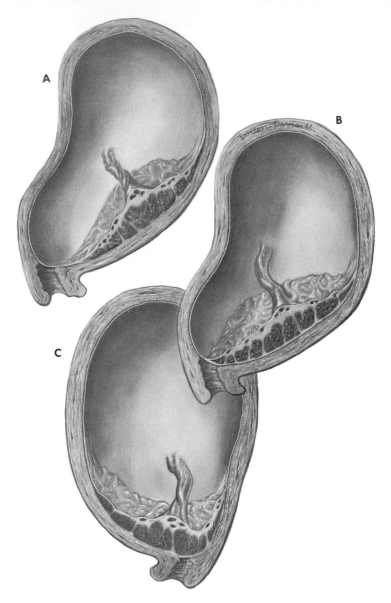

Fig. 18-5. Types of placenta previa. **A,** Low implantation. **B,** Partial placenta previa. **C,** Complete placenta previa.

have been advanced but none is proved. It occurs, however, much more frequently in multiparas, increasing with the degree of parity.

Varieties

Central, total, or complete. In central, total, or complete placenta previa the internal os is entirely covered by placenta *at full dilatation.*

Partial. In partial placenta previa the os is only partially covered.

Marginal. In marginal placenta previa the edge of the placenta comes only to the margin of the os. The term "marginal" is of no practical value because the relationship described is transitory.

Low implantation. Low implantation occurs when the placenta is in the lower uterine segment but does not encroach upon the os.

Placenta previa is best classified in terms of the area of the internal os that would be covered by placenta if the cervix were fully dilated (creating an opening 10 cm. in diameter). In other words, there is a shearing of the placental-cervical union as dilatation progresses. Theoretically, if the placental edge is palpable at the center of the internal os, about half the area of the os ought to be covered by placenta at full dilatation. This is said to constitute "50% placenta previa." In practice, however, such arithmetic precision in diagnosis is rarely achieved, and diligent efforts to determine the percentage of coverage should be avoided because they may provoke very alarming hemorrhage.

Pathology. When the placenta is attached to the lower segment, bleeding inevitably occurs as the cervix and lower segment dilate, retract, and pull away from the placenta. The lower segment cannot contract to stop the hemorrhage for two reasons:

1. It is normally relatively inactive.

2. The presence of the fetus prevents activity. Even after the fetus is delivered, the dilated inactive segment may not contract strongly enough to close the sinuses and prevent further dangerous bleeding.

Symptoms. *Painless bleeding* is the most characteristic symptom but is by no means pathognomonic. Patients with mild abruption also may bleed painlessly. The bleeding comes on suddenly, often with a gush, and usually begins after the seventh month of gestation.

After the first gush it not infrequently stops spontaneously, only to recur. The first attack seldom proves fatal. Bleeding occasionally may not occur until after labor begins.

Diagnosis

1. Painless bleeding occurs, often in gushes.

2. The cervix is softer than usual.

3. The cervical canal is more patulous, which permits palpation of the placenta by the finger.

4. Numerous methods have been employed for placental localization. The more sophisticated of these methods include angiography, amniography, radioisotopic techniques, ultrasonography, and thermography. None have succeeded in combining complete safety with precise definition of the relationship between the placental edge and the internal os. They are all useful, however, in differentiating the normally implanted from the low-lying placenta. Less complex methods have also been found to be useful.

5. The Ude cystographic method of demonstrating the relation of the fetal head to the bladder may be helpful, particularly if the separation of the two structures is so minimal that placenta previa may be excluded.

6. Soft tissue lateral roentgenograms may demonstrate the placental site.

7. Gravitational placentography may be helpful. If the presenting part lies centrally in a *standing* anteroposterior film and within 2 cm. of both the pubis and the sacral promontory in the lateral view, placenta previa does not exist (method of F. Ried, Fig. 18-6).

8. Absolute diagnosis is possible only by actual palpation of the placenta. This is done by sterile vaginal examination in the presence of a so-called "double setup." Patients suspected of having placenta previa should not be examined digitally outside of the hospital. Examination must be done in an operating room prepared for immediate abdominal or vaginal surgery with blood for transfusion at hand. Gentleness is imperative. All other possible sources of bleeding in the lower genital tract should be inspected before the area of the internal os is palpated. Placental tissue generally imparts a spongy feeling to the examining finger, but the distinction between clotted blood and the

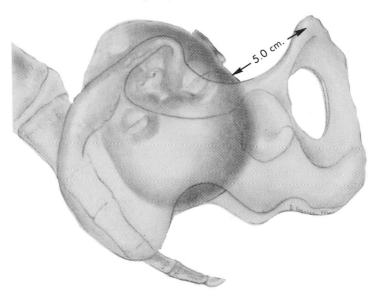

Fig. 18-6. Gravitational placentography, showing large space between the fetal head and symphysis pubis in lateral view, with patient semi-erect and the placenta situated low on the anterior uterine wall (in the gap between the symphysis pubis and the head).

placenta is not always simple for the novice. Digital examination may create such profuse bleeding that immediate delivery will become a necessity. Therefore, whenever possible, digital examination should be postponed until the fetus is clearly viable. Douching and coitus are obviously interdicted.

Treatment. *As a rule the uterus should be emptied by the most conservative method as soon as placenta previa is diagnosed.* Often, however, the potential for fetal survival can be greatly improved by postponing delivery until the fetus gains maturity. Selection of the earliest moment for a safe elective termination can be based on the assessments of intrauterine fetal maturity described in Chapter 7.

If a policy of watchful waiting is to be pursued, the patient should remain in, or close to, the hospital and emergency services and blood must be readily available.

Before labor. Before labor, with the cervix dilated to admit one or two fingers, the treatment will depend on the type of previa.

1. When the placenta is lateral or only slightly over the os:

(a) Rupture of the membranes may permit the head to press the placenta against the uterine wall and stop the bleeding.

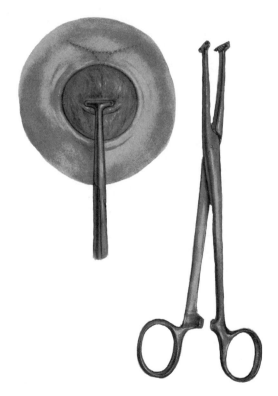

Fig. 18-7. Use of Willett forceps, which are attached to fetal scalp. (From Titus: The management of obstetric difficulties, St. Louis, The C. V. Mosby Co.)

(b) Willett scalp traction forceps (Fig. 18-7) may accelerate labor and assist in control of bleeding but may damage the scalp. Traction is provided by attaching a 2-pound weight with a cord and pulley. This treatment has, however, been largely consigned to history along with Braxton-Hicks version, use of an inflatable intrauterine rubber bag (metreurynter), and other methods of obtaining vaginal or uterine tamponade.

(c) If labor does not materialize, cautious stimulation with continuous-drip intravenous oxytocin is permissible (Chapter 23).

(d) Cesarean section has certain obvious advantages in the treatment of all but the most minor degrees of placenta previa.

2. When the placenta partially or completely covers the os, cesarean section is the only reasonable treatment. Hopefully this can be postponed until fetal viability, but if hemorrhage is significant, it must be performed regardless of gestational age or whether the fetus is dead or alive. Whether classical cesarean section or a vertical or transverse incision in the lower uterine segment is the most appropriate approach remains a moot point, but if the placenta is traversed in entering the uterine cavity, it must be done with dispatch and the cord must be immediately sought and clamped. Placental damage, before or during delivery, may result in fetal blood loss, and thus the infant's hemoglobin should be determined immediately after birth regardless of the method of delivery.

During labor. Management during labor depends on the variety of the previa, dilatation and effacement of the cervix, and the general condition of the patient.

1. If the cervix is completely dilated, forceps may be used to expedite delivery.

2. If dilatation is incomplete and the previa is lateral, rupture of the membranes may be sufficient. The presenting part will descend, compress the placenta, and stop the bleeding.

3. Under all other circumstances cesarean section is indicated.

4. The physician is especially warned against manual or instrumental dilatation of the cervix because of its unusual friability in placenta previa.

Management of third stage. Danger of alarming hemorrhage does not cease with the delivery of the infant.

1. If there is no unusual hemorrhage, the third stage of labor may be conducted in the usual manner.

2. If bleeding is profuse, the Credé method of expression should be immediately employed. If this is not effective, the placenta must be removed manually forthwith.

3. If bleeding persists after explusion of the placenta:

(a) Quickly inspect the cervix for tears.

(b) If there are no tears to account for the bleeding, the uterus should be explored digitally for the possibility of rupture of the friable lower segment. Rupture requires laparotomy for repair of the tear or for hysterectomy, depending on the circumstances.

Prognosis. Maternal mortality in modern hospitals approximates 0.1%. Fetal mortality is 15% to 20%; this may be improved somewhat as the expectant treatment of placenta previa achieves wider acceptance.

19

Pathology of the placenta, membranes, and umbilical cord

HYDATIDIFORM MOLE

Hydatidiform mole, also called vesicular mole or hydropic mole, is a degenerative disorder of the chorion occurring in the first half of pregnancy and possibly initiated by a defect in communication between the fetal and villous vasculature. It is characterized by the absence of fetal development, cystic enlargement of placental villi, and proliferation of the trophoblastic cells covering the villi. Moles are of great clinical interest because of their association with the highly malignant tumor known as choriocarcinoma or chorioepithelioma.

Incidence. Hydatidiform mole occurs about once in 2,000 pregnancies in the Western world but is five times as prevalent in Asia and parts of Africa. The recurrence rate is approximately 2%. The frequency is greatly increased in women over 45 years of age, and there are numerous reports of such moles in women in their middle fifties.

Pathology. Grossly, a hydatidiform mole is placental tissue in which chorionic villi have been converted to vesicles of varying size (1 mm. to 1 cm. in diameter) that are arranged in grapelike clusters. The total bulk of the mass varies greatly, occasionally distending the uterus to the size of a gestation of 6 months.

Microscopically, the villi show hydropic degeneration and swelling, scanty blood vessels, and proliferation of chorionic epithelium, particularly the syncytium. The majority exhibit a female sex chromatin pattern.

267

Occasionally only a portion of the placenta shows this change, and the remainder may be sufficiently normal to allow fetal development. This condition (partial molar degeneration) does not provoke the degree of concern engendered by total molar degeneration (hydatidiform mole).

Often the maternal ovaries exhibit multiple *lutein cysts*, presumably resulting from overstimulation by chorionic gonadotropin from the mole. These have been mistaken for true neoplasms and inadvertently removed. They regress after delivery and should be ignored (Fig. 19-1).

Symptoms and diagnosis

1. Bleeding, either spotty or profuse, occurs in early pregnancy and anemia is frequently noted.

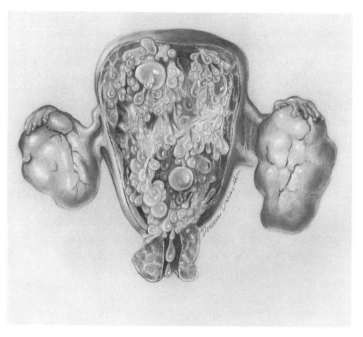

Fig. 19-1. Hydatidiform mole in bisected uterus and associated bilateral ovarian enlargement caused by multiple lutein cysts.

2. Enlargement of the uterus often goes beyond the usual size for the estimated period of gestation.

3. Bilateral adnexal masses appear—lutein cysts of the ovary.

4. Nausea and vomiting may be unusually severe.

5. Preeclampsia may appear in the second trimester, whereas in normal pregnancy it is rarely seen so early.

6. Pain is related to rapid uterine enlargement.

7. Quantitative test for chorionic gonadotropin will often show an elevated value. One must relate this to the apparent stage of pregnancy, remembering that high values occur normally near the end of the second month.

8. Care must be taken not to confuse twin pregnancy with hydatidiform mole.

9. Vesicles may be passed per vaginam; they should be recovered and examined microscopically to confirm the diagnosis.

10. Diagnosis may otherwise be made by establishing the absence of a fetal ECG pattern, the absence of a fetal skeleton

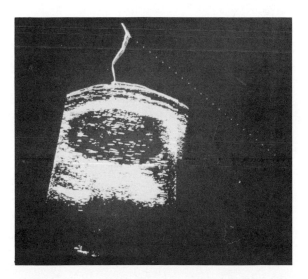

Fig. 19-2. Cross-sectional sonogram of ovoid uterine mass containing hydatidiform mole, as demonstrated by typical "speckled" appearance. (Courtesy of Dr. Louis Bartolucci, San Francisco.)

by x-ray, ultrasonography (Fig. 19-2), or by demonstrating the typical honeycomb pattern in an amniogram taken *immediately* after the intrauterine injection of 20 ml. of contrast material (Fig. 19-3).

11. Urinary estriol, plasma diamine oxidase, and serum chorionic somatomammotropin levels are all below normal.

Prognosis. The immediate outlook for the patient depends chiefly on the amount of hemorrhage, infection, or perforating

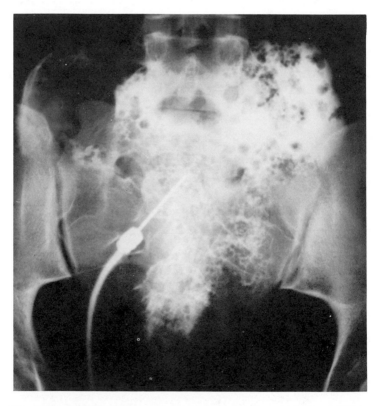

Fig. 19-3. Roentgenologic appearance of hydatidiform mole immediately after the intrauterine injection of Renografin.

trophoblastic erosion of the uterine wall. Approximately 1% of the mothers used to die from the effects of the mole. These women should be saved with proper use of blood and antibiotics. Of the women who survive the immediate dangers of the mole, probably 1% to 2% develop chorioepithelioma.

Treatment

1. Immediate evacuation of the uterus is imperative because of the great dangers from hemorrhage, infection, trophoblastic perforation of the uterus, and possibly chorioepithelioma. Often evacuation can be accomplished by stimulating the uterus with oxytocin intravenously. After spontaneous expulsion of the major portion of the mole, curettage should be done to ensure complete emptying of the cavity and to remove all placental material in contact with the uterine muscularis. The last pieces of curetted tissue are saved separately for microscopic examination because evidences of choriocarcinoma are most likely to be present in this region.

2. The uterus may be emptied from below, as in the manner of any therapeutic interruption of pregnancy, by cervical dilatation and instrumental evacuation of the molar material or by suction curettage. The latter method is preferred in that it is rapid and associated with minimal blood loss.

3. Hysterotomy may be required for the very large uterus with a relatively resistant cervix. Avoid resecting cystic ovaries observed at the time of laparotomy; spontaneous regression will occur after removal of the mole.

4. Hysterectomy may be done in selected multiparas with other indications for removal of the uterus.

Aftertreatment. Because of the danger of choriocarcinoma, a chest film should be obtained to rule out pulmonary metastases and to serve as a baseline for subsequent films.

Remaining viable trophoblastic tissues (benign or malignant) will produce human chorionic gonadotropin (HCG). After evacuation of molar tissue, most patients cease excreting HCG within 60 days. One needs to ensure that the HCG titer is falling appropriately and to institute the required investigation and treatment if it is not. Determination of the HCG titer 10, 20, 30, 45, and 60 days after molar evacuation has been recommended, with monthly determinations thereafter for a year for detection of any recurrence. Obviously, a new pregnancy should be studiously avoided so as to prevent confusion in the interpretation of any positive titer.

Immunologic pregnancy tests have been designed to have a minimum sensitivity of 3,000 to 6,000 I.U. HCG per liter of urine. Tests with greater sensitivity (for example, mouse uterine weight bioassay or radioimmunoassay) must be used in following these patients, especially after pregnancy tests have become negative.

Persistence, accentuation, or recurrence of the HCG titer requires meticulous investigation to determine its source, including chest film, liver scan, neurologic examination, curettage, and possibly even exploratory laparotomy to rule out myometrial, parametrial, or peritoneal trophoblastic extension. Persistent, repetitious, or copious uterine bleeding should be investigated by curettage, regardless of the HCG titer.

The prophylactic use of cancer chemotherapeutic agents to prevent development of choriocarcinoma appears to be effective but currently unwarranted because of the inherent risks of this therapy. However, significant abnormalities of the HCG titer are adequate indication for chemotherapy if pregnancy is not present.

CHORIOCARCINOMA (CHORIOEPITHELIOMA)

Pathology. This dark red tumor of chorionic epithelium invades uterine muscle and blood vessels rapidly and eventually perforates the uterine serosa. Microscopically, sheets of trophoblast are seen in association with hemorrhagic necrosis of the uterine musculature. Villi are absent. Metastases usually occur early in the lungs, vagina, liver, brain, and other areas. Ovarian lutein cystomas are common.

History and diagnosis. Choriocarcinoma nearly always occurs after hydatidiform mole, abortion, or term pregnancy. Irregular bleeding may be the first symptom, or a metastatic lesion may be observed before the primary tumor has been suspected. Perforation of the uterine wall may provoke massive intraperitoneal hemorrhage. Curettage and assays for chorionic gonadotropin usually will confirm the diagnosis. Radiologic study of the lungs always is indicated.

Treatment. The oral or intramuscular administration of methotrexate (Amethopterin) is the preferred treatment, although other cancer chemotherapeutic agents have also been proved to be efficacious. These are powerful agents with a limited and narrow range of safety. Renal, hepatic, neurologic, and especially hematopoietic evaluation should precede and accompany their use. These agents have produced complete remission in 50% to 75% of patients, an astounding accomplishment in the treatment of this previously lethal disease. Subsequent pregnancies are not uncommon and have not demonstrated any increased risk to the mother or fetus from the tumor or chemotherapy.

Hysterectomy, excision of localized or accessible metastases, and/or radiotherapy may be of value in certain patients.

Chorioadenoma destruens. Chorioadenoma destruens is also called malignant mole or invasive mole. It shows great trophoblastic overgrowth and deep penetration of the uterine wall, but very little tendency to distant metastasis.

The treatment is hysterectomy, since death may occur from uterine perforation and internal bleeding.

HYDRAMNIOS

Hydramnios (polyhydramnios) is the presence of an excessive quantity of fluid in the amniotic sac. The usual amount in a normal pregnancy is approximately 1 liter, but colossal amounts have been reported in some instances. A moderate excess of amniotic fluid up to 2 liters is common and of little clinical consequence; however, excessive amounts offer real clinical problems. This condition occurs in about 0.5% to 1% of pregnancies and is associated with a 25% to 30% incidence of fetal malformations. The rate of prematurity is doubled and the overall perinatal loss is above 50%.

Etiology

It appears that the placenta, membranes, cord, and fetus all play a role in the formation and absorption of amniotic fluid. Although the specific cause for excessive (or inadequate) amniotic fluid remains unknown, it should be reemphasized that a complete turnover occurs every 3 to 4 hours. Although experiments to date suggest that the turnover rate is no different in patients with normal and abnormal amniotic fluid volumes, a miniscule variation (possibly undetectable by current methods), if constant, could have an enormous effect over the weeks and months of pregnancy.

Certain abnormalities of the fetus and mother are likely to be accompanied by hydramnios, but whether any of them are etiologic factors or whether they and the hydramnios are attributable to a common cause is unknown.

1. Fetal abnormalities that frequently accompany hydramnios include the following:

    (a) Anencephalus (results in reduced fetal swallowing of amniotic fluid and thus the accumulation of excessive fluid; similarly, fetal esophageal stricture and myotonia dystrophica have both been associated with hydramnios)

    (b) Spina bifida

    (c) Ectopic bladder

    (d) Abnormalities of the fetal or cord circulation, for example, obstruction

    (e) Erythroblastosis with hydrops

    (f) Twin transfusion syndrome

2. Maternal abnormalities with hydramnios are as follows:

    (a) Multiple pregnancy

    (b) Diabetes mellitus

    (c) Preeclampsia and eclampsia

Acute hydramnios

In early pregnancy

1. Acute hydramnios in early pregnancy is rare, develops suddenly (as early as the fourth month of gestation), and is very dangerous

2. Dyspnea is distressing.

3. Cyanosis may be extensive.

4. Edema of the abdomen, vulva, and thighs occurs.

5. Pain in the abdomen and back, because of the attempted distention of an undistensible uterus, is almost unbearable.

6. The uterus is so tense and hard that the fetus cannot be felt or the heart tones heard.

7. The patient appears very sick, anxious, and exhausted and may have fever.

8. Death will occur if the uterus is not emptied forthwith.

In late pregnancy. Acute hydramnios in late pregnancy is simply a more or less rapid exacerbation of the hitherto gradually developing chronic type.

Chronic hydramnios

Chronic hydramnios is the common type of slowly developing excess of fluid that becomes apparent later in gestation.

Diagnosis

1. Palpation reveals much amniotic fluid.
2. Ballottement of the fetus is easily demonstrated.
3. *Percussion* gives a flat note.

Differential diagnosis must sometimes be made from other conditions with fluid such as:

1. *Ovarian cyst*—the history and careful examination will usually suffice; no fetus is palpable.

2. *Multiple pregnancy*—more than one fetus is felt; inasmuch as hydramnios is common with twins, the hydramnios may be easily detected and the twins missed.

3. *Ascites*—may be differentiated by shifting dullness, and no fetus is found by x-ray examination or palpation.

Symptoms and signs

1. The uterus is larger than it should be.
2. Fetal parts are indistinct and the fetal heart is heard with difficulty.

3. Dyspnea depends on the degree of distention and pressure upon the diaphragm.

4. *Cyanosis* is sometimes alarming, especially when the patient also has cardiac insufficiency.

5. Edema is purely mechanical.

6. Subjective symptoms depend largely on the rate of the accumulation of fluid. A slowly developing distention may be associated with minimal symptoms, whereas a rapidly developing distention is distressing and may even endanger life.

7. X-ray film of the abdomen shows an area of fluid haze consistent with uterine size, but associated with an under-sized fetal skeleton.

Treatment

1. Only persons with severe chronic hydramnios need special treatment. The severity of symptoms, not the degree of enlarge-

ment, is the guide. It is astonishing the amount of distention patients can endure without unusual distress.

2. Uterine paracentesis and aspiration of fluid slowly (not over 500 ml. per hour) may relieve distress, but labor usually starts promptly. There is little danger of trauma to the intestine, provided that the patient has never had abdominal surgery.

3. Puncture of the membranes via the cervical canal is the simplest method of relief, but great care should be exercised to avoid a sudden gush of fluid, which may wash out the cord.

4. Prolonged labor may be anticipated because of the lowered tone of the uterine muscle from stretching.

5. Postpartum hemorrhage is likely for the same reason.

Oligohydramnios

Deficient amniotic fluid is a very rare but real hazard early in pregnancy because:

1. The fetus is not protected.

2. Adhesion of the fetus to the amnion may occur, resulting in fetal deformity or abortion.

Low amniotic fluid volume in the third trimester (less than 300 ml.) may indicate placental insufficiency and is often associated with severe renal anomalies, pulmonary hypoplasia, and amnion nodosum.

The maximum volume of somewhat more than 1,000 ml. occurs between the thirty-eighth and thirty-ninth week, followed by a loss of about 125 ml. weekly. The weekly loss doubles after the forty-second week.

MINOR PLACENTAL PATHOLOGY
Abnormalities

Size. The size of the normal placenta averages about 15 to 20 cm. in diameter and 2.5 cm. in thickness and weighs approximately 500 grams. It may be much larger with syphilis, erythroblastosis, or congenital fetal nephrosis.

Shape. The shape is usually a flat, rounded disk but may assume bizarre forms because of an unequal blood supply to the developing placenta.

1. *Multiple lobes* more or less separated; as many as seven lobes described (placenta duplex, triplex, etc.)

2. *Placenta fenestrata* (a hole or window)
3. *Horseshoe placenta*

Important varieties

Placenta succenturiata. One or more small lobes are occasionally found in the membranes, unconnected with the main placental mass except by vessels. Succenturiate lobes are of great clinical moment since they may be left in the uterus after the third stage of labor and cause dangerous postpartum bleeding (Fig. 19-4).

NOTE: To avoid this hazard, the membranes and the edge of the fetal surface of the placenta must be inspected to be sure there are no torn vessels or nodules in the membranes at the placental border.

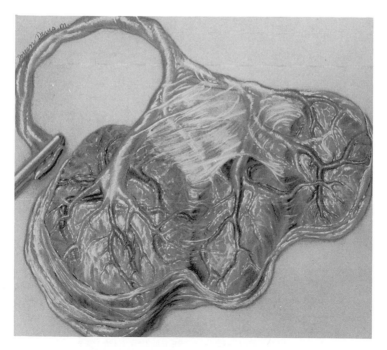

Fig. 19-4. Tripartite placenta (three lobes).

Membranous placenta. When the decidua capsularis and the villi of the chorion laeve do not atrophy as usual, a thin layer of placenta surrounds the entire ovum. The ovum usually develops normally, but the third stage of labor is complicated by failure of separation, the placenta generally requiring manual removal, and hemorrhage.

Placenta circumvallata. Occasionally there occurs on the fetal surface of the placenta an elevated fibrous ring at or near the margin, from which the membranes arise. Inside the ring the surface is normal, but the vessels disappear into the substance of the placenta at the ring. Whether this anomaly is associated with an increased incidence of abortion is debatable. Some authorities claim it leads to intermittent bleeding that may be erroneously attributed to placenta previa (Fig. 19-5).

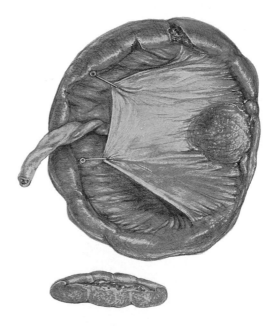

Fig. 19-5. Placenta circumvallata with succenturiate lobe. (From Titus: The management of obstetric difficulties, St. Louis, The C. V. Mosby Co.)

Diseases of placenta

Infarcts (degenerations). Recent investigations indicate that infarcts do not have a common cause or identical microscopic appearance. Some degenerations are natural biologic processes of growth, development, and senescence.

White infarcts. White infarcts are small pyramidal areas of degeneration, with their bases toward the maternal surface. They are caused by fibrinoid degeneration of the chorionic epithelium, not infarction.

Hemovillus degeneration. Hemovillus degeneration, formerly called red infarct, is the result of maternal blood clotting around a villus whose syncytium has broken away and exposed underlying connective tissue. The clot may spread to incorporate other villi and involve a considerable space in the placenta.

Authorities no longer believe that degenerative phenomena in the placenta are of clinical importance. The placenta has a large surplus physiologic capacity, so that perhaps one half of it can support fetal life.

Hematomas. If arteries or veins in the decidual basalis rupture, blood extravasates and forms a hematoma (retroplacental). An extensive process of this kind leads to *abruptio placentae*.

Large fetal vessels beneath the amnion may rupture and produce a subamniotic hematoma, which usually is small and soon organizes.

Calcification of placenta. Calcium nodules are also a consequence of degenerations occurring usually on the maternal surface. They have no clinical significance.

Tumors of placenta

Cysts. Small cysts are frequently seen; larger ones are seldom seen. They are usually derived from the chorionic membrane and hence are frequently observed on the fetal surface. They have no clinical significance.

Amnion nodosum. Mutiple nodules, each less than a centimeter in diameter and each composed of stratified squamous epithelium, are often found on the free amnion and on the fetal surface of the placenta, especially about the insertion of the cord. Their etiology and/or effect is unknown.

Fibromas. Fibromas are rare and range from the size of a small pea to several centimeters in diameter.

Myxofibromas. Myxofibromas are also rare but are found a little more often than fibromas.

Angiomas. Angiomas are infrequent and do little harm unless large enough to damage a considerable part of the placenta. Some are associated with hydramnios.

Malignant tumors. Sarcoma or carcinoma is not found *primarily* in the placenta.

Placentitis

Placentitis is customarily caused by an intrapartum infection associated with ruptured membranes and prolonged labor. Pyogenic bacteria from the vagina induce an amniochorionitis and fetal pneumonia, which may lead to fatal fetal, and even maternal, septicemia. Only under unusual circumstances should a pregnancy be allowed to go undelivered more than 24 to 48 hours after amniotic membrane rupture, especially if contractions are occurring.

Placentitis may on rare occasions result from a systemic maternal infection of nongestational etiology.

Tuberculosis

Tuberculosis of the placenta is relatively rare, but tubercles have been noted on the villi in the decidua basalis. Bacilli may be found without demonstrable tubercles. The chief clinical significance is the possibility, although uncommon, of transmission to the fetus.

Edema

Edema of the placenta is usually associated with "general dropsy" of the fetus (erythroblastosis). Occasionally it is observed with certain conditions of the mother, for example, heart disease and diabetes.

ABNORMALITIES OF UMBILICAL CORD

The umbilical cord usually is inserted upon the fetal surface of the placenta between its center and the periphery. Occasionally one of the following varieties of insertion is encountered.

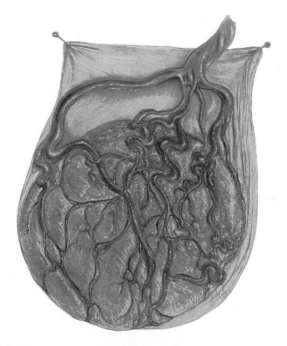

Fig. 19-6. Velamentous insertion of cord. The cord arises from the membranes some distance from the placenta. (From Titus: The management of obstetric difficulties, St. Louis, The C. V. Mosby Co.)

Battledore placenta. In battledore placenta the cord comes off the placental margin instead of near the center of the fetal surface. It has no clincal significance.

Velamentous insertion. In velamentous insertion the cord arises from the membranes some distance from the placenta (Fig. 19-6). The vessels run fanwise in an amniotic fold. The unprotected vessels are in great danger of rupture, especially if they extend across the internal os (*vasa previa*). They may be compressed between the fetal presenting part and the bony pelvis if they are low-lying in the uterus. Unanticipated intrauterine fetal death may occur in either circumstance.

Variations in length of cord. The average length of the cord is about 55 cm., but it may vary from 2 or 3 cm. to 200 cm. When too long, it may be twined about the neck or body of the fetus; occasionally it is twined so many times that the cord becomes excessively short.

When the cord is too short, consequent embarrassment of the fetal circulation may occur, with resultant intrauterine asphyxia. Theoretically, placental separation, rupture of the cord, umbilical hernia of the infant, or inversion of the uterus may also occur.

Torsion of cord. Excessive twisting is rare, but it may be sufficient to interfere with or stop the cord circulation.

Knots of cord. *True knots* may occur in the cord as a result of fetal motion, especially when the cord is long. Only rarely do they cause any difficulty, but when drawn tight, they may lead to fetal asphyxia.

False knots are developmental anomalies of the cord, so folded and adherent that they look like knots.

Varices. Varices of the cord vessels, although rare, present considerable danger of rupture of the thin vessel walls.

Tumors of cord. Tumors of the cord are so rare that only a very few cases have been reported (myxomas).

Edema of cord. Although frequently found in dead fetuses and in general dropsy (erythroblastosis) of the fetus, edema of the cord is otherwise rarely seen.

Inflammation of cord. Inflammation of the cord, like placentitis, is almost never seen in a living infant, but occasionally occurs when there is intrapartum infection with ruptured membranes.

Absence of one umbilical artery. Absence of one umbilical artery is reported in the cords of 1% of infants. As many as 25% of such infants have shown congenital malformations. Esophageal atresia, imperforate anus, renal agenesis, polycystic kidneys, chromosomal anomalies and other malformations may be associated. Whether this is a cause-and-effect relationship is not known.

20

Complications involving the generative tract

VULVA, VAGINA, AND CERVIX

External genitalia

Condylomata acuminata. Condylomata acuminata are warty growths of viral origin occurring on the cervix, vagina, and vulva (Fig. 20-1). Usually they are responsive to fulguration, excision, or repeated local application of podophyllin, dichloroacetic acid, or nitrogen mustard. Rarely their total mass attains enormous size, necessitating delivery by cesarean section to avoid hemorrhage and dissemination of the lesions.

Varices. Varices of the vulva increase during pregnancy and produce much discomfort. They very seldom rupture during pregnancy. Birth injuries may be followed by alarming hemorrhage. A snug perineal pad may relieve the discomfort and pain. A considerable degree of spontaneous resolution occurs post partum.

Abscess of Bartholin's gland. Abscess of Bartholin's gland is dangerous as a source of puerperal infection. If seen early enough to heal before labor, the abscess should be widely opened and an effective antibiotic administered.

Cyst of Bartholin's duct. Cyst of Bartholin's duct may be ignored if small. Larger cysts may be aspirated to produce temporary shrinkage, and operative excision may then be performed after delivery.

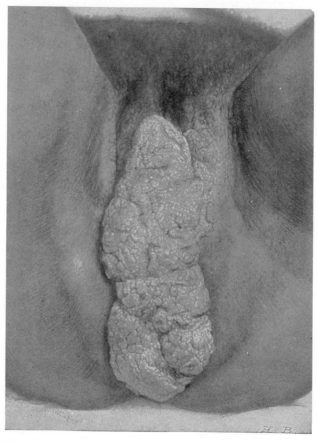

Fig. 20-1. Condylomas of vulva treated by fulguration and excision during pregnancy; normal labor. (From Stander: Williams obstetrics, New York, D. Appleton-Century Co.)

Vaginitis

Trichomoniasis. Infections from the protozoan organism *Trichomonas vaginalis* are common in pregnancy and require treatment because of discharge, burning, and pruritus. Diagnosis is made from microscopic examination of unstained secretions diluted in physiologic saline solution or from vaginal smears stained by the Papanicolaou technique. The currently popular treatment is metronidazole (Flagyl) administered orally or various trichomonacides administered vaginally. If reinfection occurs, it is wise to examine and treat the sexual partner.

Candidiasis (moniliasis). Candidiasis is a fungal vulvovaginitis caused by *Candida albicans* and is characterized by severe vulvar itching and varying amounts of watery, white, and cheesy discharge. It is particularly common in pregnancy. Diagnosis may be established by observing pseudomycelia or budding yeast cells in wet potassium hydroxide preparations or on stained slides. The fungus can be cultured on Sabouraud's or Nickerson's medium. Numerous pharmaceutic agents are recommended for therapy, particularly nystatin vaginal suppositories.

Vaginal adenosis

Vaginal adenosis, ectopic endocervical tissue within the vagina, can present as cysts, patches of red mucosa, and polypoid or ulcerative lesions, benign or malignant. In appearance, these lesions are identical to their cervical counterparts, that is, Nabothian cysts, ectropion ("erosion"), polyps, and carcinoma. Adenosis is rarely seen before puberty, is uninfluenced by pregnancy, rarely causes difficulty, and customarily does not require treatment unless symptomatic or malignant. Its incidence in the general population is unknown.

Human females exposed to diethylstilbestrol while in utero have an incidence of the effluent variety (red, granular spots or patches) approximating 30% and have also occasionally been noted to have partial transverse vaginal septa and subcutaneous pericervical fibrous collars. The latter have not as yet been observed through pregnancy and their influence on vaginal delivery is unknown. These women have also been noted to have minor anatomic variations of the cervix, most commonly involving the presence of a circular, perioral sulcus on the exocervix, plus a varying amount of ectropion. Additionally, these individuals have a higher than normal incidence of vaginal and cervical adenocarcinoma.

Cervicitis and polyps

Chronic cervicitis may occasionally occur and lead to increased vaginal discharge in pregnancy. This may be treated with sulfa

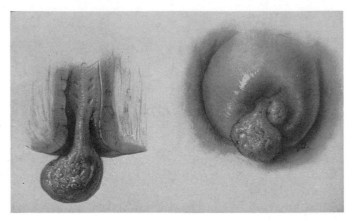

Fig. 20-2. Cervical polyp. (From Richards: Surgery for general practice, St. Louis, The C. V. Mosby Co.)

or antibiotic creams. Extensive cauterization or surgical treatment should be postponed until the pregnancy has been completed.

Cervical polyps (Fig. 20-2) may produce minor degrees of bleeding, particularly postcoital spotting. All polyps should be excised and submitted to histologic study to be certain that carcinoma does not coexist with the polyp.

Cancer of cervix uteri

An invasive, visible, and palpable carcinoma of the cervix may occasionally be encountered for the first time during routine obstetric examination. Asymptomatic patients usually have stage I lesions, which respond well to radiation therapy (Fig. 20-3). Pregnancy does not influence the cancer, nor vice versa.

External radiation is used without regard for the pregnancy in the first and second trimesters. Abortion usually occurs spontaneously toward the end of the course of therapy, and then radium is applied to complete the therapy. Occasionally curettage or hysterotomy may be required to empty the uterus. The 5-year survival rate is the same as for nonpregnant patients.

If the fetus is viable when carcinoma is discovered, delivery should be by classical cesarean section as soon as assessments

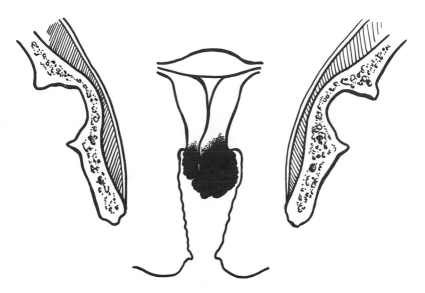

Fig. 20-3. Extensive stage I carcinoma of the cervix, which would present a major obstacle to delivery.

of the intrauterine fetus demonstrate maturation (Chapter 7), and x-ray therapy should be started as soon as the abdominal incision has healed. The uterus should be left in place for later radium placement.

The handling of cervical carcinoma in pregnancy is a problem for experts, and the average physician is well advised to refer such patients to medical centers where large numbers of patients with malignant gynecologic tumors are treated.

Carcinoma in situ of the cervix is an increasingly common lesion because the widespread application of cytologic detection to obstetric patients is disclosing these microscopic lesions. When a cytologic smear shows malignant cells, biopsy or surgical conization of the cervix should be done to determine whether the presumed cancer is strictly intraepithelial or perhaps already invasive. If the lesion is preinvasive, pregnancy may be allowed to proceed and vaginal delivery may be planned. Further therapy obviously depends on postpartum cytologic findings.

DISPLACEMENTS AND HERNIAS
Retroflexion and retroversion

In the nonpregnant woman retroflexion and retroversion of the uterus may be symptomless, but after conception the pressure of the growing uterus confined in the true pelvis causes much discomfort, pain, backache, and a heavy "bearing-down" sensation. Symptoms increase until the pregnant uterus rises above the pelvic brim, which usually occurs at the beginning of the fourth month. Abortion may occur but is not the rule. The uterus spontaneously slips past the promontory of the sacrum. When this does not take place, the uterus is *incarcerated* in the pelvis (Fig. 20-4), a most dangerous event, which may lead to abortion or to urethral compression and bladder distention, with resultant cystitis and pyelonephritis. This situation is exceptionally un-

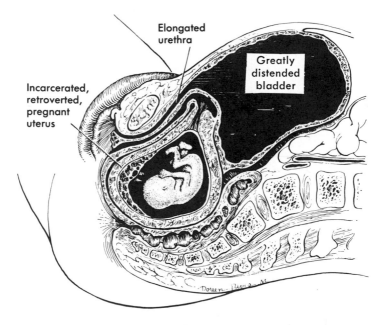

Fig. 20-4. Incarcerated, retroverted pregnant uterus. Note the elongated and compressed urethra and great distention of the bladder.

common and is almost invariably associated with severe cul-de-sac adhesions.

When the uterus is incarcerated, the urethra and neck of the bladder are compressed between the symphysis pubis and the cervix, which is pushed by the growing fundus uteri

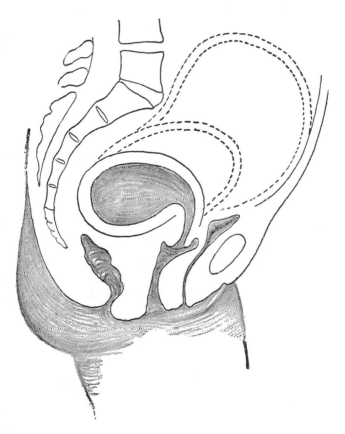

Fig. 20-5. Retroverted, adherent, pregnant uterus. Dotted lines show how the uterus grows by sacculation of the anterior wall of the uterus to accommodate the developing fetus. (From Beck: Obstetrical practice, Baltimore, The Williams & Wilkins Co.)

against or above the symphysis. The growing uterus also presses against the rectum so that defecation is difficult or impossible. Similarly the uterus is forced downward and, without sufficient support by the pelvic floor, may become prolapsed.

Diagnosis. Diagnosis is made by palpating the typically elastic soft mass of the pregnant uterus in the pelvis, by finding the cervix displaced anteriorly, plus a history of painful or difficult urination, "paradoxical incontinence," severe pelvic pain, backache, and an irresistible bearing-down feeling in the pelvis. The distended bladder, percussed and palpated above the symphysis pubis, will confirm the diagnosis. Occasionally the pregnancy will progress to term even though the retroversion persists. In this situation the anterior wall of the uterus distends and forms a sac to accommodate the fetus. The cervix is high above the symphysis, rendering normal delivery impossible because the presenting part is below it (Fig. 20-5).

Treatment

1. When a retrodisplacement is discovered in early pregnancy, it should be left alone, as treatment is rarely required.

2. If seen later, but before the fourth month, and bimanual replacement is difficult, tension on a tenaculum attached to the cervix may be of some assistance, but doing so runs the risk of cervical laceration and bleeding. The knee-chest posture may aid the maneuver.

3. Before any manipulation the bladder must be emptied slowly with a catheter. Catheterization is often very difficult, because the urinary meatus is pulled up into the vagina out of sight.

4. If repeated knee-chest posturings fail, laparotomy must be done to free adhesions and lift the uterus out of the pelvis.

Prolapse of pregnant uterus

Conception is virtually impossible with complete prolapse but is common with partial prolapse. With pregnancy the uterus usually pursues its normal course upward into the abdominal cavity and the pregnancy goes uneventfully to full term. When the uterus does not ascend, its increasing growth may result in incarceration in the pelvis, and it may be forced into increased prolapse entirely outside the body.

Treatment. When a prolapsed uterus is seen early enough, it should be replaced and held by a ring pessary until its size will retain it. When the pessary is inadequate, the patient must stay in bed until the uterus is big enough to be retained by the pelvic brim. If the hypertrophied cervix appears outside the vulva, meticulous cleanliness must be observed to prevent infection.

Vaginal enterocele

Vaginal enterocele is a hernia containing intestines protruding into the vagina behind the cervix. It usually gives little trouble during pregnancy. During labor it can be controlled by reduction and by being held up until the presenting part has passed. Operative cure will be required later.

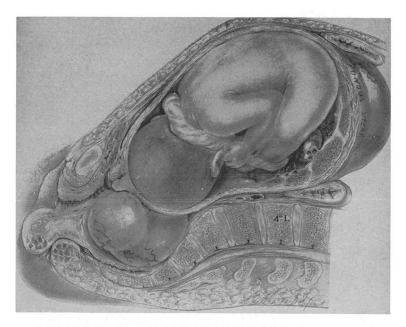

Fig. 20-6. Fibromyomas obstructing labor. (From Titus: The management of obstetric difficulties, St. Louis, The C. V. Mosby Co.)

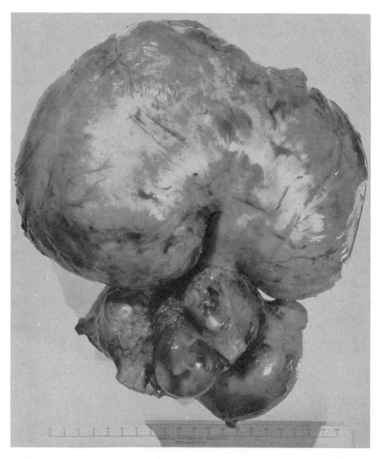

Fig. 20-7. Large uterine myomas in early pregnancy. Note the fetus in the sac above the center of the ruler. (From Titus and Willson: The management of obstetric difficulties, St. Louis, The C. V. Mosby Co.)

Other hernias

Inguinal, femoral, ventral, and umbilical hernias may usually be controlled by trusses or bandages until after delivery. Eventually they usually require surgical correction.

Gynecologic or other surgical operations may be performed during pregnancy, but unless urgent it is better to await delivery and puerperal recovery.

MYOMAS OF UTERUS

Myomas (Figs. 20-6 to 20-8) may affect pregnancy in the following ways:

1. Interfere with conception (especially submucous tumors)
2. Promote abortion
3. Produce dystocia by blocking the pelvis
4. Lead to abnormal fetal presentations
5. Interfere with uterine contractility in labor (inertia) and after delivery (postpartum hemorrhage)
6. Interfere with placental separation

Pregnancy may cause myomas to increase in size and produce pressure symptoms. Degenerative changes may occur in the

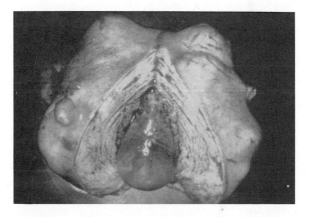

Fig. 20-8. Multiple myomas with gestation 8 weeks. Incarcerated uterus was removed because of urinary obstruction.

tumors and produce pain, fever, and mild leukocytosis, or the pedicle of a subserous tumor may undergo torsion. If symptoms are severe and prolonged, exploratory laparotomy may be required.

Tumors in the pelvis that would appear to be mechanical obstructions to delivery will not infrequently rise out of the pelvis as pregnancy advances.

Treatment. Although all pregnant women with myomas require constant observation, very few will need operation. The physician should defer operation until near full term when he can better determine the possibilities of spontaneous labor or the necessity of cesarean section. If the latter is required, the tumors may be simultaneously enucleated if not too large and numerous. If the uterus is extensively involved, it is better to allow full resolution of the pregnancy changes before initiating myomectomy.

TUMORS OF OVARY

Cystic ovarian masses large enough to cause trouble in pregnancy occur about once in 300 gestations. These tumors may undergo torsion, rupture, or lead to dystocia in labor. Obviously many such tumors escape detection prior to labor because the enlarging uterus masks the presence of the ovarian mass.

Symptoms. Often there are no symptoms or only moderate pelvic discomfort. However, when the cyst grows to considerable size, the combined masses of the tumor and the pregnancy may cause severe pressure symptoms. The usual accidents that accompany ovarian cysts in nonpregnant women are more likely to occur in pregnancy. These are torsion of the pedicle, rupture, and, in the case of a malignant neoplasm, metastases to adjacent peritoneal surfaces.

Diagnosis. Diagnosis is easy when the cyst remains in the pelvis, but it may be missed entirely when it has ascended into the abdomen, is relatively small, or the uterus has enlarged enough to conceal the cyst behind it.

In differentiating between myomas and cysts it must not be forgotten that tense cysts may be mistaken for myomas, and soft degenerating myomas may feel as soft as cysts, especially when pregnancy exists.

Treatment. An ovarian cyst or tumor discovered during pregnancy should in most instances be promptly removed, especially if it is firm and over 5 to 6 cm. in diameter. The desirability of witholding surgical exploration until after the third month of gestation, lest abortion be provoked, is debatable. The decision for or against operation would be simpler if the physician could determine the microscopic diagnosis preoperatively and assure the patient that the lesion is not malignant. Regretfully, this is not possible. Similar indecision abounds when ovarian tumors are first discovered rather late in pregnancy. If the tumor is in the pelvic cavity, there are obvious advantages to the combination of elective cesarean section and excision of the ovarian mass, provided that one is justified in waiting for fetal maturity. There is no general rule that may be applied successfully to the management of all ovarian tumors in pregnancy.

In the puerperium twisted pedicle, with subsequent necrosis, gangrene, and peritonitis, is particularly likely to occur.

Other obstructing masses

Rarely complications of pregnancy and labor are attributable to pelvic ectopic kidney and to tumors of the bladder, bowel, vagina, and retroperitoneal tissues.

MALFORMATIONS OF GENITAL TRACT

The genital tract is formed by fusion of the müllerian ducts of the embryo. The upper portions of the ducts do not fuse but remain separate to form the fallopian tubes. The uterus is derived from the middle parts of the ducts, and the vagina represents the lowest portion.

When the ducts fuse, there is a septum between them, which normally disappears, leaving the cavities of the uterus and vagina. Therefore, there are two types of deformities:

1. Failure of the ducts to fuse
2. Persistence of the original septum

These two types tend to appear together. There may be partial or complete failure of fusion or partial or complete persistence of the septum; hence, there may be any degree of either or both deformities (Fig. 20-9).

Uterus unicornis unicollis. This is a uterus with a single-horned fundus and a single cervix, the product of unilateral development.

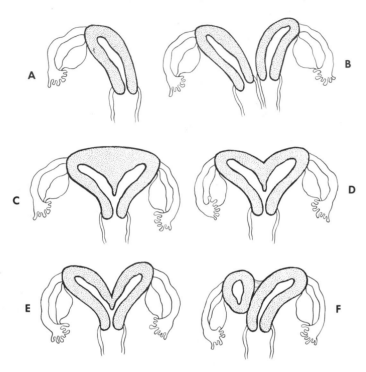

Fig. 20-9. Abnormal uterine development. **A,** Unicornis unicollis. **B,** Bicornis bicollis (didelphys). **C** to **E,** Bicornis unicollis (bicornuate) with nearly complete septum showing possible variations of external contour. **F,** Unicornis unicollis with noncommunicating rudimentary horn.

Uterus bicornis bicollis (uterus didelphys). This is a uterus with two independent fundi and two cervices, the product of bilateral development and, typically but not always, a total lack of uterine fusion.

Uterus bicornis unicollis (bicornuate uterus). This is a uterus with two fundal canals and a single cervix. The fundal canals are of varying length depending on the length of the intervening septum. The septum may persist partially (subseptus) or completely (septus) and, on occasion, may continue downward sufficiently to divide the canal of the single cervix as well (hemi-cervix). The exterior contour of the uterus may be normal, heart-shaped (arcuate) or deeply divided.

Rudimentary horn. Complete development of the fundus and cervix may occur on one side, with only partial development occurring on the other. The latter is designated as a rudimentary horn. Its size is highly variable. Its lining may or may not respond to ovarian hormones and its canal may or may not communicate with the canal on the opposite side, or with the vagina.

Double vagina. Lack of fusion in the vaginal area results in two totally separate vaginal barrels with a double introitus and a separate cervix in each vault. Fusion with persistence of the original septum results in a vaginal barrel with a complete or incomplete longitudinal septum associated with a single introitus. Twin cervices are common, but not always seen.

Complete or partial transverse vaginal septa may also be seen.

Clinical significance

1. Pregnancy in a rudimentary horn may lead to spontaneous rupture and intraperitoneal hemorrhage. Therefore, if the diagnosis can be made with reasonable certainty, the pregnant horn should be amputated promptly.

2. The closer the uterine and cervical development approximates normality, the better the organ functions obstetrically.

3. The deeply divided bicornuate uterus is a poor performer because of the deformed myometrium; there is a high incidence of abortion, premature labor, and uterine dysfunction with this anomaly. Malpresentations tend to increase the need for cesarean section, and the incidence of retained placenta is about 10%. Observation of the abdominal contour in the third trimester of pregnancy may suggest uterine anomalies that can be confirmed by hysterogram postpartum. Patients with positive hysterograms should have intravenous pyelography because of the high incidence of associated urinary tract anomalies.

4. Both the hemicervix and the true double cervix often dilate poorly, and cervical dystocia leads to cesarean section in about two out of three patients.

5. The poorest obstetric results have been associated with complete doubling of the uterus and with unilateral development.

6. The problems of longitudinal and transverse vaginal septa

usually are solved permanently by excision of the septum at the time of the first delivery.

7. Often malformations are not suspected until trouble arises or until the discovery is made more or less accidentally. Therefore, the physician should suspect and carefully investigate all patients with unusual types of dysmenorrhea, anomalous menstruation, and retained menstrual blood.

8. Whenever a vaginal septum (double vagina) is discovered, the physician should always suspect other genital tract deformities.

Labor

1. Dystocia is frequent, but so many women deliver normally that is wise to avoid hasty and early interference.

2. The nonpregnant horn may offer the same mechanical obstruction as any other tumor, but this is by no means the rule.

3. Postpartum hemorrhage is always a potential danger because of the defective uterine muscle. Oxytocics should be given to prevent bleeding.

21

Preeclampsia, eclampsia, and hypertension in pregnancy

In the past it was customary to group various hypertensive disorders, particularly those arising rather late in gestation or early in the puerperium, under the illogical and ambiguous heading "toxemia of pregnancy." However, no toxin has yet been demonstrated, and it seems unwise to perpetuate this phraseology as a synonym for *preeclampsia,* which is a syndrome or symptom-complex peculiar to pregnant and puerperal women. It is characterized by hypertension, proteinuria, and edema, and occasionally by convulsions and coma. When convulsions or coma develop, the diagnosis is changed to *eclampsia.*

Because hypertension is a prominent feature of preeclampsia-eclampsia, or the eclamptogenic syndrome, it is difficult to differentiate chronic hypertension of whatever cause from preeclampsia in women first seen beyond the twentieth week of gestation, especially when the level of blood pressure prior to pregnancy is unknown. Women with antecedent hypertension may develop a fulminating vasculorenal syndrome that appears to be preeclampsia superimposed on the underlying chronic disorder. Many schemes for classifying hypertensive disorders in pregnancy have been proposed or are still being studied by various committees, but these are merely expressions of ignorance regarding etiology.

The relative frequencies of preeclampsia and chronic hypertensive disease vary widely from place to place, depending perhaps on who makes the diagnoses and on the proportion of black patients in the sample. It is commonly said that black women are more susceptible to preeclampsia than are white women, but this may reflect their lack of proper prenatal care and diet.

Eclamptogenic disease or chronic vascular disease, or both, occur in 5% to 7% of pregnant women in the United States. Of the total number with these disorders, approximately 65% have preeclampsia or eclampsia, and 35% have vascular disease with or without superimposed acute toxemia.

PREECLAMPSIA

Diagnostic features. The cardinal signs are *hypertension, proteinuria,* and *edema* appearing in the last trimester of pregnancy. These three features of preeclampsia may be detected promptly by diligent prenatal examination. Indeed, the detection of preeclampsia in its incipient stage is one of the outstanding accomplishments of modern prenatal care.

Efforts to differentiate between mild and severe forms of preeclampsia on the basis of a few rigid criteria are of relatively little prognostic value and should be discouraged.

Hypertension. A systolic pressure of 140 mm. Hg and a diastolic pressure of 90 mm. Hg are considered to be the upper limits of normal. Occasionally, however, pressures below these levels may be associated with preeclampsia, and any persistent rise in pressure (30 mm. Hg or more) usually is significant. The diastolic value is a more reliable guide to preeclampsia and may exceed 90 mm. Hg when the systolic reading is not alarmingly high.

Proteinuria. Proteinuria varies enormously, depending on the severity of the disease process. In the mildest form of preeclampsia only a trace of protein will be detectable in the urine. With more severe disease, 6 to 8 grams or more per liter may be demonstrated by the Esbach precipitation technique, and a 4+ qualitative reaction will be obtained.

Edema. Edema may be noted by the patient in the form of swollen ankles, face, or fingers. This retention of water in the tissues is accompanied by abnormal gains in weight. A gain of more than 1 pound a week may indicate impending preeclampsia. Weight changes should be followed with great care, since this simple measurement is often an early warning of future trouble. Generalized edema may or may not be present and is not required for diagnosis. In cases of fulminating preeclampsia, on the other hand, water retention may be extreme and such patients may gain 10 pounds or more in a week.

Other signs and symptoms of preclampsia are headache, epigastric pain, visual disturbances, and oliguria. These phenomena are explainable on the basis of anatomic lesions demonstrable by gross and microscopic examination post mortem. Presumably these morphologic abnormalities are reversible in the patients who recover.

Headache. Headache, frontal or occipital, may be indicative of impending convulsions. Postmortem examination of the brains of eclamptic persons usually shows thrombosis and fibrinoid necrosis of small vessels, as well as microscopic or gross hemorrhages. Edema is frequently reported, but Sheehan has questioned its presence in the brains of persons examined promptly after death.

Epigastric pain. The origin of epigastric pain is not clear; it may be attributable to stretching of the liver capsule by small hemorrhages, or possibly it is of central origin.

Visual disturbances. Visual disturbances from slight blurring to complete blindness occur. The retina may show localized arteriolar spasms or general constriction, edema of the disk, and rarely detachment. Hemorrhages and exudates are indicative of chronic vascular disease.

Oliguria. Oliguria is presumably the result of both pathologic and physiologic changes in the kidneys. The renal lesion includes the following:

1. Swelling of the endothelial cell cytoplasm (Fig. 21-1)
2. Increase in the number of intercapillary cells
3. An amorphous deposit between the basement membrane and the cytoplasm of the endothelial cells.

These changes reduce or even obliterate the capillary lumen. Such lesions have been found by electron microscopy in renal biopsies even from patients with the mildest preeclampsia. Therapy seems to have no effect on the lesion, but it clears rather rapidly after delivery.

Although renal blood flow is about the same as in nonpregnant women, it is below that for pregnant women prior to the final few weeks of pregnancy. The glomerular filtration rate is

Epithelial cell nuclei   Epithelium

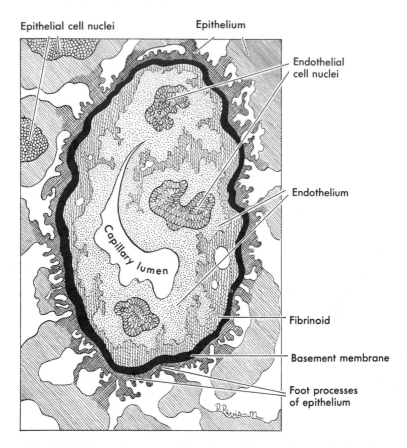

Endothelial
cell nuclei

Endothelium

Fibrinoid

Basement membrane

Foot processes
of epithelium

Capillary lumen

Fig. 21-1. Schematic reproduction of an electron micrograph, showing renal glomerular capillary in a woman with preeclampsia. Note swelling of endothelial cells and greatly narrowed lumen, but normal basement membrane.

decreased in preeclamptic patients. This presumably leads to retention of sodium because there is not a corresponding reduction in tubular reabsorption of sodium.

Physiologic and biochemical changes. Generalized arteriolar spasm is a prominent feature of preeclampsia and explains many of the pathologic lesions observed in various organs, but there is no proof that an abnormal vascular tree is responsible for the disease. Despite widespread vascular spasm, there has been no demonstration of reduced rates of blood flow in liver, brain, arm muscles, and skin.

Water retention is an outstanding feature of preeclampsia and usually is the first manifestation of trouble. None of the usual factors in edema formation can be cited as the primary cause.

Retention of sodium also is noted in these patients, possibly because of the ability of steroid hormones to increase renal tubular reabsorption of sodium. However, sex steroids appear to be diminished in preeclamptic women, and sodium retention is perhaps better explained by reduced glomerular filtration, as previously noted.

Uric acid concentration in the blood usually is increased because of diminished uric acid clearance by the kidneys.

The carbon dioxide combining power of the blood may be reduced in the most severe cases of preeclampsia, particularly after the convulsive seizures of eclampsia, because of increased serum lactic acid.

Serum protein and blood sugar values are not regularly altered in any characteristic fashion.

Etiology. The etiology is not known. Many attractive hypotheses have been advanced, but few, if any, have stood the test of time. Currently the uterine ischemia theory has the greatest support. Briefly stated, the uterine blood supply may be impaired by mechanical or nervous factors, such as the size of the uterus at term (particularly in a primigravida), multiple pregnancy, hydramnios, and chronic hypertensive vascular disease. Hypoxia at the placental site results in the release of protein substances that may in various ways produce both antidiuretic and hypertensive effects, as well as capillary thromboses and proteinuria. It seems clear that the hypertension of preeclampsia is not neurogenic, but is of humoral origin. Though increased concentrations of pressor compounds have not yet been found in the plasma of women with preeclampsia, their arterial systems exhibit an increased responsiveness to such substances (such as vasopression, norepinephrine, angiotensin). Presumably this leads to generalized vasoconstriction and hypertension. Increased vascular responsiveness may be related to increased concentration of sodium in the extracellular mucopolysaccharides of the arterial wall. The situation has been likened to a vicious circle, or a chain of events that once initiated is self-perpetuating and will persist until the circle is broken by the termination of pregnancy. Signs or symptoms may be reduced or masked by the use of drugs, but the more severe forms of preeclampsia or eclampsia cannot truly be eliminated prior to delivery.

Although the responsible chemical agents have not been identified, the present popularity of the uterine ischemia hypothesis results in part from its ability to explain certain prominent features of pregnancy toxemia:

1. Lower incidence in multiparas
2. Worsening of toxemia during labor
3. Higher incidence in pregnancies associated with overly distended uteri
4. Higher incidence in latter part of pregnancy
5. Its limitation to human beings whose upright posture impairs uterine circulation

Endocrine disturbances related to changes in the pituitary gland, adrenal glands, and placenta, as well as dietary deficiencies, have received much attention in recent years, but at the moment these etiologic possibilities are far from proved.

Treatment. Early detection of preeclampsia depends on close antepartum observation, especially in certain categories of patients presumably predisposed to this disorder. Predisposing factors are nulliparity, familial history of preeclampsia, multiple fetuses, diabetes, hypertension, hydatidiform mole, and fetal hydrops. Whether preeclampsia can really be prevented is uncertain, but its progression to the severe form and to eclampsia can usually be arrested.

Ambulatory treatment is permissible only for patients whose blood pressures do not exceed 140/90 mm. Hg and whose edema and proteinuria are minimal. Bed rest in lateral recumbency usually promotes effective diuresis. Small doses of phenobarbital every 8 hours may encourage the patient to restrict physical activity. Claims that salt restriction, with or without diuretic therapy, reduces the incidence of severe preeclampsia are not entirely convincing, and restriction of dietary sodium is now condemned as vigorously as it was advocated 20 years ago. Probably pregnant women should be allowed to salt their food to taste. Patients with possible incipient preeclampsia should be examined twice weekly, and labor should be induced as soon as the condition of the cervix is favorable.

Hospital treatment is indicated if the blood pressure exceeds 140/90 mm. Hg, significant proteinuria (1+ or greater) develops, or weight increases repeatedly more than 3 pounds a week. A definite and detailed program of observations and treatment should be started. In addition to complete bed rest, this program includes the following:

1. Daily weighing and determination of fetal heartbeats
2. Blood pressure determination every 4 to 6 hours
3. Recording of fluid intake and urinary output
4. Daily urinalysis, with quantitative estimation of protein and examination for casts
5. Retinoscopy at frequent intervals
6. Hematocrit and/or hemoglobin determination
7. Phenobarbital, 30 to 60 mg. every 6 hours
8. Daily determinations of blood urea nitrogen, uric acid, and plasma carbon dioxide content (in the more severe cases).

The treatment of mild preeclampsia is chiefly in the interest of the fetus, with the hope that further intrauterine life will improve the chance of survival after birth. Urinary or plasma estriol determinations may be helpful in assessing fetal status, and fetal biparietal measurements with ultrasound techniques may indicate the rate of fetal growth. Treatment of severe preeclampsia is largely in the maternal interest, that is, prevention of eclampsia and its possible fatal consequences. Whether a pregnancy is permitted to continue to the point of apparent fetal maturity depends on the maternal response to therapy. Even in the face of apparent improvement, continued hospitalization is desirable because the disease may very suddenly worsen.

Delivery. Termination of pregnancy is the only definitive treatment for preeclampsia. The length of the preliminary period of medical treatment will vary according to the severity of the situation, the stage of the pregnancy, and the ease with which delivery may be effected. Generally speaking, if the pregnancy has advanced to the thirty-fourth week, there is little to be gained for the fetus by waiting longer. When the cervix is favorable for membrane rupture and oxytocin stimulation, labor should be induced by this means. If there is no prospect of prompt delivery by the vaginal route, cesarean section under local or regional anesthesia is the procedure of choice.

In the face of severe or so-called fuminating preclampsia, it is particularly desirable to get the patient delivered if a definite improvement is not achieved after 24 hours of conservative therapy.

Prognosis. The immediate maternal prognosis depends on whether eclampsia develops, since preeclampsia ordinarily is not a fatal disorder. Fetal mortality is around 5% to 6% and depends largely on the severity of the disease and the degree of prematurity inflicted upon the infant by deliberate preterm delivery. The incidence of prematurity in preeclamptic patients has been about 18% in recent years.

ECLAMPSIA

In addition to what has just been said about preeclampsia, there are a few statements that must be made regarding the patient who has progressed to the point of clonic and tonic *convulsions*. Eclampsia has become quite a rare disorder, except in areas where much of the prenatal care still is inadequate. The initial convulsion may appear before labor, during labor, or in the puerperium (usually within 24 hours after delivery) and is followed by a varying period of coma. Other convulsions may follow at irregular intervals, with or without recovery of consciousness after each attack. Rarely, prolonged coma and death occur after a single seizure.

The typical patient with eclampsia will exhibit severe hypertension, rapid and stertorous respiration, pronounced proteinuria, hematuria, urinary casts, oliguria or anuria, and massive edema. Patients dying of eclampsia exhibit extensive *pulmonary edema*. Occasionally death occurs suddenly from cerebral hemorrhage.

Postmorten examination reveals characteristic lesions in the liver, kidneys, brain, lungs, and heart. Most of the lesions are small necrotic, hemorrhagic areas surrounding thrombosed arterioles. The arterioles may be occluded by fibrin plugs produced when excessive amounts of thromboplastin are released into the circulation.

It appears that the typical lesion of eclampsia is an arteriolitis in precapillary arterioles, probably provoked by vasospasm. Damage to vascular walls leads to local necrosis and hemorrhage. Support for this viewpoint has been provided by observations of functioning vessels in the retina, conjunctiva, and fingernail bed.

Differential diagnosis. A convulsion in a pregnant woman is not always indicative of eclampsia. The eclamptic seizure may be stimulated by epilepsy, hysteria, brain tumor, encephalitis, uremia, or certain chemical poisonings.

Treatment. Although most authorities advise prompt termination of pregnancy in a woman with fulminating preeclampsia, the superimposition of a convulsion usually calls for the institution of a fairly complicated program of medical management. Whether this attitude is justifiable is a debatable matter, but unfortunately there are no modern statistics to support or refute the suggestion that prompt delivery may be desirable for the eclamptic patient who is seen during or immediately after the initial seizure. To be sure, the results of cesarean section for eclampsia were poor in the early years of this century. It cannot be said, however, that they would be poor today with suitable anesthesia, sedation, and control of shock and infection. Since the advent of a convulsion is not always correlated with the clinical severity of preeclampsia, it is at least theoretically illogical to condemn operative delivery in eclampsia and advise it for fulminating preeclampsia.

Medical management has at least four broad objectives:
1. Sedation to prevent further convulsive seizures
2. Promotion of diuresis to decrease generalized edema
3. Alleviation of generalized vasospasm
4. Correction of hemoconcentration

Morphine and magnesium sulfate have been widely used to depress the central nervous system, but there are certain physiologic objections to the use of these agents, and they have been replaced very largely by barbiturates.

Magnesium sulfate, which is believed to block neuromuscular transmission by altering the metabolism of acetylcholine, has been given both intravenously and intramuscularly to control convulsions. It is presumed also to lower the blood pressure by reducing vascular reactivity and tone. Various dosage schedules have been recommended, but arguments persist in the current literature as to what regimen is best. Overdosage must be guarded against by observing urinary output (at least 100 ml. in 4 hours), respiratory rate, and presence of patellar knee-jerk reflex.

A popular dosage scheme is 4 grams of magnesium sulfate in 20% solution injected intravenously in about 4 minutes. Then 10 grams in 50% solution are injected deeply into each buttock. If convulsions do not cease in 15 minutes, a second 4-gram dose is given. Every 4 hours 5 grams of magnesium sulfate in 50% solution are injected into alternate buttocks if urinary output, respiratory rate, and patellar reflexes are satisfactory. This program is continued for 1 day after delivery, which is effected as soon as possible after control of convulsions. A similar regimen is advocated by some for severe preeclampsia with intense headache, considerable hyperreflexia, and epigastric pain.

Many other drugs have been used to control hypertension, particularly protoveratrine, hydralazine (Apresoline), reserpine, and methyldopa hydrochloride (Aldomet). No single agent is universally acknowledged by obstetricians to be both useful and safe, and persons who have had no experience in the use of such drugs should obtain appropriate consultation.

Sodium amobarbital (Sodium Amytal) or thiopental sodium (Pentothal Sodium) may be given intravenously and sodium phenobarbital intramuscularly. Dilantin may be used as a specific anticonvulsant.

Dextrose solutions given intravenously (5% to 20% in distilled water, never in saline solution) provide calories and may promote diuresis, but extreme care must be taken not to administer excessive fluid to a patient with inadequate kidney function.

To prevent aspiration of vomitus during a convulsion or during anesthesia at delivery, nothing is given orally. A mouth gag to prevent injury to the tongue and a tracheotomy set should be at the bedside. An indwelling catheter is desirable for accurate determination of urinary output.

Diuretic agents, such as hydrochlorothiazide, may be given intravenously every 6 hours if there is considerable edema. These drugs usually enhance the action of hypotensive agents. Mercurial diuretics should be avoided because of their toxic effects.

Blood pressure may be lowered by conduction anesthesia (continuous catheter caudal, or lumbar epidural).

The administration of oxygen and digitalis may be beneficial in selected patients.

The practitioner is referred to the larger standard obstetric texts for full details of therapeutic plans for the conservative handling of eclampsia.

Delivery. When convulsions and coma have been absent for a day or more, it is wise as a rule to effect delivery. Some eclamptic patients of course will go into labor spontaneously and deliver during the course of medical therapy. The others eventually are delivered vaginally or by cesarean section, depending on whether the cervix is favorable for induction of labor with amniotomy and oxytocin. Regional anesthesia, such as pudendal block, is preferable for vaginal delivery. Spinal anesthesia is undesirable because it may cause severe hypotension. If cesarean section is to be done, local, epidural, or caudal anesthesia may be instituted initially and thiopental added after the fetus has been removed.

Obviously eclamptic patients require diligent postdelivery care, involving control of blood pressure, irritability, and renal excretion. Rapid improvement is the rule, and medications may be reduced in amount or discontinued over 48 to 96 hours. Transient exacerbation about the third postpartum day is not uncommon.

Prognosis. Maternal mortality from *eclampsia* probably is around 10% to 15% in the United States, and fetal mortality approaches 50%. Maternal mortality may be much higher (approximately 35%) in the most severe form of eclampsia, with many convulsions, persisting coma, fever, and greatly elevated pulse and respiratory rates. Anuria and pulmonary edema are grave signs, and if cerebral hemorrhage occurs, the outcome is likely to be fatal. It is difficult to predict the course of events in each patient. Some severely ill patients may recover; others with seemingly mild eclampsia may exhibit rapid progression of the disease and die.

ULTIMATE PROGNOSIS FOR PATIENTS WITH ECLAMPSIA

Patients with eclampsia usually recover promptly after delivery, with return of normal blood pressure and disappearance of proteinuria and edema. The best available evidence suggests that eclampsia in the first pregnancy does not cause chronic hypertension. The remote mortality in these patients is the same as in unselected women. The remote mortality in multiparous eclamptics is considerably greater, but undoubtedly many of these women had antecedent hypertension.

With suitable prenatal care, the chance of eclampsia reappearing in a subsequent pregnancy is extremely small. However, 25% to 30% of eclamptic patients will show some variety of hypertensive disease in subsequent pregnancies. There is no evidence that waiting several years between pregnancies is beneficial, particularly because increased age and weight are unfavorable factors in pregnancy. Likewise, about one third of all women who have suffered from preeclampsia will have a repetition of edema and proteinuria, but seldom does the disease recur in its severe form. Long-term follow-up of women who had eclampsia in the first pregnancy shows that the prevalence of hypertension is not increased over that in unselected women matched for age and race.

HYPERTENSIVE DISEASE WITH AND WITHOUT PREECLAMPSIA

A considerable number of women with chronic hypertensive vascular disease or essential hypertension become pregnant. As would be expected, many of these women are in the older age group and are multiparas, and quite a few are also obese. Other than hypertension, signs and symptoms are not remarkable unless the vascular disease is far advanced. As pregnancy advances into the second trimester, some hypertensive patients show a *fall* in blood pressure.

Hypertensive disease may be associated with the production of small infants, and occasionally placental infarcts are present to explain the inadequate fetal nutrition. Abruptio placentae is common, occurring in the last few weeks of pregnancy in about 3% to 4% of these patients. It is desirable to deliver these patients, if feasible, somewhat ahead of the expected date of confinement to avoid late fetal death in utero from placental abruption.

In recent years improved care of the hypertensive pregnant

woman has resulted in a sharp reduction of fetal mortality. A British study shows a fetal loss of 8%, whereas 20 years earlier a comparable figure in the same area was 32%.

At least 15% and possibly more of hypertensive gravidas will suffer in the last trimester from superimposed preeclampsia. The onset may be gradual, but often it is fairly rapid, with appearance of edema, pronounced proteinuria, oliguria, nitrogenous retention, retinal exudates, and hemorrhages. Blood pressure assumes a higher level, 30 mm. Hg or more above its previous value. At this point the problem becomes that of treating preeclampsia (see previous discussion). In this group of patients fetal loss has been about 50%.

When a woman with chronic hypertensive disease develops preeclampsia, she is very likely to repeat the performance in a subsequent pregnancy. Such patients should be advised against attempting further pregnancies. Those who become pregnant despite such advice must be seen at very frequent intervals, and interruption of pregnancy should be effected as soon as adverse signs and symptoms appear. Impaired renal function and cardiac failure must be anticipated. When therapeutic abortion is necessary because of hypertensive vascular disease, some form of surgical sterilization also is indicated.

Pregnancy should be discouraged in women with essential hypertension and, in addition, one of the following:

1. Two or more episodes of preeclampsia
2. Untreated diastolic blood pressure of 110 mm. Hg or higher
3. Organ involvement (enlarged heart, retinopathy, previous cerebrovascular accident)
4. Renal involvement with proteinuria

22

Medical and surgical disorders complicating pregnancy

Any disease observed in nonpregnant women may be contracted during pregnancy or may exist prior to conception. Thus the list of disorders with which pregnancy may coexist is enormously long, but only the more common problems are mentioned here. It is important to know whether a particular disease is likely to be made worse by pregnancy, and whether the disease may jeopardize the pregnancy. Answers to these questions obviously will determine the desirability of terminating the pregnancy. When a disease exists before pregnancy and pregnancy is contraindicated, some reliable form of contraception should be provided. Unfortunately, contraception often is overlooked by physicians not fully conversant with reproductive physiology, or patients may ignore advice that is given rather casually.

ACUTE INFECTIOUS DISEASES
Rubella (German measles)

Women who have rubella in the first or second trimester of pregnancy often give birth to infants with malformations, particularly cataracts, microcephaly, cardiac lesions, and deaf-mutism. In addition, retarded intrauterine growth, abortion, premature delivery, fetal and neonatal death, and mental retardation have been reported. Early embryonic processes are injured by rubella virus in about 50%, 25%, and 10% of patients in the first, second, and third months of pregnancy, respectively. When the infection occurs as late as the fourth month, the incidence of fetal defects is only about 4%.

An unequivocal clinical diagnosis of rubella cannot be made easily, but one should determine immediately after *exposure* whether the pregnant woman is susceptible or immune. The hemagglutination inhibition test (HAI) for antibodies against rubella virus can be done promptly in most localities. If an initial test, done within a few days after exposure, is positive, it is likely that immunity exists as a result of past infection. When the first test is negative, a second specimen taken 2 to 4 weeks later should show a significant antibody titer if the mother has been infected (even though her infection was clinically inapparent).

If the antibody test is negative and the mother presumably susceptible, the question arises whether to give immune serum globulin. Because this material may abort clinical symptoms without preventing viremia, it probably should not be used routinely but reserved for women who would not consider therapeutic abortion if frank rubella should develop during the first trimester.

Vaccination of the pregnant woman is contraindicated, but a woman with a negative HAI test may be vaccinated if there is assurance that she will not become pregnant for at least 2 months. All pregnant women should be tested for rubella antibodies at the first prenatal visit. If a question of exposure to rubella arises in a woman with a negative test, seroconversion from a negative to a positive test within a few weeks indicates recent infection and raises the question of termination of the pregnancy.

It has been recommended that rubella-susceptible women be vaccinated immediately post partum, while still in the hospital. Effective contraception must be provided, of course, to prevent fetal infection in a subsequent pregnancy that might otherwise appear within a few months. Transplacental passage of live, attenuated rubella-vaccine virus has been demonstrated in abortion specimens.

Rubella virus may persist in the fetus throughout pregnancy; infants with the congenital rubella syndrome may excrete virus and thus are contagious. Nurses caring for such infants have contracted rubella.

Measles (rubeola)

Most women are immune to measles, and therefore this disease is rare during pregnancy. It may cause abortion or premature labor, and the disease may be transmitted to the fetus.

Pregnant women who have not had measles in childhood and who are intimately exposed to the virus probably should receive prophylactic gamma globulin. It is obviously desirable to avoid the numerous complications and difficulties attendant upon the hospitalization and delivery of a woman with florid measles. Women who have never had measles and who are contemplating pregnancy probably should receive measles vaccine. The teratogenic effect of measles virus appears to be very slight.

Chickenpox (varicella)

Though varicella is rare in women of childbearing age, there are reports of serious fetal deformities after contracting maternal varicella in the first trimester. Skin, bone, and muscle defects and chorioretinitis and hydrocephalus have been noted, as well as growth retardation. Pregnant women exposed to varicella should avoid other pregnant women and infants during the potential incubation period of 2 to 3 weeks. It is not established that gamma globulin given to a pregnant varicellar woman will prevent or modify the disease in the fetus.

Influenza

Influenza is a serious complication of pregnancy, particularly when pneumonia develops. Abortion and premature labor may occur, but there is no conclusive evidence that the influenza virus produces congenital anomalies. Recent pandemics of Asian influenza have produced many maternal deaths. Because the incidence rate for the disease appears to be higher in pregnant women, they should be protected with influenza vaccines.

Smallpox

Vaccination has made smallpox extremely rare. Abortion and premature labor are common when the disease is severe. The baby may or may not contract smallpox in utero. Primary vaccination for smallpox should be avoided during pregnancy lest it produce generalized vaccinia of the fetus and lead to abortion. Revaccination (within 10 years) during pregnancy is permissible.

Mumps (epidemic parotitis)

Mumps rarely complicates pregnancy, but it has been reported to cause abortion or premature labor, or even fetal death, if infection occurs late in pregnancy. Microcephaly and hepatomegaly have been seen in children whose mothers had mumps during pregnancy, but the teratogenic effects of mumps virus are not well established. Hyperimmune mumps gamma globulin may be useful for both prophylaxis and amelioration of symptoms.

Gonorrhea

Acute gonorrheal infections acquired during pregnancy usually are limited to the lower genital tract. Salpingitis is unlikely to occur after the third month, when the chorion laeve fuses with the parietal decidua to obliterate the endometrial cavity. Asymptomatic infections may involve lower genital tract, lower urinary tract, and rectum. If untreated, these may lead to infection of the sexual partner, gonorrheal ophthalmia in the infant at the time of delivery, salpingitis after delivery, and gonococcal arthritis. Gonococci should be identified by culture of material from the endocervix and lower anal canal.

Penicillin is the treatment of choice in most instances, and there are various regimens for administering it either intramuscularly or orally. Erythromycin, tetracycline, and kanamycin are useful in women sensitive to penicillin. Kanamycin has no effect on *Treponema pallidum* and thus does not alter the course of syphilis.

Herpesvirus hominis infections

Herpes simplex virus, type II, produces herpetic ulcers of the external genitalia, vagina, and cervix. Intranuclear inclusion bodies may be seen in smears stained by the Papanicolaou method. The virus spreads to the fetus usually by direct contact in the genital tract during delivery. Because the virus may be lethal in the newborn, cesarean section is advisable whenever the mother has had a genital infection within 3 weeks of rupture of the membranes or labor.

Typhoid fever

Despite improved water supplies and increased public health activities, typhoid fever remains a menace in some localities. The typhoid bacilli are known to be transmitted through the placenta to the fetus. This accounts for the high incidence of fetal deaths and consequent abortion or premature labor.

CHRONIC INFECTIOUS DISEASES
Pulmonary tuberculosis

Pregnancy does not exert a harmful effect on pulmonary tuberculosis. Transmission to the fetus through a tuberculous placenta is possible but extremely rare. Babies of tuberculous mothers should be removed at birth from the infectious environment.

Treatment. The ultimate outcome for the tuberculous pregnant woman depends on the stage of the tuberculosis and the application of modern methods of treatment with streptomycin, para-aminosalicylic acid, and isoniazid, just as in the nonpregnant patient. Pneumothorax and thoracic operations are not contraindicated. Some authorities still believe that therapeutic abortion is justifiable, but most of them limit their indications to first-stage tuberculosis and pregnancies in the first trimester.

Women with active tuberculosis should avoid pregnancy. Contraception should be practiced until the tuberculosis has been inactive for at least 2 years. A program of skin testing and chest x-ray examinations should be established for all prenatal patients to detect unsuspected disease, and possible reactivation of treated tuberculosis must be anticipated by diligent examination in subsequent pregnancies.

Syphilis

Modern methods of detecting and treating syphilis have sharply reduced the incidence of congenital syphilis, once a major cause of perinatal mortality, but the problem is by no means solved. Untreated syphilis contracted prior to pregnancy often causes midtrimester abortion after fetal death in utero. Syphilis acquired at the time of conception or early in pregnancy tends to produce premature delivery of a fetus with congenital syphilis. Maternal infection contracted in the second half of pregnancy may or may not be transmitted to the fetus.

Diagnosis. Because more than three fourths of known syphilitic pregnant women do not show clinical evidence of the disease, its positive diagnosis can only be made by the serologic Wassermann test (or one of its modifications). This is a sufficient argument for the application of the test to all pregnant women. Although syphilitic lesions are infrequently found in pregnant women, when they do appear they have a tendency to become more extensive; for example, ulcerations, particularly in the pelvic region, may be larger and deeper and condylomas more widespread than in nonpregnant women. Material from such lesions should be searched for *Treponema pallidum* by microscopic dark-field techniques.

Every pregnant woman should have a serum test for syphilis at the first prenatal visit. Those with positive tests should have additional laboratory studies (such as the *Treponema pallidum* immobilization test and fluorescent treponemal antibody-absorption test) and should be seen by an expert in the management of syphilis. Though there are numerous explanations for false positive tests, in the interests of the fetus such serologic results must be explored thoroughly in order to reach a valid decision for or against therapy.

Treatment. Some form of penicillin G administered intramuscularly is used as a rule. There are numerous treatment schemes requiring 8 to 9 days for completion. Erythromycin administered orally has been used for patients sensitive to penicillin.

A successfully treated mother may be susceptible to a subsequent syphilitic infection. It is important, therefore, to treat the sexual partner and to observe the gravida closely for evidence of reinfection. Occasionally a pregnant woman known to have been exposed to infectious syphilis does not develop stigmas of the disease, or they are so minimal they escape notice. In such instances it is unwise, from the standpoint of the fetus, to procrastinate about therapy until clinical or laboratory evidence appears.

Those who have received adequate antisyphilitic treatment prior to pregnancy need not be retreated if serologic tests are negative and if no clinical or serologic relapse develops. When in doubt, retreatment should be carried out for the sake of the fetus.

The serologic status of the infant should be determined at birth, but a positive blood test does not prove that the infant is syphilitic. If the mother's serum test for syphilis is positive at delivery, the newborn's test also will be positive. Potentially syphilitic infants must be followed carefully with serial serum tests for 4 to 6 months. A rising titer indicates congenital syphilis and treatment should be started with penicillin G.

Malaria

Even in malarial areas malaria is not usually a serious complication in pregnancy. Only the most virulent types of the disease ever cause abortion or premature labor. About 10% of the offspring of infected women have plasmodia in their cord blood. The parasites are not transmitted through breast milk. Malarial relapses are common in pregnancy and in the puerperium. Pregnancy is not a contraindication to the use of any of the common antimalarial drugs. However, some of the newer agents have anti–folic acid activity and may provoke megaloblastic anemia.

Listeriosis

Maternal listeriosis is said to be a cause of abortion in some parts of the world. The term fetus may be infected transplacentally or by organisms in the lower genital tract of the mother.

In the mother listeriosis is associated with vaginitis, urinary tract infection, enteritis, and meningitis. *Listeria monocytogenes* may be identified by culture or by complement fixation test, and the organisms are sensitive to erythromycin, penicillin, and tetracycline.

Toxoplasmosis

Toxoplasmosis is a protozoal disease that may cause repeated abortion. Infected term infants may be stillborn or may exhibit a pathognomonic tetrad of chorioretinitis, cerebral calcification, hydrocephalus or microcephaly, and psychomotor disturbances. The infected mother usually presents no recognizable sign of the disease, and it has never been reported in siblings.

Current or previous infection may be demonstrated by a positive intradermal toxoplasmin skin test. Various serologic tests are used to demonstrate active toxoplasmosis. There is no very satisfactory treatment, but sulfadiazine and pyrimethamine have been advocated.

IMMUNIZATION DURING PREGNANCY

The relatively large number of vaccines now available has created much confusion regarding their use in pregnant women. Live virus vaccines should not be given except when susceptibility and exposure are highly probable and the disease to be prevented poses a greater threat than vaccination to the woman or her fetus. Susceptibility may be established by a reliable history or, if available, by serologic testing. During pregnancy it is preferable to reduce exposure than to vaccinate with live virus, and travel in areas endemic for plague, yellow fever, or smallpox should be forbidden unless the woman has been vaccinated previously. Obvious sanitary precautions may decrease the likelihood of exposure to typhoid, cholera, and hepatitis.

Pregnancy may alter the complication rate in certain infectious diseases. With tetanus, the high morbidity and mortality (60%) do not change during pregnancy. Tetanus toxoid is indicated for pregnant women whose immunity has been allowed to lapse. The mortality from smallpox, however, is significantly higher (up to 90%) in pregnant women, and the paralysis of poliomyelitis is said to occur more frequently during pregnancy.

In each instance the physician must assess the vaccine he plans to use, determining its effectiveness and its potential for complicating pregnancy. Current information and advice may be obtained from the U.S. Public Health Service's Center for Disease Control, Immunization Branch, Atlanta, Georgia 30333.

HEART DISEASE IN PREGNANCY

The heart has an extra load during gestation because of the many factors that create extra work for it. The increased circulatory activity is demonstrated by increases in cardiac output, blood volume, pulse rate, and venous pressure in the lower extremities. Concurrently, blood viscosity, circulation time, and arteriovenous oxygen difference are diminished. The normal heart compensates for all these demands, but if it is damaged, insufficiency may develop. Unless pregnant women with heart murmurs have a history of myocardial insufficiency or have decompensation, they usually endure pregnancy and labor very well. The incidence of valvular heart disease in pregnant women is 1% or 2%. Congenital lesions account for about 10% of the total number.

Diagnosis. In normal pregnancy systolic heart murmurs that are functional are quite common, and accentuated respiratory effort may be mistaken for dyspnea. The standard criteria for the diagnosis of heart disease are (1) a diastolic, presystolic, or continuous murmur; (2) cardiac enlargement; (3) loud systolic murmur, especially if associated with a thrill; and (4) severe arrhythmia.

Prognosis. The prognosis in such patients is much better than has been generally supposed, especially when the patient is carefully watched throughout pregnancy.

Decompensation accounts for nearly three fourths of the deaths, most of them occurring during pregnancy and increasing as gestation advances, particularly after the seventh month. Mendelson reported a maternal death rate of 15% in 137 patients with heart failure. These facts and the not infrequent favorable results from the modern treatment of heart failure again emphasize that many lives can be saved by early diagnosis and treatment.

The pregnancy does not alter the pathologic condition in the heart. The effect is only deleterious to the heart muscle by virtue of the overload. It may be said in general that the prognosis depends on the following:

1. The character of the lesion
2. The presence or history of cardiac embarrassment or decompensation
3. The care with which the patient is observed
4. The earliest possible detection of beginning failure
5. Prompt and thorough treatment of the slightest evidence of decompensation

Although modern knowledge of heart disease has added materially to the more successful management of the patient with a damaged heart in pregnancy, there still is insufficient knowledge to measure accurately the ability of the heart to carry the extra load of pregnancy.

Functional classification of organic heart disease

It will be impossible in the limited space of this synopsis to give the details of the classification of organic heart disease. The reader is referred to works on the heart for complete data. (Only headings are given here.)

Class 1—Patients with cardiac disease who have no limitation of physical activity.

Class 2—Slight limitation of physical activity. Ordinary exercise may produce palpitation, dyspnea, and anginal pain.

Class 3—Considerable limitation of activity. Less than ordinary exercise produces symptoms.

Class 4—Unable to undertake any physical activity without discomfort. There are symptoms of insufficiency even at rest.

This classification gives an approximate estimate of the prognosis and helps in determining the treatment in each group.

Treatment. One must recognize at once that no classification can, unerringly, demark one group from its nearest neighbor. Some overlapping is inevitable. However, it offers a good working basis for determining treatment. The essential requirements in all groups consist of more frequent prenatal visits, constant watchful attendance during labor, immediate digitalization at the earliest evidence of heart distress, and immediate delivery when medication fails, if circumstances permit.

Class 1

Treatment of class 1 patients is chiefly prophylactic against possible decompensation.

1. More watchful prenatal care than usual is necessary; infections should be treated promptly and specifically.

2. Observation should be redoubled during the latter weeks of gestation. Even these patients with mild heart disease should be hospitalized for observation during the last week before the expected time of delivery.

3. Adequate rest is required—10 hours at night and a half hour after each meal.

4. Spontaneous delivery is the rule. Forceps delivery, after complete dilatation of the cervix, may be used to relieve the strain of the second stage of labor.

5. Therapeutic abortion or cesarean section is not indicated.

Class 2

1. Treatment is essentially the same as in class 1.

2. The patient should enter the hospital 2 weeks before the expected delivery because of the greater likelihood of decompensation.

3. Heart medication is more often needed.

4. Since labor and its sequelae may stir up a transient bacteremia, prophlyactic antibiotic therapy should be given during labor and in the early puerperium to prevent endocarditis.

5. Local or regional anesthesia is preferable, and oxygen should be given freely during labor and in the early puerperium.

6. It is desirable for the patient to remain in the hospital for a week after delivery and to be assured adequate rest at home thereafter. Women who have shown little or no distress during pregnancy or labor sometimes collapse after delivery. Postpartum hemorrhage, puerperal infection, and thromboembolism may be very serious complications in a patient with heart disease. Postpartum tubal sterilization should be delayed at least a few days, until it is obvious that the patient is afebrile, not anemic, and able to undertake limited exercise. Those who are not sterilized should be given explicit contraceptive advice.

Class 3

1. The patient should spend 1 day of every week in bed.

2. If failure develops during pregnancy, the patient must remain in the hospital throughout the rest of the pregnancy.

3. Since decompensation will occur in about one third of these patients, therapeutic abortion may be given some consideration if carried out in the first trimester. The decision to abort is made only after thorough investigation of the patient's total life situation. Women who have had cardiac failure in a previous pregnancy are likely to decompensate again and probably should be aborted if surgical treatment of the lesion is not feasible.

Operation for mitral stenosis is advised for women with progressive disability in the first half of pregnancy and for those who progressed from class 2 to class 3 in a previous pregnancy.

4. Vaginal delivery always is desirable.

Class 4

In the event of decompensation, any form of delivery is associated with a mortality of about 50%. Therefore, the physician's entire attention must be directed toward correction of the cardiac failure. After reversion to a class 3 status, most of these patients can be delivered vaginally.

The length of labor is believed by many to be shortened, but there is insufficient evidence to support or deny this.

Congenital heart disease

In general, women with noncyanotic congenital defects and low pulmonary artery pressures do quite well under good management. Women with cyanosis have a high maternal mortality as well as a high rate of fetal and perinatal loss. Those with tetralogy of Fallot and Ebstein's anomaly are in an intermediate position, perhaps because they do not have pulmonary hypertension. About 2% of infants born to women with congenital heart disease have congenital cardiac defects themselves (about six times the usual incidence).

Bacterial endocarditis

Although this disorder may occur during pregnancy, it is more likely to appear in the puerperium. Hence, at the time of either abortion or delivery the patient with rheumatic heart disease should be given prophylactic antibiotics. Endocarditis should be considered in any cardiac patient with fever.

When the disease appears during pregnancy, medical treatment produces results about as favorable as those in nonpregnant women.

Heart surgery and pregnancy

Pregnancy is becoming rather commonplace in women who have undergone heart surgery. These operations should be done prior to childbearing, although corrective surgery can usually be performed with no increased maternal risk during the first trimester. However, the fetal loss rate has been about 33% when surgery is undertaken during pregnancy.

In a woman with an adequate mitral valvuloplasty the risk of pregnancy is minimal, and the temporary hemodynamic burden does not adversely affect long-term prognosis. All valvuloplasty patients should be given prophylactic protection against bacterial endocarditis at the time of delivery. In most patients with valve prostheses the risks of pregnancy are low, but complications related to malfunction of a valve and to anticoagulants have been reported.

Heparin should be used for anticoagulation late in pregnancy because it does not cross the placental barrier, as do the lower molecular weight oral anticoagulants. The latter should be discontinued 4 to 8 weeks before delivery, to allow the fetus to correct its prothrombin deficiency before the trauma of labor. Oral anticoagulants are believed to be potentially teratogenic during the first 8 weeks of pregnancy.

A patient who has had total correction of a congenital defect before developing pulmonary hypertension or myocardial deterioration can go through pregnancy without difficulty. In instances of only partial correction, prognosis for both mother and fetus depends on the severity of the residual hemodynamic abnormality. Antibiotic prophylaxis against bacterial endocarditis at delivery should be provided to most patients who have had operations for congenital lesions, particularly after repairs with synthetic patches, grafts, prostheses, or homografts.

There is at least one report of successful term pregnancy after a coronary bypass operation. No increase in maternal or fetal risk has been noted in women with permanent artificial pacemakers.

OTHER CIRCULATORY PROBLEMS
Phlebitis and phlebothrombosis

Phlebitis and phlebothrombosis are rare in pregnancy, but they may be serious because of the danger of embolism. Anticoagulant therapy has been used successfully without the production of postpartum hemorrhage, but its status is debatable. Thromboses in superficial varicose veins of the leg are common and rarely serious.

Varicosities and hemorrhoids

Varicosities from interference of the return circulation from the lower extremities are common and often distressing. Relief usually occurs after the use of elastic stocking, cotton elastic bandage, or support by adhesive plaster. They may be cured by injection or operative treatment. Vein stripping may be done between the fourth and seventh month of pregnancy. Operation during pregnancy should be limited to women with incompetent veins before onset of pregnancy and those with previous phlebitis and severe sequelae. Although complete eradication of incompetent veins requires more time and diligence in pregnant than in nonpregnant patients, small incompetent varices or perforators are less likely to be overlooked during pregnancy.

Varicosities of the vulva and vagina sometimes rupture, followed by dangerous hemorrhage. Active treatment is not wise, but considerable comfort may be derived from a soft perineal pad held lightly by a T-bandage.

Hemorrhoids are very common, annoying, and progressive during pregnancy. Palliative bland ointments and heat may give considerable relief. Hemorrhoidectomy should be done if bleeding is persistent, but unless the situation is fairly extreme, it is wise to defer operative therapy until after delivery.

Pulmonary embolism

Despite varicose veins, hypercoagulability, and increased venous pressure in the lower extremities during pregnancy, pulmonary embolism is uncommon. When embolism does occur, it is usually massive, and autopsy often shows evidence of prior embolism that had not been suspected. Pulmonary embolism, however, occurs in a large percentage of those patients with overt thrombophlebitis, and it is a major cause of maternal death. In addition to routine diagnostic procedures, radioactive isotope lung scans and pulmonary angiography often are helpful.

Protection against further embolization during the remainder of the pregnancy and postpartum should be provided by anticoagulant therapy and venous interruption. Coumarin derivatives cross the placenta, and numerous instances of fetal death have been reported. Though heparin is safer for the fetus, its prolonged administration beyond 10 to 14 days is difficult. Venous interruption should be done by ligating or placing a Teflon clip on the inferior vena cava just below the level of the right renal vein. If a pelvic source of embolism is suspected, the ovarian veins also must be ligated.

BLOOD DISEASES IN PREGNANCY
Anemia

The definition of anemia is somewhat arbitrary, but in the main it may be said that anemia exists in a nonpregnant woman whose hemoglobin is less than 12 grams per 100 ml, and in a pregnant woman with a hemoglobin value below 10 grams per 100 ml. The mean value in healthy pregnant women in mid-pregnancy is 11.5 grams, and at term it is somewhat over 12 grams. The lowering of hemoglobin levels during pregnancy in women who are not deficient in iron or folate is attributable to a relatively greater expansion of plasma volume compared to the increase in hemoglobin mass and volume of red cells. The frequency of anemia during pregnancy depends on whether supplemental iron is taken.

Iron-deficiency anemia is the commonest variety. The maternal need for iron created by pregnancy is about 800 mg., with 300 mg. committed to the fetus and placenta and 500 mg. to expand the maternal hemoglobin mass. Since this amount usually exceeds available iron stores, iron-deficiency anemia will develop unless exogenous iron is absorbed from the gastro-intestinal tract during pregnancy. Many women begin pregnancy with low iron reserves resulting from loss in previous pregnancies, menstruation, diet poor in iron, and other sources of chronic blood loss. The fetal demands for iron then produce a true anemia (depletion of reserve iron) that may appear first at varying stages of gestation. The erythrocytes are usually normocytic and slightly hypochromic. Serum iron is below 60 μg per 100 ml. Treatment consists of 1 gram of ferrous sulfate daily divided into three doses to promote maximal absorption. Iron may be given intramuscularly when oral iron is not tolerated or absorbed. Transfusion of blood is not an efficient or particularly safe means of supplying iron.

Anemia from acute loss of blood may be associated with abortion, ruptured tubal pregnancy, placenta previa, abruptio placentae, or postpartum hemorrhage. After correction of serious hypovolemia, the residual anemia should be treated with iron rather than with further transfusions.

Anemia with chronic infection has normocytic or slightly microcytic erythrocytes. The serum iron concentration is decreased and serum iron-binding capacity is not much below the normal nonpregnant range. There is decreased erythropoiesis coupled with slightly increased destruction of red cells. This form of anemia is refractory to treatment with iron, but it is advisable to give iron and folic acid to offset any deficiency induced by pregnancy.

Megaloblastic anemia (macrocytic anemia, or pernicious anemia of pregnancy) is the result of a deficiency of folic acid. The symptoms are anorexia, nausea, vomiting, mental depression, and diarrhea. The hemoglobin may drop to extremely low levels in severe cases, yet the fetus usually is not adversely affected. Spontaneous remissions occur after delivery. History of malnutrition or chronic infection is common. Bone marrow biopsy establishes the diagnosis (abnormal megaloblasts), and serum iron values are high. Treatment consists of folic acid, 15 mg. per day, plus iron. Megaloblastic anemia caused by lack of vitamin B_{12} during pregnancy is very rare. There is no reason to withhold folic acid during pregnancy lest one cause neurologic lesions in women with unrecognized Addisonian pernicious anemia.

Aplastic or hypoplastic anemia is a rare but grave complication of pregnancy. The bone marrow is noticeably hypocellular, and there is usually thrombocytopenia and leukopenia. The major risks are hemorrhage because of thrombocytopenia, and infection. Termination of pregnancy may sometimes result in remission.

Thalassemia is characterized by moderate reduction in hemoglobin, hypochromia, and microcytosis. In *beta thalassemia minor* the synthesis of the beta chains of globin is impaired and the A_2 hemoglobin fraction is elevated. This disorder results from the combination of an abnormal autosomal gene from one parent and a normal allelic gene from the other. The homozygous condition, *beta thalassemia major* (Cooley's anemia), is usually fatal during childhood. There is no specific therapy for thalassemia minor during pregnancy and the outcome usually is satisfactory. Iron and folic acid may be of value.

Sickle cell disease is a group of genetically determined blood disorders in which abnormal types of hemoglobin occur, such as hemoglobin S and hemoglobin C, and is seen predominantly in persons of Negroid descent. About 9% of American Negroes show the sickle cell trait (hemoglobin pattern S-A), but less than 1% have true sickle cell anemia with hemoglobin pattern S-S, lifelong anemia, and repeated crises of abdominal and bone pain. Bone pain crises may occur in the nonpregnant but are more frequent in pregnancy, particularly during the last trimester, during labor, and in the puerperium. Marrow embolism may develop during a bone pain crisis, and fat droplets can be identified in the circulating blood.

The structural intricacies and great numbers of hemoglobin variants discovered in recent years have made the consideration of hemoglobinopathies a complex subject beyond the understanding of the average physician. Likewise, there is as yet very little objective information on which to base conclusions regarding the maternal and fetal effects resulting from abnormal hemoglobin syndromes. With the availability of hemoglobin electrophoresis it became necessary to discard much of the information on sickling diseases in pregnancy and redefine the complications associated with SS disease, SC disease, CC disease, and the thalassemia syndromes. Recent studies suggest that the highest rates of maternal complications and reproductive wastage occur with hemoglobin SS disease and AC disease and are associated with a sharp increase in urinary tract infection during pregnancy.

Leukemia

Leukemia occurs infrequently and may or may not be made worse by gestation. Chemotherapy should be avoided in early pregnancy because the effective drugs have abortifacient and teratogenic properties. Radiation of liver or spleen is feasible if the uterus is shielded, but radioisotopes must be avoided during pregnancy. No authentic case of transmission of leukemia to the fetus has been reported.

Thrombocytopenic purpura

Thrombocytopenic purpura is not seriously modified by pregnancy, and postpartum hemorrhage, contrary to expectation, has not been the rule. Splenectomy may be done even during pregnancy. Cortisone may be helpful.

Hodgkin's disease

There is no evidence that pregnancy makes Hodgkin's disease worse. There is some evidence of transmission from mother to fetus. Roentgentherapy may be used if the fetus is adequately shielded. However, extensive radiologic diagnostic studies and intensive radiation therapy to wide areas are potentially very hazardous to the fetus, and thus it is usually desirable to interrupt an early pregnancy prior to such treatment.

DISEASES OF URINARY SYSTEM
Acute glomerulonephritis

This disorder is characterized by the sudden appearance of hematuria, edema, and hypertension in a previously normal person, usually from infection with a strain of group A streptococcus. It is extremely rare in pregnancy and treatment is the same as in the nonpregnant patient. If symptoms persist more than 2 weeks, termination of pregnancy may be advisable. Women with healed acute hemorrhagic nephritis may safely undertake additional pregnancies.

Chronic glomerulonephritis

This produces progressive destruction of renal glomeruli, and eventually symptoms of renal insufficiency and hypertensive cardiovascular disease. The patient with mild chronic glomerulonephritis in an inactive form may tolerate pregnancy satisfactorily. In those patients with more marked degrees of nephritis, renal function usually becomes worse as pregnancy advances, and for these women therapeutic abortion and sterilization should be considered. In each patient the situation should be evaluated by an internist with special training in renal physiology.

Patients with proteinuria as their only manifestation of chronic nephritis generally tolerate pregnancy well. This is not true with hypertension over 160/100 mm. Hg. Interruption of pregnancy is indicated when nitrogen retention supervenes, but major surgical procedures may be hazardous when the non-protein nitrogen level is above 75 mg.%. In such instances it may be preferable to continue hospitalization and hope that abortion will occur spontaneously. Renal dialysis is reported to be helpful in this situation.

A rare form of chronic renal disease, the *nephrotic syndrome,* is occasionally seen during pregnancy and may be confused with preeclampsia because it is associated with edema and massive proteinuria. Most women with this disorder can be carried successfully through pregnancy, but infections and thromboembolic phenomena are common.

Pyelonephritis

Infections of the urinary tract are very frequent during pregnancy. The predominant organism is *Escherichia coli,* but staphylococci, streptococci and *Proteus vulgaris* are not uncommon. Bacteriuria without symptoms may be demonstrated in 1% to 2% of pregnant women, and 6% to 8% of all prenatal patients are likely to have significant bacteriuria (at least 100,000 colonies per milliliter) during pregnancy or early in the puerperium. Bacteriologic screening of urine is mandatory for all women with a history of urinary tract infection, instrumentation of the urinary tract, or symptoms of infection, however minimal. In this way inapparent bacteriuria may be discovered and treated before it leads to severe acute pyelonephritis in late pregnancy or to chronic pyelonephritis in later life.

Acute urinary tract infection during pregnancy usually is a characteristic event involving urinary frequency and urgency, dysuria, chills, fever, backache, and tenderness over the involved kidney. Diagnosis is confirmed by demonstration of leukocytes and bacteria in the urine and identification of the bacteria in urine cultures. The distinction between pyelonephritis and appendicitis occasionally is difficult to make; salpingitis and cholecystitis also should be considered in the differential diagnosis.

Treatment

1. Oral sulfonamides or nitrofurantoin usually are sufficient for the minimal infections in ambulatory patients.

2. Acutely ill patients should be hospitalized to receive appropriate antibiotics, parenteral fluids, and analgesics. Tetra-

cyline should be avoided because it may produce yellow deciduous teeth in the infant.

3. Ureteral catheterization may be required to establish drainage in a kinked ureter. Nephrostomy rarely is necessary to salvage the kidney.

FOLLOW-UP CARE. Every patient with pyelonephritis during pregnancy must be observed until all evidences of urinary tract disease have been eliminated. At least one intravenous pyelogram should be obtained, preferably after involution of the tract postpartum, to uncover or exclude any organic lesion. Recurrence of pyelonephritis in subsequent pregnancies is common.

Chronic pyelonephritis of long standing, with symptoms of renal insufficiency, usually is not improved by antimicrobial therapy. One may need to terminate pregnancy to prevent further irreversible damage to the kidneys. As in other chronic progressive renal disorders, maternal and fetal prognosis depends on the extent of renal destruction. With expert care, fetal viability may be achieved.

Polycystic disease of the kidney

If the disease has not progressed to hypertension, proteinuria, and azotemia, the prognosis is good. With normal renal function and mild hypertension, pregnancy poses the same risk it does in women with other varieties of chronic hypertension.

Renal and ureteral calculi

Renal lithiasis is more common in pregnancy than at other times because of urinary tract stasis and hypercalciuria resulting from ingestion of extra calcium and vitamin D. Small stones enter the ureter and cause characteristic symptoms during their passage to the bladder. Retrograde manipulation with a catheter may dislodge the stone and encourage it to pass into the bladder. If pain persists and progressive hydronephrosis develops, the stone must be removed by extraperitoneal ureterolithotomy.

Pregnancy after nephrectomy

Pregnancy after nephrectomy is usually uneventful unless the remaining kidney cannot carry the extra load, especially when toxemia or renal infection develops; then the pregnancy may need to be terminated. Diligent prenatal care is necessary to detect any renal inefficiency early.

Acute tubular necrosis

This is the major cause of acute renal failure during pregnancy. It results from ischemia after severe blood loss, sudden intravascular hemolysis, severe sepsis, or combinations of these problems, most of which are preventable. Renal function usually returns to normal after healing occurs, and thus future pregnancies are not contraindicated.

Renal cortical necrosis

Renal cortical necrosis is rare and usually occurs after septic abortion, abruptio placentae, or severe toxemia. Oliguria or complete anuria develops, and the general picture is that of acute renal failure.

Pregnancy after renal transplantation

In general, pregnancy should be deferred for at least 1 year after successful transplantation of a kidney from a living relative and for 2 years after a cadaver transplant. Stable renal function is a prerequisite for conception. Unless the graft has descended into the true pelvis, vaginal delivery is feasible. The immuno-suppressive agents used in these patients are potentially teratogenic, but low doses of azathioprine and corticosteroids thus far appear not to have been harmful. The risk of maternal infection obviously is increased in this group of patients. Renal transplantation has created a new group of high-risk pregnancies offering many challenges to the perinatologist. Though the transplant patient is one who has been ill for years, a successful pregnancy in such a woman may be a gratifying emotional experience for both patient and physician.

DISEASES OF DIGESTIVE TRACT AND LIVER
Dental caries

There is no evidence that pregnancy causes or aggravates dental caries or that caries may be avoided by adding extra calcium to the diet. Routine dental care is advisable during pregnancy as at all other times.

Heartburn, (pyrosis, acid stomach)

Heartburn or pyrosis often is very annoying in pregnancy. It appears to be associated with a feeble gastroesophageal sphincter that does not respond to increased intragastric and intra-abdominal pressure, and reflux of gastric contents into the esophagus occurs.

Antacids containing aluminum or magnesium hydroxide may be helpful. Some patients are improved by the use of neostigmine hydrobromide, 15 mg every 4 to 8 hours orally, which presumably increases peristalsis and prevents reflux of gastric secretions into the esophagus.

Gastric (peptic) ulcer

Gastric or peptic ulcer is very uncommon in pregnancy, but vomiting of pregnancy may aggravate the lesion. Exacerbation may occur in the puerperium because of the stresses of motherhood. Medical treatment is the same as in the nonpregnant woman.

Appendicitis

Inflammation of the appendix occurs about once in 2,000 pregnancies. Diagnosis is more difficult during gestation because of the enlarged uterus and the higher position of the appendix. Pregnancy should not affect the decision to operate. Abortion is rare unless the appendix is ruptured. Hypoxia and hypotension must be avoided during operation. Other than local tenderness, a recent abdominal scar is not a problem during labor and vaginal delivery. Mortality from appendicitis in the pregnant woman is essentially that associated with surgical delay.

Intestinal obstruction

Mechanical intestinal obstruction is rare, but when it does occur, immediate operation is indicated. Usually it is related to previous abdominal surgery. The enlarging uterus displaces intestines sufficiently to stretch adhesions; other causes of obstruction are volvulus, intussusception, or incarceration of intestinal loop in a hernia.

Paralytic (adynamic) ileus, another cause of intestinal obstruction, occurs in mild form for a few days after normal delivery and particularly after cesarean section. It may occur also with severe pyelonephritis or with any situation that leads to infection or hemorrhage in the peritoneal cavity.

Gallstones and cholecystitis

Progressive symptoms of gallstones may render operation necessary, but if feasible, it should be postponed until a reasonable time after delivery. During advanced pregnancy only cholelithotomy may be feasible, deferring cholecystectomy to a later date.

Severe cholecystitis and choledocholithiasis are rather uncommon in pregnancy despite the propensity of women to develop gallstones. Symptomatic relief may be obtained with meperidine and atropine.

Pregnancy seems to favor formation of gallstones by providing increased cholesterol for excretion into bile, as well as atony and delayed emptying time of the gallbladder. Biliary colic may be less frequent in pregnancy because the duct is atonic, and a stone may pass along to the intestine within a few days.

Acute infectious (viral) hepatitis

Acute infectious hepatitis, a viral disease, is not uncommon in pregnant women, but it does not differ from hepatitis in the nonpregnant women. Abortion and premature labor occur occasionally. Apparently congenital malformations in the fetus are not associated with the virus of hepatitis. Most hepatitis is the result of ingesting contaminated food or water, but *serum jaundice* (long-incubation hepatitis) occasionally is seen in pregnant women 2 to 4 months after infusion of blood or plasma containing the virus. It is uncertain whether the infectious agents causing viral hepatitis, such as Australia antigen, cross the placenta and reach the fetus. However, hepatitis transmitted from mother to fetus has been reported.

Other causes of jaundice. *Recurrent cholestatic jaundice of pregnancy* is a benign disorder of the last trimester characterized by severe itching and elevation of serum alkaline phosphatase. It clears soon after delivery but recurs in about half of subsequent pregnancies. The mild cholestasis may be related to high levels of certain steroids produced in pregnancy. Premature labor is common.

Obstetric acute fatty liver (obstetric acute yellow atrophy), usually seen only during the last 6 weeks of gestation, is accompanied by severe vomiting, epigastric pain, and intense jaundice. Stillbirth is common, and the mother may expire from hypoglycemia, hemorrhage, or superimposed infection. Whenever feasible, labor should be induced.

Ulcerative colitis

When pregnancy and active ulcerative colitis coincide, more than half the patients have a sharp exacerbation during pregnancy and after delivery. The onset of colitis during pregnancy often is disastrous. Therapeutic abortion may be desirable in fulminating colitis resistant to all treatment.

Regional enteritis (Crohn's disease)

This disorder is not adversely affected by pregnancy. The risk of abortion, premature labor, stillbirth, and congenital anomaly is not increased. In a survey of married women with Crohn's disease, about one third were sterile.

Spontaneous rupture of the liver

This produces upper abdominal pain and signs of hemorrhagic shock. About 75% of patients with this problem have preeclampsia or eclampsia. Management consists of treatment of shock, control of hepatic bleeding from the large hematoma beneath Glisson's capsule, and termination of pregnancy.

NEUROLOGIC DISEASES

Only those few neurologic diseases that have some particular relation to childbearing are discussed.

Neuritis

Polyneuritis of pregnancy, from lack of thiamine, occurs occasionally with pernicious vomiting or chronic alcoholism in early pregnancy.

Traumatic neuritis is rare, but it may occur after injury to the sacral plexus in difficult deliveries.

Neuralgia

Neuralgic pains, though common, are usually not serious, but sometimes they are quite intractable.

Brachialgia statica dysesthetica is a numbness and tingling of fingers of both hands, with temporary local anesthesia. It is believed to be caused by the stretch on the brachial plexus resulting from abnormal droop of the shoulders, and some women complain of this during each pregnancy.

Epilepsy

Convulsions during pregnancy always make one think of eclampsia; therefore, the differential diagnosis is very important. The history of previous attacks and the presence or absence of the characteristics of eclampsia will clear any confusion. Treatment of epilepsy is the same as in nonpregnant women. Although the attacks are often made worse by pregnancy, therapeutic abortion is seldom necessary.

Several reports have shown that the incidence of congenital malformations among the infants of epileptic mothers is two to three times higher than usual, and this has been attributed to the use of anticonvulsant drugs. The increased incidence of cleft lip and cleft palate has been particularly striking.

Multiple sclerosis

Multiple sclerosis is a rare complication that usually is not affected by pregnancy and seldom is an indication for therapeutic abortion. Some of these patients have relatively painless labors. Although in some cases the condition seems to be aggravated by pregnancy, even in nonpregnant women multiple sclerosis is characterized by numerous exacerbations and remissions.

Poliomyelitis

Pregnant women appear to be slightly more susceptible to poliomyelitis than nonpregnant women. When the disease begins in the first trimester, abortion is common (40%), but the incidence of fetal death is much less when the mother is afflicted in the second or third trimester.

Vaginal delivery usually is possible. Cesarean section is

indicated for patients with severe bulbar-spinal complications requiring respirators and tracheotomy.

Paralytic poliomyelitis may occur in the infant, but only when the mother has had the disease near term and was delivered shortly after the onset of the infection.

Pregnant women should be vaccinated against poliomyelitis or, if already protected, may have their immunity increased by a booster dose. Oral live poliovirus vaccine (Sabin) and also the Salk vaccine appear to be safe for both the mother and the fetus.

MENTAL ILLNESS IN PREGNANCY
Simple emotional problems

Pregnancy, labor, and the puerperium may place severe strain on the patient's emotional stability. Numerous superstitions and bits of misinformation may emerge, and the physician must be willing to listen effectively, supply facts as needed, and repeatedly provide reassurance to both the patient and the husband. The prophylactic approach to emotional problems in pregnancy is the subject of a vast current literature, but this sort of material is not easily condensed to fit a synopsis. The student is referred to the larger textbooks and to the many small books intended for the patient and her husband. In most communities there are prenatal classes sponsored by civic or hospital groups or by private physicians to foster discussion of antenatal and postnatal problems.

Psychosis in pregnancy

Psychosis requiring psychiatric consultation occurs in about 0.2% of pregnant and puerperal women. Somewhat more than half the psychotic episodes occur in the first 2 weeks after delivery. Pregnancy itself does not cause psychosis unless the patient is in some way predisposed to a psychotic response to a stressful situation.

Whether therapeutic abortion is helpful in selected instances of mental illness is a highly controversial issue. Decisions in this realm are not likely to be entirely meaningful until much more is known about the causation of mental disorders. Suicidal threats are commonplace among women with unwanted pregnancies, but the incidence of successful suicide is notably low.

Puerperal psychosis, or postpartum psychiatric syndrome, appears to have a psychologic rather than physiologic basis. It consists largely of feelings of shame, confusion, and helplessness, and may appear even after adoption of an infant. The usual precipitating factor seems to be conflict in assuming the mothering role, and may arise out of the patient's ambivalent identification with her own mother, who failed to serve as an adequate model.

About half the patients show features of schizophrenia, and 40% are manic-depressive. Psychotic episodes often are repeated in successive pregnancies. Prophylactic psychotherapy is indicated for those who show major personality problems early in pregnancy.

METABOLIC DISORDERS
Thyroid diseases

Hypothyroidism. The precise relationship of thyroid hypofunction to the maintenance of pregnancy is not fully understood. If there are adequate medical grounds for a diagnosis of hypothyroidism and if therapy with thyroid substance has been established, treatment probably should be continued throughout the pregnancy. Thyroid hormone replacement should be complete, but there is no need to increase the usual dose, since the daily hormonal utilization is not increased during pregnancy. If dessicated thyroid or one of the synthetic mixtures is prescribed, the free thyroxine index can be used to evaluate the adequacy of replacement.

Pregnancy is rare in myxedematous women, and the incidence of spontaneous abortion is increased in the presence of hypothyroidism. Theoretically, hypothyroidism should improve in pregnancy, and fetal goiters should occur when maternal function is greatly depressed.

Colloid goiter. Simple colloid goiter, if unassociated with hypothyroidism, has no effect on pregnancy.

Hyperthyroidism. Because the symptoms of this disorder—nervousness, emotional instability, intolerance to heat, tachycardia, and thyroid enlargement—are common findings in normal pregnancy, the diagnosis depends largely on laboratory tests. The most reliable procedure is measurement of the free serum thyroxine concentration. The presence of ophthalmopathy, pretibial myxedema, and positive test for long-acting thyroid stimulator (LATS) imply Graves' disease.

Treatment of thyrotoxicosis in pregnancy should control maternal disease without endangering the fetus. The use of radioiodine therefore is contraindicated. Propylthiouracil or methimazole (antithyroid drugs) are relatively safe, but the maternal free thyroxine concentration should be kept in the high normal range, and one must be alert to the development of leukopenia.

Preparation for surgical management (subtotal thyroidectomy) includes a short course of antithyroid drugs and administration of iodide for about 10 days. Hypothyroidism after operation is common and should be anticipated and promptly treated.

Inheritance of thyroid diseases is well established. The possibility of thyroid dysfunction in the newborn may be suggested by the free thyroxine index of cord blood at birth. Women with Graves' disease may produce infants with thyrotoxicosis because long-acting thyroid stimulator crosses the placenta. Its activity persists for an appreciable time in the newborn.

Adrenal disorders

Addison's disease is uncommon in pregnancy. If hyperemesis does not occur, women with Addison's disease do well while pregnant, but they may require special supportive therapy during labor and in the immediate puerperium.

Adrenocortical hyperfunction (Cushing's disease) associated with pregnancy is extremely rare, as is pheochromocytoma (medullary hyperfunction).

A few cases of pregnancy in women treated for *congenital adrenogenital syndrome* have been reported and more may be expected as girls who have been treated with cortisone enter the childbearing age. Thus far no teratogenic effects of steroids have been seen in newborn infants. It is estimated that a treated patient has a 1 : 100 to 1 : 200 chance of producing an infant with adrenocortical hyperplasia, which is related to an autosomal recessive gene.

Diabetes mellitus and pregnancy

Before the availability of insulin, the combination of pregnancy and diabetes often precipitated diabetic acidosis and coma, and the fetal wastage from abortion or stillbirth was enormous. Though insulin has reduced the maternal mortality rate to a level similar to that for nondiabetics, and though juvenile diabetics now become fertile adults, excessive perinatal mortality is still a major problem.

Metabolic abnormalities peculiar to diabetes may occur many years before the onset of clinical symptomatology. This state of prediabetes can be converted into clinical diabetes by certain stresses, one of which is pregnancy. Thus the class A diabetic is a patient who develops an abnormal glucose-tolerance curve for the first time during pregnancy and whose offspring are subjected to metabolic abnormalities that increase fetal and neonatal mortality. The obstetrician may discover patients destined to develop diabetes by screening with an appropriate test all prenatal patients with (1) glycosuria, (2) familial diabetes, (3) previous stillbirth, (4) infants over 9 pounds at birth, (5) habitual abortion, or (6) excessive obesity.

White's classification of obstetric patients with diabetes is helpful in comparing various groups of patients with respect to prognosis and response to treatment. Briefly, the classification is as follows:

A. Patients requiring no insulin and minimal dietary control

B. Disease began in adult life; duration under 10 years; no vascular disease

C. Disease of long duration; onset between the ages of 10 and 19 years; some vascular disease

D. Diabetes over 20 years' duration; disease began before 10 years of age; considerable vascular disease, with retinitis and proteinuria

E. Patients with radiologic evidence of calcified pelvic arteries

F. Patients with nephritis

Glycosuria is easily detected with Tes-Tape or Clinistix, which are specific for glucose. A positive reaction is not attributable to pentosuria, fructosuria, or lactosuria, which is seen often in late pregnancy and during lactation. Patients with glycosuria should have as a screening procedure a blood sugar determination 2 hours after ingestion of 100 grams of glucose. Those with abnormal tests should have a standard glucose tolerance test. Many class A diabetic patients are detected in this manner.

A normal glucose tolerance test early in pregnancy is no assurance that the same patient will react normally closer to term.

Influence of diabetes upon pregnancy

1. Abortions, premature labors, and intrauterine and neonatal deaths occur in approximately one fourth of all diabetic pregnancies.

2. Preeclampsia or eclampsia occurs four or five times more often than in pregnant nondiabetic patients.

3. Excessive-sized infants are common, resulting in mechanical difficulties in labor and often necessitating cesarean section.

4. Hydramnios and congenital malformations are common.

5. Fetal hypoglycemia and anoxia are common in the neonatal period.

Influence of pregnancy upon diabetic patient

1. There is enlargement of the islets of Langerhans and hyperinsulinemia in normal pregnancy but decreased ability of peripheral tissues to use insulin (possibly a response to excess growth hormone). However, increasing amounts of exogenous insulin are required by the patient who cannot elevate her own natural output of insulin, for example, the juvenile diabetic.

2. A few diabetic patients require less insulin than usual during pregnancy; the reason for this is not known.

3. Vomiting in the first trimester interferes with dietary regulation and promotes acidosis.

4. The activity of labor may deplete glycogen reserves.

5. Puerperal hypoglycemia may be anticipated.

6. Puerperal infection of any sort may result in acidosis and coma rather quickly.

Treatment. Diabetic patients require extremely close supervision during pregnancy by an obstetrician and internist. Visits should be made every 2 weeks in the first two trimesters and weekly thereafter. Fractional urines should be tested frequently for glucose, acetone, and albumin. *The diabetes must be rigidly controlled* by diet and insulin.

Frequent hospitalization may be needed for regulation of diabetes, treatment of infections, weight reduction, and finally for the careful planning that precedes delivery.

About 3 or 4 weeks before the calculated date of delivery,

induction of labor may be considered to circumvent the possibility of intrauterine fetal death as term approaches. If the cervix is favorable and the infant is estimated to weigh 3,000 grams or more, membrane rupture and oxytocin infusion may be undertaken. Before inducing labor it is wise to obtain radiologic evidence of fetal age (distal femoral epiphyses usually visible at 37 weeks) and of an adequate maternal pelvis.

If early vaginal delivery is not feasible, cesarean section should be considered when one or more of the following are present:

1. Manifest diabetes, classes B to F, known to exist before pregnancy, with or without retinal and renal evidence of degenerative phenomena

2. Preeclampsia or hypertension

3. Inability to maintain good control of the diabetes

4. An excessively large fetus

5. Any valid obstetric indication for section

When prompt delivery does not seem urgent, watchful waiting is practiced until conditions are suitable for vaginal delivery or until an indication for cesarean section appears.

Adequate pediatric care for the newborn infant of a diabetic mother is essential, and arrangements for this should be made well in advance of delivery. Hypoglycemia and hypoxia require special attention, and this is best obtained by giving these infants the type of care usually provided for premature babies.

Prognosis. With proper care and full cooperation of the patient, maternal death attributable to obstetric factors should be preventable. Perinatal mortality may be reduced to 10% in frank diabetic patients by diligent attention to the details of maternal and fetal management; it may be as low as 5% for the prediabetic group.

Diabetic patients in classes E and F should be discouraged from attempting pregnancy. The fetal loss in these women has been very great, and those with severe renal disease may require therapeutic abortion as a lifesaving measure.

MISCELLANEOUS CONDITIONS
Pruritus and dermatoses

Either abdominal or generalized pruritus distresses some pregnant women and interferes with sleep. The usual treatment is local application of antihistaminic drugs and the use of sedatives if necessary.

Papular dermatitis of pregnancy is an itchy, generalized eruption of crusted erythematous papules. It clears rapidly after delivery, and treatment is symptomatic.

Molluscum fibrosum gravidarum resembles skin tags. The lesions appear on the sides of the neck, on the upper chest, and beneath the breasts. They usually disappear a few months post partum.

Herpes gestationis is peculiar to pregnancy and is manifested by vesicular, bullous, and pustular lesions that are intensely itchy and cover extensive areas. It usually but not invariably disappears soon after delivery and may recur in another pregnancy. Treatment with adrenocortical steroids has been advised, but occasionally therapeutic abortion may be indicated.

Disseminated lupus erythematosus

Women with systemic lupus without renal disease or hypertension may undertake pregnancy during remission without undue risk. Most patients in remission at the beginning of pregnancy remain so through the postpartum period. Exacerbations occur most often after delivery. Although it appears desirable for women with disseminated lupus erythematosus to avoid pregnancy, there is some doubt that therapeutic abortion is helpful, although it is often advised.

Breast cancer

Breast cancer frequently is masked by pregnancy changes, and thus the diagnosis may be delayed until the lesion is rather advanced. However, pregnancy does not appear to influence the tumor otherwise, and therapeutic abortion does not improve the prognosis. The treatment most commonly advised is radical mastectomy.

The 5-year survival rate for stage I breast cancer found during pregnancy and treated by radical surgery is about 65%. For stage II tumors the survival rate is less than 10% even with surgery and postoperative radiotherapy.

Drug addiction during pregnancy

Addictive drugs apparently do not greatly impair fertility. Most pregnant addicts use heroin and methadone, sometimes supplemented by barbiturates, tranquilizers, or marijuana. Many patients seek detoxification during pregnancy, but there is a high rate of recidivism, and some mothers have been detoxified two or more times during a single pregnancy.

Women on heroin will quickly develop withdrawal symptoms after delivery (nausea, tremors, abdominal pain, and yawning) and are likely to leave the hospital within the first day unless placed on a methadone detoxification schedule. Obstetrical complications are premature labor, preeclampsia, breech presentation (related to high incidence of premature infants), and short labors. About 70% of infants born of addicted mothers show some evidence of withdrawal symptoms or narcotism. They exhibit irritability, tremors, diarrhea, vomiting, fever, high pitched cries, sneezing, respiratory distress, and hyperreflexia. Congenital anomalies are not increased. An extensive study of pregnancy among women in a methadone maintenance treatment program revealed no serious effects in the neonatal period, provided that no other drugs (alcohol, tranquilizers, hypnotics) were involved.

23

Dystocia caused by
faulty uterine action

Labor is a contest between the forces of expulsion and the resistance of the birth canal. In normal labor the expulsive forces win over natural, ordinary opposition. However, when the contractions are inefficient or when the bony pelvis and soft parts offer unusual resistance, labor becomes difficult and *dystocia* develops. Dystocia literally means "difficult birth" in the sense that there is some sort of mechanical difficulty impeding delivery.

Normal labor is marked by continued progress in either cervical dilatation, fetal descent, or both. Any significant cessation of progress should alert the obstetrician to evaluate the situation and to institute appropriate diagnostic investigation or treatment, or both.

DYSTOCIA CAUSED BY DEFICIENT
FORCES OF EXPULSION

Primary inertia or dysfunction. Primary inertia or dysfunction exists when the contractions are inefficient from the beginning of labor. In other words, there is prolongation of the latent phase of labor (Chapter 10), and some form of therapy may be required to develop the active phase. It is undesirable to set definite time limits for the persistence of uterine dysfunction and to declare arbitrarily that active treatment must be instituted after a specific time has elapsed. Seasoned obstetric judgment is required for the successful management of patients with this problem. Undue prolongation of either the first or second stage of labor results in increased perinatal mortality.

There are two types of uterine activity that result in dysfunction:

1. *Hypertonic* contractions may exhibit reversal of gradient (midsegment stronger than fundus) or asynchronism of impulses starting in cornual areas. Fetal distress may appear.

2. *Hypotonic* contractions exhibit a normal pattern of gradient from the fundus to the cervix but very low amplitude (under 15 mm. Hg). The uterus is indentable even at the peak of the contraction. Fetal distress is uncommon.

Hypertonic contractions occur most often in the latent phase of labor, are painful, and respond poorly to oxytocin. Either expectant management or heavy sedation is recommended. Productive contractions often develop after a short interval of sleep. Hypotonic dysfunction in the latent phase may be indistinguishable from false labor. Either rest with moderately heavy sedation or stimulation of uterine activity with exogenous oxytocin should be initiated. In either variety, the patient should not be allowed to become exhausted or dehydrated.

The recommended method for administering oxytocin is by continuous intravenous drip, 5 units in 1,000 ml. of 5% glucose solution. A screw clamp, dropmeter, or constant infusion pump must be used to regulate the flow. The rate of flow should be adjusted to produce contractions every 2 to 4 minutes, lasting no longer than 60 seconds. Excessive and sustained contractions must be avoided. This is readily accomplished by adhering to the following technique:

1. Start the infusion with dextrose solution alone.

2. Adjust the drip rate to less than 5 drops per minute.

3. Add oxytocin to the dextrose solution in the concentration noted above and *mix thoroughly.*

4. Stand at the bedside and continually monitor the contractions while increasing the drip rate slightly every 10 to 15 minutes until the desired uterine response is achieved.

5. If an undesiredly rapid flow is required to produce appropriate contractions, the concentration of oxytocin may be increased and the drip rate proportionately diminished. The antidiuretic effect of oxytocin occurs at dose levels above 0.045 unit per minute.

Secondary inertia. Secondary inertia occurs when previously normal and effective contractions become infrequent, short, weak, or stop entirely.

The inefficiency of the uterine muscles in inertial dystocia may be caused by the following:

1. Poor tone from overdistention
2. Feto-pelvic disproportion
3. Emotional factors
4. Premature use of analgesics and conduction anesthesia
5. Maternal exhaustion

In most instances, however, the cause of inertia is not apparent. It tends not to be repetitive in subsequent labors.

Treatment. The diagnostic ability of the physician is often severely taxed to determine the cause of the inefficiency.

1. Be certain about the status of the cervix and the fetal position; these should be checked by vaginal examination.

2. Roentgen pelvimetry may disclose pelvic contraction or abnormality of fetal position or presentation. If any of these exists, cesarean section may be required.

3. Membranes may be ruptured artificially if the cervix is at least 4 cm. dilated and the fetal head is in the pelvis.

4. Oxytocin may be used as a stimulant if there is no evidence of feto-pelvic disproportion.

5. *Rest* is the treatment for delayed labor caused by maternal exhaustion or hypertonic dysfunction. Rest means not merely pain relief, but *sleep*.

Morphine (15 mg.) and a sedative will usually ensure sleep, which to be of real value should persist for several hours. The patient awakens refreshed, regular contractions soon recur, and delivery is usually normal. Oxytocin stimulation should be initiated without delay if progressive labor fails to develop.

6. If oxytocin stimulation fails to effect vaginal delivery, cesarean section must be performed. If intrapartum fever exists, massive antibiotic therapy should be started prior to operative delivery. About 5% of women with hypotonic dysfunction will fail to respond to oxytocin. To prevent fetal and possible maternal sepsis, delivery should be effected by whatever means necessary within 24 hours after rupture of membranes in labor.

Extraperitoneal cesarean section used as a device to prevent puerperal peritonitis is no longer widely employed. Similarly, Dührssen's incisions in the partially dilated cervix to permit delivery by forceps are no longer recommended in dysfunctional labor.

Patients requiring treatment for primary or secondary inertia should be treated prophylactically with continuous-drip intravenous oxytocin for several hours postpartum to avoid uterine atony and hemorrhage.

SHORT LABOR CAUSED BY EXCESSIVE CONTRACTIONS

Precipitate labor. Precipitate labor usually follows excessively forceful contractions and minimal resistance from the soft parts. Deep lacerations often occur. Otherwise there is seldom any harm done to the mother, except in the unusual event of amniotic fluid embolism (Chapter 29). But the fetus may suffer from anoxia (frequent, strong contractions), cerebral trauma, or from the consequences of being born unattended.

By definition, a precipitate labor is one that lasts 3 hours or less. About 15% of labors fall into this category.

When this sort of labor is recognized in a hospital, appropriate anesthesia should be instituted and preparations should be made for immediate delivery under controlled conditions. Procrastination on the part of attendants may result in delivery under less than ideal circumstances with unnecessary maternal and fetal trauma.

ANNULAR UTERINE STRICTURES

In obstructed labor, the active fundal portion of the uterus retracts as the passive lower segment balloons increasingly to accommodate the fetal mass. A depressed, contractile ring develops at their juncture and appears to rise as labor progresses. This sign of impending uterine rupture is termed *Bandl's pathologic retraction ring*. It is only seen in neglected labor, and immediate cesarean section is required.

Constriction rings are annular spastic strictures occurring at any level of the uterine wall, most commonly in the lower segment. They do not change position as labor advances, and they are usually associated with ineffective uterine contractions. They are believed to arise as a result of inappropriate oxytocin or manual stimulation and the majority are palpable only on the uterine interior. Amyl nitrite inhalation, intravenous administration of epinephrine, or deep anesthesia may relieve the localized spasm and allow delivery, but, in general, cesarean section is required.

FAILURE OF UTERINE CONTRACTION

Missed labor. In missed labor for some strange reason labor begins and soon stops without proceeding to delivery. The fetus dies and remains unexpelled for weeks, months, or even years, undergoing various kinds of degeneration, and if the membranes are ruptured, putrefaction occurs.

The cause of the inexplicably dormant uterus has never been satisfactorily explained. As soon as the diagnosis is made, the uterus should be emptied.

Missed labor is very rare. Abdominal pregnancy must be considered whenever labor has ceased and the fetus has died.

24

Dystocia caused by abnormal fetal position or development

In some instances dystocia may be attributed to abnormal development of the fetus or to a faulty position or presentation; either or both of these factors interfere with the normal mechanisms of expulsion.

PERSISTENT OCCIPUT POSTERIOR POSITION

The mechanism of labor in posterior positions of the occiput has already been described (Chapter 11). In about 5% of patients rotation of the fetal head fails to occur, particularly in women with anthropoid and android pelves. Inadequate flexion of the head often is associated with persistence of the posterior position. Such persistence is one of the common causes of inertial or protracted labor.

Management. There are two obvious solutions to this problem, after allowing a reasonable time for spontaneous rotation to occur in the second stage.

1. The physician may attempt delivery by forceps in the occiput posterior position, aided by deep mediolateral episiotomy or a midline incision that has deliberately included the anal sphincter and lower anterior rectal wall (episioproctotomy).

2. He may attempt manual rotation. If this fails, as it usually does with a molded head, forceps rotations should be performed with the Kielland instrument, followed by extraction with this or with a more conventional instrument. The Scanzoni rotation maneuver also is widely used (Chapter 31).

Operative rotation is the more popular procedure, although the fetal mortality is about the same in the absence of rotation. Delivery without rotation usually requires more traction over a longer period of time.

Secondary uterine inertia often accompanies the posterior position of the occiput. When inertia is coupled with some degree of cephalopelvic disproportion, labor may be unusually prolonged, and excessive molding of the fetal head may occur. Tentorial tears and intracranial hemorrhage are not uncommon and result in fetal death. Although nearly all infants presenting occipitoposteriorly ultimately can be delivered vaginally, the physician may question the advisability of risking fetal death instead of choosing delivery by cesarean section after a reasonable trial of labor. There are no simple rules to guide the physician in the management of the more bothersome occipitoposterior positions. Radiologic study of the pelvis during labor may be helpful, but the conclusions reached from films touch upon only one facet of the problem. Rupture of the membranes may be salutary and should be performed if the head is engaged. Analgesia should be minimal, and conduction anesthesia, if used, should be started late to avoid initiating secondary inertia. General support of the mother with intravenous infusions of glucose and water must not be overlooked.

BREECH PRESENTATIONS

The incidence of breech presentations is 2.5% to 3.5% of deliveries. If only full-term fetuses are considered, the former figure is more nearly correct for a large series of infants. Breech presentation is more common in multiparas than in primigravidas.

Diagnosis. In diagnosis the same maneuvers and methods are used as in cephalic presentation, but the differential points are as follows:

1. The hard mass of the head is in the fundus uteri.

2. The softer breech is at the pelvic brim (unless engagement exists).

3. The fetal heart tones are at the level of the navel or above.

4. The vaginal or rectal findings are as follows:

(a) A mass softer than the head is felt along with the hard sacrum and tubera ischii.

(b) The buttocks, anus, and external genitalia may be distinguishable by palpation.

(c) It is not always easy to distinguish a breech from a face presentation.

5. Roentgenologic diagnosis should be employed when in doubt.

Types

Complete breech. In the complete breech the feet may be palpable alongside of the buttocks (Fig. 24-1).

Frank breech. In the frank breech no small parts are palpable per vaginam. The legs and thighs are extended with the feet near the face (Fig. 24-2).

Footling. In the footling presentation one foot is prolapsed (Fig. 24-3).

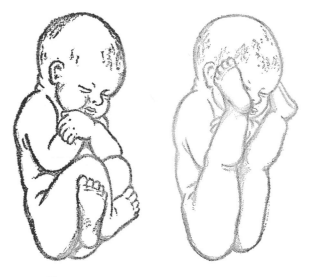

Fig. 24-1   **Fig. 24-2**

Fig. 24-1. Complete (full) breech. (From Beck: Obstetrical practice, Baltimore, The Williams & Wilkins Co.)

Fig. 24-2. Frank breech. Note extended legs and feet near the face. (From Beck: Obstetrical practice, Baltimore, The Williams & Wilkins Co.)

Double footling. In the double footling presentation both feet are prolapsed.

Incomplete foot or knee. One foot or knee presents.

Etiology. Breech presentation is habitual in some women. Various factors are associated with this position and thus are said to interfere with the more common adaptation of the fetal head to the lower uterine segment. Breech position is common with hydramnios, hydrocephalus, placenta previa, prematurity, and partial uterine septa.

Three mechanisms. First of all one must remember that there are

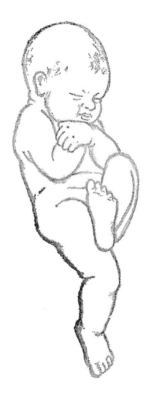

Fig. 24-3. Footling. (From Beck: Obstetrical practice, Baltimore, The Williams & Wilkins Co.)

three successively larger parts of the fetus that must go through all of the various steps of the mechanism: (1) the breech, (2) the shoulders, and (3) the aftercoming head.

Breech mechanism

ENGAGEMENT

1. The anterior hip is directed toward the iliopectineal eminence.

2. The posterior hip is directed toward the sacroiliac articulation.

INTERNAL ROTATION

1. The anterior hip is the lower one.

2. Therefore, it strikes the pelvic floor first and rotates internally to the symphysis pubis.

BIRTH OF BREECH

1. By lateral bending of the body the posterior hip is born over the perineum.

2. Then the anterior hip slips from behind the symphysis.

3. Then the legs and feet are born.

EXTERNAL ROTATION. The back turns forward as the shoulders adjust themselves to the pelvis.

Shoulder mechanism

1. The anterior shoulder rotates internally to the symphysis pubis.

2. The posterior shoulder is born over the perineum (Fig. 24-4).

3. The anterior shoulder now slips from behind the symphysis pubis where it was stemmed.

Aftercoming head mechanism

1. The head engages in the pelvic oblique diameter opposite to that used by the breech and shoulders.

2. The head rotates internally into the anteroposterior pelvic diameter, with the nape of the neck under the symphysis pubis.

3. The chin, mouth, nose, and forehead emerge in order over the perineum.

4. The occiput then slips from behind the symphysis pubis.

5. *Posterior rotation of the head* may occur but happily this is rare.

(a) The abdomen instead of the back is anterior.

(b) The face is under the symphysis.

(c) Birth may take place in two ways:

(1) The infant may be born with the nose behind the sym-

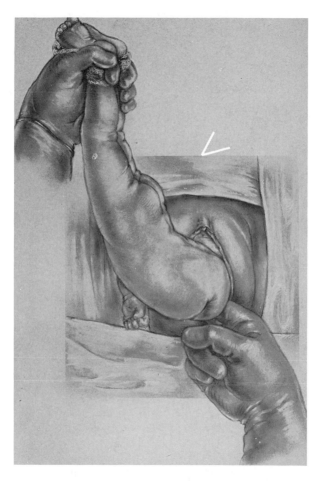

Fig. 24-4. Breech extraction, delivery of the posterior shoulder. Fingers are passed over the shoulder and down along the infant's arm. (From Titus: The management of obstetric difficulties, St. Louis, The C. V. Mosby Co.)

physis and the head flexed; the vertex, bregma, and brow successively are born over the perineum, which is greatly stretched and usually deeply torn.

(2) When the head is extended and the chin is stemmed at the symphysis, the occiput may be brought over the perineum by rotating the exteriorized portion of the fetus over the symphysis onto the maternal abdomen.

Management. There are certain dangers and difficulties that must be kept in mind constantly.

1. The prognosis for the mother as to mortality is good, but lacerations are common.

2. The gross fetal mortality of 12% to 14% is largely the result of associated prematurity. Nonetheless, a fetal mortality three times that of vertex presentation occurs on the basis of the presentation alone and the style of delivery necessitated.

(a) Pressure upon the cord by the body and aftercoming head embarrasses the fetal heart.

(b) Prolapse of the umbilical cord is common with complete or incomplete (one foot down) breech. The presenting part fails to fill the lower uterine segment, and the cord may find its way into the cervical canal and thence to the vagina. Vaginal examination should be performed immediately after spontaneous membrane rupture and frequently thereafter. Regular and preferably constant monitoring of the fetal heart rate also should be instituted.

(c) Cerebral hemorrhage is much more frequent than in cephalic presentation.

3. Conversion to a vertex presentation may be tried late in pregnancy. When engagement exists or the membranes have ruptured, any attempt at conversion is unwise. In early labor the irritability of the uterus renders external version difficult or impossible. Breech presentations tend to recur after conversion.

4. "Watchful expectancy" is the key to successful breech delivery. Let the breech be expelled spontaneously to the umbilicus. Then by the Smellie-Veit-Mauriceau maneuver (Fig. 24-5) complete the delivery of the shoulders and head quickly but deliberately (Chapter 31). It is important that the cervix be fully dilated before attempting any vaginal delivery. This is particularly true when the infant is premature, for the relatively larger head may be trapped by an incompletely dilated cervix.

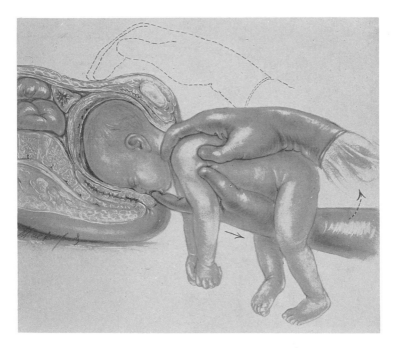

Fig. 24-5. Breech extraction, delivery of the head. The Mauriceau maneuver for delivery of the head. Dotted hand outline shows how the operator's or an assistant's hand may be used for pressure above. (From Titus: The management of obstetric difficulties, St. Louis, The C. V. Mosby Co.)

5. When the usual methods of delivering the head are difficult, the specially designed Piper forceps (or ordinary forceps) for the aftercoming head may be used (Fig. 24-6). This technique has the additional advantage that once the forceps are applied, the mouth of the fetus is usually exposed to the exterior, allowing both bulb aspiration of the oral pharynx and fetal breathing. Time is no longer of the essence once a fetal airway is available. A scrubbed and gowned assistant is mandatory in this circumstance and should be present at every breech delivery.

6. Whatever method of breech delivery is employed, it is wise to do a deep midlateral or midline episiotomy to facilitate the delivery of the shoulders and aftercoming head.

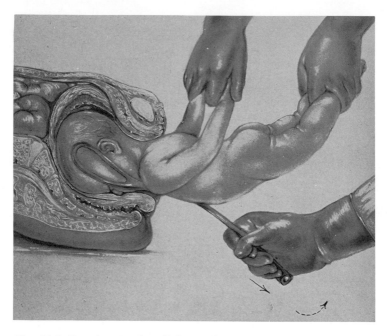

Fig. 24-6. Breech extraction. Delivery of the aftercoming head with the Piper forceps. The arms and legs are held by an assistant. Note how the construction of the forceps facilitates flexion of the head. (From Titus: The management of obstetric difficulties, St. Louis, The C. V. Mosby Co.)

7. Cesarean section is advised in the presence of pelvic contraction, a large fetus, and often for a primigravida over 35 years of age. Obviously this decision must be made before the second stage of labor because there is no possibility of turning back after the breech delivery is in progress. Prenatal x-ray pelvimetry is often employed to facilitate this decision.

FACE PRESENTATIONS

When the head is completely extended, the face presents. It is the most frequent of the various deflections of the head. When deflection is extreme, the birth is usually not very difficult.

1. The chin presents.

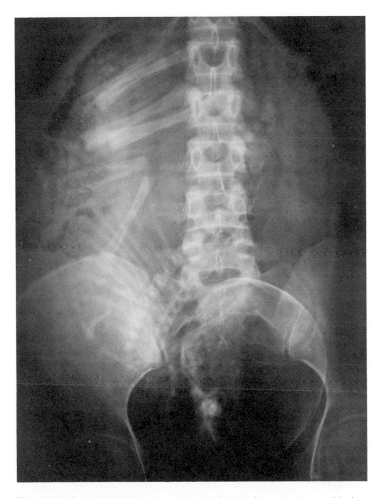

Fig. 24-7. Roentgenologic appearance of term fetus in utero with face presentation. (Courtesy Community X-Ray Division, Stanford University Hospital, Stanford, Calif.)

2. The head is fully extended, with the occiput against the back (Fig. 24-7).

3. The back is not arched as in vertex presentations but has a double curve, with the chest protruding on one side and the lower back on the other.

4. The *incidence* is about 0.3% of labors.

5. Except for such an obvious cause as fetal thyroid tumor, the *etiology* is unknown. It is seen in multiparas, with anencephalic fetuses, and in instances of contracted pelvis.

6. *Engagement* is usually in the right oblique (the longest available) diameter; hence, face presentations are more frequently L.M.A. or R.M.P.

Left mentoanterior positions

Diagnosis. The same methods of examination for left mentoanterior positions are employed as in vertex presentations, but for lack of space only differential points will be mentioned.

1. The chin is pointing to the left iliopectineal eminence.

2. Behind the chin are the mouth, nose, eyes, and orbital ridges.

3. The back is to the right posterior.

4. The chest is left anterior.

5. The fetal small parts are easily palpable at left front.

6. Of utmost importance is finding the distinctive cephalic prominence on the right, the same side as the back. When the head is flexed (L.O.A.), the prominence is always opposite the back.

7. The point of maximum intensity of the fetal heart is on the left because the chest is forced in that direction by extension of the head.

8. Vaginally, the mouth, nose, zygomas, and orbital ridges should be distinguishable. The mouth forms a triangle with the zygomas as opposed to the straight line formed by the anus and ischial tuberosities in breech presentation.

9. Roentgen pelvimetry and fetography should be performed to establish or rule out pelvic contraction or fetal anomaly. In face presentations the incidence of inlet contraction or at least borderline disproportion is about 35%.

Mechanism

1. Full extension is likely not to occur until labor begins, when the force of contractions and the resistance of the pelvic brim complete it.

2. The mechanism is the same as in L.O.A. positions, except that extension exists instead of flexion and the head is born by flexion instead of extension. Otherwise the chin goes through the same mechanism as does the occiput in vertex labors.

3. The head cannot be born unless the chin rotates to the symphysis pubis (Fig. 24-8), therefore:

(a) *Persistent* posterior chin or one rotating to the hollow of the sacrum cannot be born because the neck is not long enough (Fig. 24-9).

(b) *Fortunately, however, 99% of chins directed posteriorly rotate to the front spontaneously or can be artificially rotated.*

4. Birth:

(a) The chin is temporarily stemmed under the symphysis.

(b) Then the head is born by flexion, the chin emerging first and then, in order, the mouth, eyes, orbital ridges, brow, bregma, and the occiput.

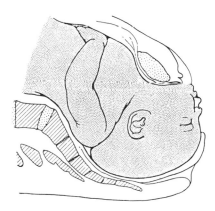

Fig. 24-8. Face presentation, chin rotated anterior. The head will be born by flexion. (Redrawn from Bumm.)

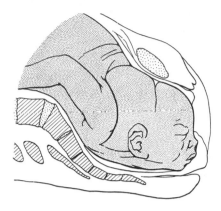

Fig. 24-9. Face presentation, chin rotated posteriorly. Infant cannot be born. Further extension is impossible, and the neck is not long enough to permit birth in this position. (Redrawn from Bumm.)

5. The same factors that produce the caput succedaneum cause swelling and distortion of the face.

Management

1. *Fortunately most face presentations will be born spontaneously if left alone* because the diameters of the head are favorable. The suboccipital-bregmatic diameter (the most favorable of the head diameters) and the trachelobregmatic diameters are very similar and may be shortened by molding.

2. Even when the chin is posterior, it usually rotates to the front.

3. Because of the increased downward push on the pelvic floor prior to flexion of the head, deep lacerations are common unless an extensive episiotomy is employed.

4. Forceps may be used as with vertex deliveries when the chin is anterior. They should be applied to the sides of the face along the occipitomental line.

5. Fetal mortality is increased and is about 14% overall. The mortality for term fetuses is 4% or 5%.

6. Conversion to other presentations may be attempted, but it is not commonly successful and is not recommended. The

methods available subject the fetus and the maternal tissues to excessive risk and undue trauma.

7. When the face is on the pelvic floor and the chin fails to rotate (which will be rare), manual rotation may be attempted.

8. If the chin persists posteriorly, delivery is accomplished by cesarean section.

9. When the fetus is dead and the chin is posterior, cesarean section or perforation and extraction with the cranioclast may be performed.

BROW PRESENTATIONS

Brow presentations (Fig. 24-10) occur when flexion fails and extension is incomplete. Labor is much more difficult than with face presentations because longer diameters of the head are involved in the mechanism of labor. Molding of the fetal head must necessarily be greater and more complications occur unless spontaneous conversion to a face or occipital presentation develops.

1. Brow presentations are rare, occurring only once in 1,500 to 2,000 labors.

2. The head is partially extended, but the forces of labor usually convert it to a face presentation by completing the extension, or less frequently to an occipital presentation with complete flexion.

3. When these conversions fail a "persistent brow" exists.

4. As with face (chin) presentations the most likely positions are left anterior or right posterior.

Diagnosis

1. The abdominal palpatory findings are much the same as those in face presentations but are less definite.

2. The cephalic prominence is on the same side as the back but is less prominent.

3. By vaginal examination the following can be determined:

(a) The large anterior fontanel is palpable.

(b) The frontal suture runs from it toward the face.

(c) The anterior part of the sagittal suture runs toward the occiput.

(d) The coronal suture extends from it laterally in both directions at right angles to the frontal and sagittal sutures.

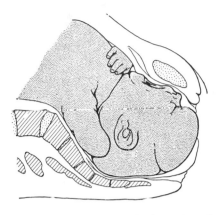

Fig. 24-10. Brow presentation. (Redrawn from Bumm.)

(e) Toward the face only the orbital ridges, eyes, and root of the nose are palpable. The tip of the nose, mouth, and chin are beyond reach.

Mechanism

1. *Engagement* is possible only after extensive molding because the mento-occipital diameter (13.5 cm.) is the largest diameter of the fetal head and usually must be shortened.

2. The brow rotates anteriorly and the head is born by considerable flexion; the brow, sinciput, and occiput emerge in order over the perineum; then the lower face, mouth, and chin slip from under the symphysis pubis.

Management

1. The labor is likely to be prolonged and difficult unless the child is small.

2. Inasmuch as brow presentations early in labor offer the possibility of becoming chin or occipital presentations, the physician may await this event for a reasonable time, or he may attempt conversion.

3. In a primigravida with persistent brow presentation, cesarean section may be the only procedure that will assure a living infant and an unruptured uterus. In a multipara with a large fetus and persistent brow presentation, abdominal delivery

also may be desirable. This recommendation seems particularly valid if the physician agrees with the concept that cephalopelvic disproportion is a factor in the production of the abnormal presentation.

SHOULDER PRESENTATIONS

The diagnosis of shoulder presentation is readily made by abdominal inspection and palpation. Vaginal examination reveals the ribs, scapula, clavicle, axilla, and occasionally a prolapsed hand and arm.

The presumed causes of *transverse lie* are pelvic contraction, placenta previa, prematurity, hydramnios, multiple pregnancy, and a greatly relaxed abdominal wall. It is much more common in multiparas. Cord prolapse occurring after spontaneous membrane rupture is a common complication.

Spontaneous delivery of a full-term infant in a transverse presentation is practically impossible. As the uterine contractions continue, the shoulder becomes firmly impacted in the pelvis; the lower uterine segment is stretched to the point of rupture. In rare instances an infant of moderate size, usually dead, may be delivered spontaneously by a mechanism called *spontaneous evolution*. This consists of shoulder impaction with prolapse of the arm, stretching of the neck to allow emergence of the shoulder under the pubic arch, extreme lateral flexion to bring about delivery of the thorax and breech, and finally spontaneous or manual delivery of the aftercoming head.

Treatment. Transverse lie is best handled by cesarean section. Attempts to convert the fetus to a longitudinal position seldom are successful.

When a patient with transverse lie is first observed with the cervix fully dilated, membranes intact, and the fetus small, internal podalic version and extraction may prove feasible in the hands of an experienced physician. In general, however, cesarean section should be employed freely and early in labor in the majority of patients. Fetal mortality is formidable with any other variety of management. Elective cesarean section prior to labor should be seriously considered in all transverse presentations once the fetus has achieved maturity (Chapter 7).

A neglected transverse lie of an infant with a severely impacted shoulder and intrauterine infection should be treated in a multipara with large doses of antibiotics and cesarean hysterectomy. Decapitation used to be recommended but few modern obstetricians have had any experience with this operation, and the danger of uterine rupture is appreciable.

COMPOUND PRESENTATION

In compound presentation an extremity prolapses alongside the presenting part, and both enter the pelvic canal simultaneously. Most commonly a hand or an arm comes down with the head.

Less commonly one or both lower extremities will prolapse alongside the head, or a hand may prolapse beside a breech. Prolapse of the umbilical cord occurs in about one fourth of compound presentations.

The prolapsed part seldom interferes with labor. If an entire arm is down, it probably should be pushed up while the head is being depressed by fundal pressure. When the cord prolapses, the problem then becomes one of managing the cord abnormality (see discussion at end of chapter).

EXCESSIVE DEVELOPMENT

An infant at birth rarely weighs more than 5,000 grams, although there are well-documented instances of much larger infants having been born through the vagina. It is common practice to designate newborn infants weighing over 4,000 grams as "excessive sized," and about 5% of infants are in this category.

It is unusual for a normal fetus weighing less than 10 pounds (4,500 grams) to cause dystocia in the average pelvis. In overly developed fetuses the harder head may not mold readily, but it is ordinarily the large shoulders that create difficulties.

Excessive development may be attributed to:
1. Maternal diabetes
2. Large size of one or both parents
3. Multiparity of the mother.

The physician must be prepared to estimate the approximate size of the fetus in utero. With a little practice at palpation, combined with attempts to impress the head into the pelvis, the size can be estimated with fair, but inconsistent, accuracy.

Ultrasonography can be of significant value in this estimation and is far superior to manual approximations.

Treatment

1. If gestation has unquestionably gone beyond term, the fetus is unusually large (over 8 pounds—3,600 grams), and the pelvic diameters are normal by x-ray measurement, it is wise to attempt a medicinal induction of labor. Failing in this, another medicinal induction combined with artificial rupture of the membranes may be attempted, provided that the fetal head is engaged and the cervix is soft and dilatable.

2. *Shoulder dystocia,* a frequent problem with large fetuses, may be overcome by applying pressure to the fundus from above, or by rocking the anterior shoulder from side to side through the mother's abdominal wall, with the hope that the shoulders will find a more favorable diameter for descent.

3. A second maneuver (Rubin) to overcome shoulder dystocia is adduction of the more accessible shoulder (usually the posterior), pushing it *toward* the anterior fetal thorax to reduce the transverse diameter of the shoulders. This also turns the fetus on its long axis in such a direction that the opposite shoulder tends to adduct toward the anterior chest wall (Fig. 24-11). By this maneuver 180-degree rotation may allow egress of the shoulder anteriorly. Continuation of this corkscrew maneuver, or reversal, may then allow the opposite shoulder also to be delivered anteriorly.

4. A third maneuver is to attempt to deliver the posterior arm by introducing a hand along the infant's chest, grasping the posterior hand or forcarm, and sweeping it across the chest and anterior shoulder. If successful, 180-degree rotation and repetition of the maneuver will allow delivery. Deep episiotomy, or episioproctotomy, is of great aid.

5. When the baby is dead, cleidotomy is useful in overcoming shoulder dystocia.

6. Cesarean section may be necessary for delivery of a large fetus even after an attempt has been made to deliver vaginally by forceps. Obviously, whenever a fetus is believed to weigh about 9 pounds or possibly more, the very best obstetric judgment must be exercised to decide whether a trial of labor is to be permitted and, if so, when to resort to cesarean section in the event

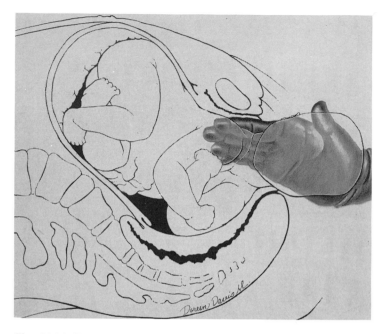

Fig. 24-11. Rubin's adduction maneuver to reduce the transverse diameter of fetal shoulders.

of inadequate progress toward vaginal delivery. Pronounced shoulder dystocia with a huge fetus is something to be avoided.

GROSS FETAL MALFORMATIONS
Double monsters (conjoined twins)

Although congenital anomalies are numerous and may involve virtually every part of the body, relatively few have obstetric significance in the sense that they may complicate the course of pregnancy or create mechanical problems at delivery.

Double monsters vary widely, from those in which two well-developed bodies are separate except for a minor superficial connection to those in which only a small part of the body is duplicated or in which an amorphous mass is attached to the outside of an otherwise normal body.

Twins that are reasonably complete may share in common the following areas of the body: anterior, posterior, cephalic, or caudal. Such twins are called, respectively, *thoracopagus* (xiphopagus), *pygopagus, craniopagus,* or *ischiopagus.* *

Delivery of many monsters is easy because of their small size (rarely full term) and mobility at the point of union. Craniotomy or amputation of the presenting head of a dicephalic monster may be necessary in order to deliver the remainder. Delivery may be less complex when the breech presents, however, as the aftercoming heads often spontaneously engage and deliver successively without difficulty.

Acardius

An acardius is a monster that is usually one of a pair of single-ovum twins, with the other having developed normally. An acardius possesses a rudimentary heart or no heart at all. The monster may have recognizable human form only at one end (acephalus or acormus), or be simply an unrecognizable nodular mass with attached umbilical cord (amorphus).

Anencephalus

An anencephalus is a monster with an imperfectly developed head from which a large part of the brain and skull is absent. Pituitary hypoplasia and hypoadrenalism are regularly seen. Well over 50% of the cases are associated with hydramnios and maternal urinary estriol excretion is invariably low (< 4 mg. per day). Suspicion is aroused by the absence of a well-defined fetal head on abdominal palpation and is confirmed by x-ray examination (Fig. 24-12). Ultrasonography may also be used. Abnormal presentations and shoulder dystocia are common. The deformity is incompatible with life and the majority of these fetuses expire before or during labor. Prolonged gestation occurs commonly when the pregnancy is otherwise uncomplicated.

The incidence of anencephaly appears to vary geographically and is especially high in Ireland and Scotland. In the United States incidence rates in reports from various sectors have ranged

---

*For details of these and numerous other varieties of monsters see Potter, E. L.: Pathology of the fetus and infant, Chicago, Year Book Medical Publishers, Inc.

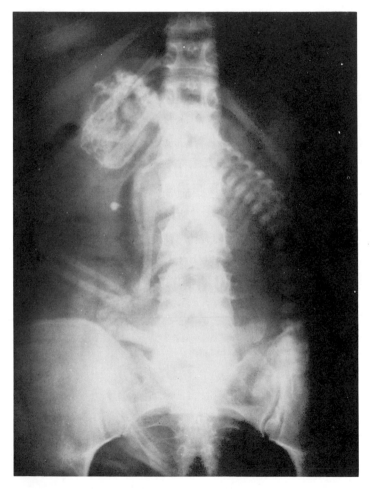

Fig. 24-12. Radiograph of pregnant uterus containing anencephalic fetus. Note absence of cranial portion of the fetal skull.

from 1 in 500 to 1 in 5,000 births. The usual female-to-male ratio is about 3:1. Both genetic and environmental etiologic factors are suspected and the recurrence rate is about 5%.

Attempts may be made to shorten gestation by oxytocin infusion or by the transabdominal drainage of amniotic fluid. The latter is particularly successful if hydramnios is present and the method may be augmented by the intra-amniotic instillation of hypertonic saline.

Early diagnosis of recurrence, with allowance for elective termination of pregnancy prior to 20 weeks of gestation, may be made by ultrasonographic visualization and by detection of elevated alpha-fetoprotein levels in amniotic fluid.

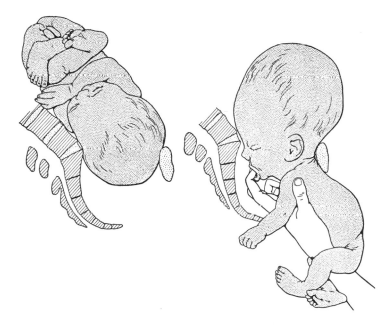

Fig. 24-13. Hydrocephalus, showing forecoming head (left) and aftercoming head (right). In either case, delivery is impossible without perforating the head. (Redrawn from Bumm.)

Hydrocephalus

A hydrocephalic fetus presents a large head with cerebral ventricles grossly distended by cerebrospinal fluid, commonly 500 to 1,500 ml. at term. Serious dystocia is the rule. Associated defects (particularly spina bifida and myelomeningocele) are common and hydramnios is present in about 10% of cases. The incidence is approximately 1 in 2,000 births and the fetal mortality approximates 70%. The cranium is tense, thin, and indentable and reveals widely spaced fontanels. Diagnosis may be confirmed, if necessary, by x-ray or ultrasonographic examination.

Engagement of the head rarely occurs (Fig. 24-13) and craniotomy or drainage by puncture with a spinal needle or trocar either transabdominally or transvaginally is definitely indicated for delivery whether presentation is vertex (two thirds of cases) or breech (one third of cases). The delivery of a presenting breech with obvious spina bifida should instantly alert the obstetrician to the immediate potentiality of hydrocephalus if he has not entertained this diagnosis previously. The head may be decompressed at any point in labor and decompression is probably most advantageous when performed early.

Rupture of the uterus may occur if the condition is unrecognized or labor is prolonged without cephalic decompression. Rarely the hydrocephalic head will burst prior to delivery.

ENLARGEMENT OF FETAL BODY
General dropsy (erythroblastosis)

Occasionally a fetus affected with general dropsy or erythroblastosis is so large that spontaneous delivery is impossible. Extraction of the shoulders and trunk offers most of the difficulty.

Congenital cysts and tumors

Retention of urine causes distention of the abdomen and consequent dystocia. Congenital cystic kidneys sometimes become tumors of great size.

Other rare causes of enlargement of the fetal body include tumors of the abdominal organs, lipomas and angiomas, dermoid cysts and teratomatous tumors about the perineum and sacrum, umbilical hernia, and spina bifida.

If dystocia is conspicuous in any of these conditions, delivery can be accomplished only after opening the fetal body to allow escape of fluid or after removing at least a portion of the offending tumor. Cesarean section is generally the preferred method for delivery if diagnosis antedates attempts at extraction.

PROLAPSE OF UMBILICAL CORD

Prolapse of the umbilical cord (Fig. 24-14) may be caused by any factor that interferes with acute adaptation of the presenting part to the superior strait, for example:

1. Abnormal presentation (breech, shoulder, face, and compound)
2. Multiple pregnancy
3. Premature rupture of the membranes and a small fetus
4. Contracted pelvis
5. Hydramnios

The physician may distinguish between *presentation* and *prolapse* of the cord. When the cord presents, it is merely palpable through the cervix. But when truly prolapsed, a loop protrudes

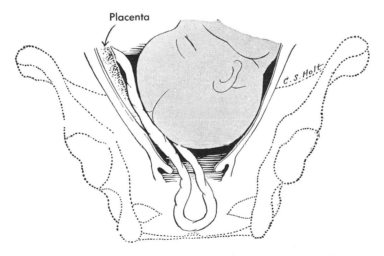

Fig. 24-14. Prolapse of the umbilical cord. Note pressure of head upon the cord, endangering fetal circulation. (From Falls and McLaughlin: Obstetric and gynecologic nursing, St. Louis, The C. V. Mosby Co.)

into the vagina or even beyond the vulva. *Occult prolapse* is the presence of the cord along the side of the presenting part. It may or may not be palpable. The potential clinical result is the same for all; compression of the cord between the presenting part and the bony pelvis. Unless this is effectively counteracted, embarrassment of the fetal circulation may occur, leading ultimately to fetal asphyxia and death. The incidence of prolapsed cord is about 1 in 200 deliveries.

Signs and symptoms. Occasionally the patient may feel the cord slide out over the vulva. More commonly, the cord is felt vaginally by the examining physician. Diagnostic abnormalities of the fetal heart rate develop, which can readily be detected if continuous electronic heart rate monitoring is underway. These may readily be missed, however, and the diagnosis may be made only after fetal death, if only intermittent auditory or Doppler auscultation is employed.

Prognosis. Perinatal mortality is 20% to 30%. Labor is not affected.

Treatment. Treatment depends mainly on the degree of dilatation of the os and to a lesser extent on the presentation of the infant.

If the cord prolapses under the observation of the obstetrician and if the cervix is completely dilated and no obvious disproportion exists, the infant can usually be saved by completing the delivery at once, by forceps if the head is engaged, and in breech presentations by extraction.

If the cervix is only partially dilated, the potential for survival of the infant is reduced. In this case:

1. Place the mother in knee-chest or deep Trendelenburg position at once, and keep the fetal head out of the pelvis with pressure from below per vaginam. Very occasionally the cord may be pushed back into the uterus, but unless the presenting part promptly engages, the cord will prolapse again.

2. While keeping the presenting part out of the pelvis, prepare for immediate cesarean section, but proceed with the operation only if the fetal heart is regular and strong. The risk of cesarean section should not be inflicted on the mother if the fetus is clearly dead.

25

Dystocia caused by contracted pelvis

Significant shortening of one or more of the internal diameters of the bony pelvis is known as pelvic contraction, and this may be associated with pelvic dystocia. Pathologic changes in the structure and dimensions of the pelvis may be congenital, or may be due to malnutrition, injuries, disorders of the spine or hip joints, and tumors. Gross physical defects in the patient, or unusual gait, may suggest the possibility of contracted pelvis. Prolonged labor and difficult delivery in a previous pregnancy may have been the result of unrecognized abnormality of the bony pelvis.

The diagnosis of pelvic contraction usually can be made or suspected by clinical examination of the pelvis, but occasionally radiologic examination is required for confirmation. (The details of pelvic mensuration, or pelvimetry, are given in Chapter 9.) It is customary to consider the spatial diminution as occurring at the inlet of the pelvis, in its midportion at the level of the ischial spines, and at the outlet or level of the ischial tuberosities. Diminished diameters may be demonstrated at one, two, or all three of these levels (Fig. 9-7).

INLET CONTRACTION (PLATYPELLOID PELVIS)

The pelvic inlet is contracted if the anteroposterior diameter is 10 cm. or less or if the greatest transverse diameter is 12 cm. or less. When the diagonal conjugate diameter is less than 11.5 cm., one may assume that the anteroposterior distance is under 10 cm.

Etiology. Anteroposterior inlet contraction may be caused by rickets, spondylolisthesis, or other orthopedic or traumatic abnormalities. The etiology of transverse inlet contractions is less well known. Some pelves are generally small without showing obvious bony abnormalities and are often spoken of as *generally contracted*. Fortunately, for unknown reasons, women with generally contracted pelves tend to have accommodatingly smaller fetuses. Still others exhibit merely an anteroposterior contraction (simple flat pelvis), presumably of congenital origin. Osteomalacia, from severe calcium deficiency, may lead to substantial reduction in pelvic capacity and conversion of a normal gynecoid inlet into a compressed triradiate pattern.

Complications during pregnancy. In extreme degrees of anteroposterior inlet contraction the uterus may be prevented from rising out of the pelvis by the overhanging sacral promontory. Late in pregnancy the contraction may interfere with descent of the fetal head, and the uterine fundus will then remain at its maximum height throughout the last month of gestation. Malpositions of the fetus and prolapse of the umbilical cord are common.

Mechanism of labor. The mechanism of labor and the possibility of spontaneous birth depend chiefly on the degree of contraction, but other factors must be considered, for example, size and hardness of the head, malleability (molding), and the power of the expulsive forces, all of which are factors difficult to determine accurately. Greatest reliance must be placed upon determining the degree of contraction by pelvic measurements.

1. In anteroposterior inlet contraction, the head must enter the flattened pelvis transversely because of the short conjugate and the longer transverse diameter.

2. When the obstetric conjugate is below 9 cm., the biparietal diameter of the normal head (9.25 to 9.5 cm.) cannot enter the pelvis unless there is some compensating mechanism.

3. Entry is accomplished by the following mechanisms:

(a) The head slides laterally so that the smaller bitemporal diameter (8 cm.) is related to the obstetric conjugate.

(b) Uterine contractions force the anterior part of the head into the pelvis, and the back of the head is forced proportionately upward; that is, the head becomes somewhat deflexed. This explains the high incidence of face presentations with inlet contractions.

(c) The small fontanel is felt per vaginam with difficulty, and the large one is felt with unusual ease.

4. Because of the normal anteflexion of the uterus, the *anterior parietal bone usually presents* (anterior asynclitism).

5. The sagittal suture lies transversely and near the sacral promontory.

6. The posterior parietal bone is forced tightly against the promontory, whereas the anterior parietal is forced past the symphysis.

7. After this is accomplished, the posterior parietal bone slides slowly down into the pelvis over the sacral promontory. The sagittal suture gradually moves forward toward the symphysis pubis.

8. The pressure on the parietal region is sometimes so great that a definite curved tracing is seen on the scalp, marking the course of the head past the promontory. When the head has passed the pelvic brim, no further trouble is encountered if the contraction is limited to the inlet.

9. When the posterior parietal bone presents (posterior asynclitism), the mechanism is reversed. The sagittal suture lies near the symphysis, the posterior parietal bone is gradually forced past the promontory, and the anterior parietal bone slips by the symphysis, whereas the sagittal suture progresses backward toward the sacrum.

When the breech presents, there are additional problems:

1. The cord, legs, and arms may prolapse because of the poor fit of the buttocks into the distorted pelvic brim.

2. Often the aftercoming head is delivered with great difficulty, if at all.

Complications during labor

1. Labor is prolonged not only by the small pelvis but also because the cervix does not dilate readily.

2. The membranes are likely to rupture prematurely.

3. With ruptured membranes, the presenting part must serve as the dilator. Dilatation is delayed because the pelvis holds it back until molding permits the descending head to contact the cervix.

4. Molding requires a long time even after the cervix is dilated, especially when the pelvis is flat and generally contracted or when the pelvic canal is small throughout.

5. The uterine contractions commonly fail because of the long labor (secondary inertia).

6. Women with generally contracted pelves frequently have poor contractions from the beginning (primary inertia).

7. Rupture of the uterus may occur because of prolonged labor and considerable thinning of the lower uterine segment.

8. Prolonged pressure on the soft tissues between the head and the pelvis may cause fistulas.

9. Rupture of the symphysis pubis, especially with injudicious use of forceps, may occur.

Dangers of labor to the infant are the following:

1. Intrapartum infection attributable to the ascent of bacteria through prematurely ruptured membranes may occur.

2. Prolapse of the umbilical cord is common.

3. Intracranial hemorrhage from prolonged pressure and molding may occur.

4. An excessively large caput succedaneum not infrequently leads to the error of thinking that the head is lower in the pelvis than it really is, and forceps may be applied too soon.

5. Excessive molding causes extensive overlapping and consequent tears of the tentorium and brain hemorrhage.

6. Fractures of the skull are rare unless forceps are used injudiciously. Depression fractures are very serious, causing brain pressure, and should be surgically corrected.

Prognosis of labor. Probably no mature infant can be delivered safely through the vagina if the obstetric conjugate diameter is less than 8.5 cm. The outcome is difficult to predict in the borderline pelvis with an obstetric conjugate between 8.5 and 10 cm. Obviously other factors must be considered, such as previous labor at term, size of the infant, presence or absence of inertia, and general pelvic architecture. Roentgen pelvimetry just before or early in labor will be helpful in deciding whether to deliver at once by cesarean section. The results of attempts to engage the fetal head by impressing it into the pelvis via fundal or direct pressure may aid in this decision. If this testing maneuver causes the lowest portion of the fetal head to descend to a point below the ischial spines, one can assume that inlet disproportion does not exist. If doubt still exists, a "trial labor" of 3 to 4 hours may determine whether engagement of the head will occur. This is a reasonable approach whenever the pelvic diameters below the inlet are normal or perhaps even quite large.

Breech and face presentations with contracted inlet often lead to fetal disasters, and in such situations cesarean section should be freely employed.

Treatment of labor. Treatment of labor will depend on the degree of contraction and the history of previous labors.

No simple rules can be established to fit all situations. If the outlook for safe vaginal delivery is not good, cesarean section is done either electively or after a reasonable "trial labor." Probably 80% to 90% of fetuses will be delivered vaginally without great difficulty. But if progress in labor should cease, cesarean section is the wisest recourse.

Analgesic drugs should be used sparingly, if at all, because of the high incidence of inertia.

Fetal heads must not be driven through contracted inlets by the use of oxytocin.

Forceps are not to be applied to high or floating heads.

True conservatism consists of doing the right thing at the right time; for example, it is radical to interfere in moderate degrees of contraction if progress in cervical dilatation and fetal descent is occurring, but, on the other hand, it is conservative to do a cesarean section when the obstetric conjugate is 8.5 cm. because the necessity for conserving fetal life demands it.

MIDPELVIC CONTRACTION

Average midpelvic measurements are as follows:

1. Interspinous (transverse), 10.5 cm.

2. Anteroposterior (lower symphysis to junction of fourth and fifth sacral vertebrae), 11.5 cm.

3. Posterior sagittal (midpoint of interspinous line to same point on sacrum), 5 cm.

When the interspinous measurement is below 9 cm. and the posterior sagittal measurement is below 4 cm., one may anticipate dystocia with a fetus of average term size.

Accurate midpelvic measurements are obtainable only by radiologic methods. Women with unusually prominent ischial spines or with contraction of the intertuberous diameter at the outlet should have x-ray mensuration.

In white women midpelvic contraction is more common than inlet contraction and leads to transverse arrest of the fetal head and difficult midforceps extractions. Whenever possible, it is wise to permit the uterus to push the biparietal diameter past the interspinous obstruction. When the perineum is bulging, one may be fairly certain that the largest part of the head has passed the obstruction, and low forceps delivery then may be quite simple. Keen judgment is required to determine when such patients must be delivered by cesarean section, lest the infant be lost through the combined effects of prolonged labor and damaging midforceps delivery.

The *vacuum extractor* has been advised for selected patients with midpelvic contraction because it occupies less space than obstetric forceps and usually maintains good flexion of the fetal head (Chapter 31).

CONTRACTED OUTLET (FUNNEL PELVIS)

Outlet contraction alone is rather rare. It is nearly always associated with narrowing at the midpelvic level and converging side walls. An android pelvis is likely to have a small outlet because the intertuberous diameter is relatively short and the rather straight sacrum is inclined forward to complete the funneling effect (Fig. 25-1).

When the transverse diameter of the outlet between the tuberosities of the ischium (normally 10 or 11 cm.) is 8 cm. or less, the outlet is contracted and the pubic arch (angle) is narrowed so that the infant's head cannot fit into it but is forced back toward the tip of the sacrum. If there is enough room in the hindpelvis, the head may pass the outlet. To determine if there is adequate room, the posterior sagittal diameter (7 to 8 cm.) must be measured. It extends from the level of the transverse diameter to the tip of the sacrum (not the coccyx, which is movable).

Experience has shown that when the sum of the transverse and posterior sagittal diameters is 15 cm. or more, the head can usually pass the outlet (Thoms' rule). Measurements may be made with the crossed arms of the Breisky pelvimeter (Fig. 25-2) or with the Thoms' (Fig. 9-5) or other outlet pelvimeter especially devised for the purpose.

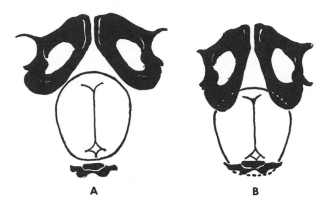

Fig. 25-1. A, Funnel pelvis with a narrow subpubic arch (angle) but with a posterior sagittal diameter long enough to permit the head to pass the tip of the sacrum. **B,** Funnel pelvis with a very narrow arch and a posterior sagittal diameter so short that the head cannot pass the tip of the sacrum. (From Beck: Obstetrical practice, Baltimore, The Williams & Wilkins Co.)

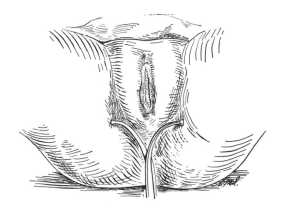

Fig. 25-2. Measuring the transverse diameter of the outlet with the Budin or Breisky pelvimeter. (From Titus: The management of obstetric difficulties, St. Louis, The C. V. Mosby Co.)

Treatment. First make certain that the initial measurements of the intertuberous and posterior sagittal diameters are accurate. Inexperienced examiners are likely to take the intertuberous measurement too far forward on the pubic rami. If the intertuberous measurement is less than 8 cm., x-ray pelvimetry probably should be obtained to determine the status of the midpelvis, which is likely to be contracted.

Unequivocal contraction of the pelvic outlet is, of course, an indication for cesarean section. In most instances of borderline contraction, a deep episiotomy will facilitate delivery and prevent the third degree laceration of the perineum that frequently occurs with funnel pelvis.

LESS COMMON TYPES OF DEFORMED PELVES

Osteomalacic pelvis. Osteomalacic pelvis is extremely rare in America. In this type of pelvis the bones lose their mineral deposits (chiefly calcium) in adult life.

Pelvic distortion is so great that childbirth is usually impossible except by cesarean section.

Dwarf pelvis

1. A *hypoplastic* dwarf is only a tiny person symmetrically developed. The pelvis is of normal shape, but all of the diameters are short. The pelvis is generally contracted.

2. A *cretin* dwarf has hypothyroidism, short, deformed long bones, and a generally contracted pelvis.

3. A *chondrodystrophic* pelvis is caused by chondrodystrophia fetalis; the pelvis is flattened.

Dwarfs who become pregnant require cesarean section.

Nägele's pelvis. Nägele's pelvis is obliquely contracted because of underdevelopment or absence of one sacral ala (Fig. 25-3). The other ala may be normal, but cesarean section is practically always indicated.

Robert's pelvis. Robert's pelvis is transversely contracted. Both alae of the sacrum are absent, rendering the pelvis too narrow for childbirth (Fig. 25-4).

Assimilation pelvis. In assimilation pelvis the last lumbar vertebra (sometimes more) is fused into the sacrum, thus increasing its depth (Fig. 25-5).

Split pelvis. In split pelvis the pelvic bones do not unite at

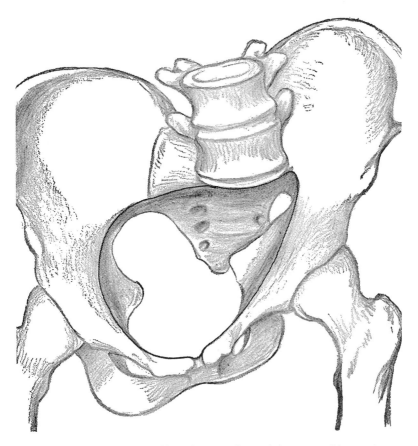

Fig. 25-3. Nägele's pelvis. Note absence of sacral ala on one side, causing unequal lateral contraction. (From Beck: Obstetrical practice, Baltimore, The Williams & Wilkins Co.)

the symphysis. Other failures of development, such as exstrophy of the bladder, are likely to accompany this deformity.

Kyphotic pelvis. When the kyphosis is high in the dorsal region, the pelvis is seldom affected. The nearer the kyphosis approaches the pelvis the more likely is pelvic deformity. Funnel

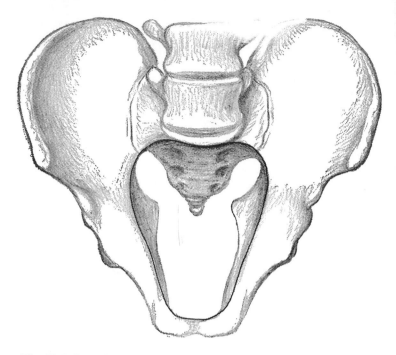

Fig. 25-4. Robert's pelvis. Note very narrow alae on both sides, causing symmetric lateral contraction. (From Beck: Obstetrical practice, Baltimore, The Williams & Wilkins Co.)

pelvis usually accompanies low kyphosis because the sacrum is rotated forward and the tuberosities and spines of the ischium approach each other. When the kyphosis is very low, the spine may hang over the pelvic inlet enough to prevent the presenting part from entering.

Malpositions are common because the abdominal cavity is constricted because of the closeness of the ribs to the pelvis. A pendulous abdomen is common. Because of the large inlet the presenting part easily enters but cannot get out because of the funnel pelvis.

The treatment depends almost entirely upon the capacity of the outlet, but cesarean section often is indicated.

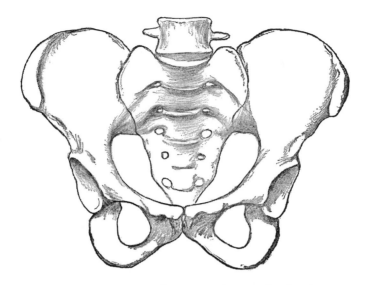

Fig. 25-5. Assimilation pelvis. The last lumbar vertebra has been trans-formed (assimilated) into the sacrum as the first sacral vertebra. (From Beck: Obstetrical practice, Baltimore, The Williams & Wilkins Co.)

Kyphorachitic pelvis. The effects of kyphosis and rickets may counterbalance each other. Thus a patient with conspicuous vertebral deformity may have a fairly normal pelvis. However, with a high kyphosis the pelvic changes are largely rachitic.

Scoliotic pelvis. Unless the scoliosis (Fig. 25-6) is caused by rickets, little, if any, pelvic deformity results, and if rickets is the cause, the problem is chiefly one of a rachitic pelvis.

Spondylolisthetic pelvis. In spondylolisthetic pelvis the last lumbar vertebra is dislocated forward on the sacrum, which may prevent the presenting part from entering the pelvis. The degree of displacement determines the prognosis. When the distance from the under edge of the symphysis pubis to the dislocated vertebra ("pseudoconjugate") is 8 cm. or more, spontaneous delivery may be possible.

Deformities from unilateral lameness. When one leg is lame, the constant limping puts undue force upon the good side,

causing asymmetric distortion of the pelvis or *coxalgic pelvis*.
It may be due to:

1. Hip disease
2. Dislocation of the femur
3. Poliomyelitis
4. Clubfoot, etc.

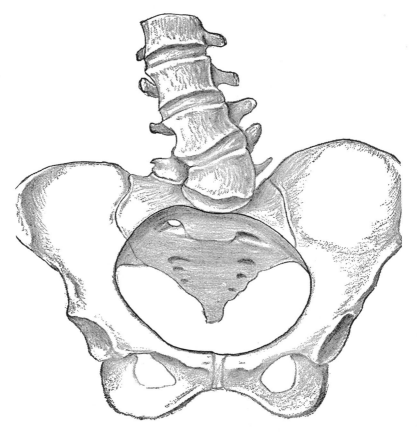

Fig. 25-6. Scoliotic pelvis. (From Beck: Obstetrical Practice, Baltimore,
The Williams & Wilkins Co.)

Bilateral lameness. Bilateral lameness resulting from luxation of both femurs is not very likely to cause deformities that interfere with labor. Widening of the inferior strait results.

Bone tumors and fractures. Very rarely exostoses or bony tumors may be large enough to shorten the pelvic diameters. Fracture, when there is pronounced dislocation, may do the same.

26

Problems of the third stage of labor

POSTPARTUM HEMORRHAGE

Postpartum hemorrhage is the most common cause of major blood loss in obstetrics and accounts for one fourth the maternal deaths in the hemorrhage category (including placenta previa, abruptio placentae, abortion, uterine rupture, and ectopic pregnancy).

Blood loss exceeding 500 ml. is generally considered postpartum hemorrhage. When blood losses are measured carefully, it is found that nearly all women lose 500 to 600 ml. of blood in the 24-hour period beginning with delivery, although major hemorrhages (over 1,000 ml.) are rather uncommon. Women may survive losses of larger amounts of blood, but their ultimate recovery is retarded. Although some women may bear the loss quite well, the effect on the individual patient will depend more on her initial blood volume and general condition than on the actual quantity lost. A woman already exhausted by prolonged labor or weakened by disease may succumb after bleeding 1,000 or 1,500 ml., whereas a woman in good condition sometimes bears this amount or more with impunity, but it is decidedly unsafe to run the risk of such a loss.

Etiology. Postpartum hemorrhage is chiefly caused by:

1. Atony of the uterine muscle (etiologic in 9 out of 10 cases)

2. Partially separated placenta or retention of individual cotyledons

3. Deep tears of the birth canal, particularly the cervix

4. Prior complications, such as abruptio placentae, placenta previa, or rupture of the uterus

5. Placenta accreta (partial)

6. Uterine tumors

An atonic uterus cannot constrict the endomyometrial blood vessels. The cause of the atony is not always obvious, but the usual precipitating factors are failure of the placenta to separate, deep general anesthesia, prolonged labor from inertia, distention of the uterus by multiple pregnancy, large fetus or hydramnios, multiparity, and myomas of the uterus.

As long as the placenta is firmly attached to the uterine wall, hemorrhage cannot take place because no vessels have been torn. But when the placenta is partially detached, the uterus cannot contract uniformly and constrict the sinuses, so that hemorrhage occurs. This is called *third-stage bleeding.* Incomplete separation is usually due to the improper management of the third stage of labor, particularly too early and too energetic an attempt at expression of the placenta. The retention of isolated cotyledons or placenta succenturiata may interfere with contraction and retraction of the uterus in precisely the same manner as the partially separated placenta.

The bleeding may occur during or after the third stage of labor; in the former it is usually due to tears or partial separation and in the latter to tears, atony of the muscle, or retention of placental remnants.

Diagnosis. Diagnosis usually is easy, but if the hemorrhage is concealed, an enormous amount of blood may accumulate. Concealed hemorrhage seldom occurs in a properly watched patient.

If the bleeding commences immediately after the birth of the infant, it is usually due to tears or to partial separation of the placenta.

If the hemorrhage persists after the uterus is empty and well contracted, a tear should be suspected, sought for, and sutured. For proper exposure and expeditious repair, an assistant is usually necessary. If vagina and cervix are intact, digital exploration for uterine rupture should be performed.

When the uterus does not retract and contract firmly after expulsion of the placenta or remains contracted only by constant kneading, the cause is either atony or retained remnants of the placenta. To determine if remnants are retained, a careful examination of the placenta should be made in every patient as a routine procedure. A large defect on the maternal surface means a retained portion, whereas torn vessels at the margin of the placenta on the fetal surface means that a placenta succenturiata has been left behind.

Treatment. With proper management of the third stage of labor, postpartum hemorrhage should be extremely rare. *Prophylaxis* is the keynote in the treatment.

Prophylactic. The most important prophylactic measures are as follows:

1. Ensure hemoglobin of 12 gram % or more at term by prenatally diagnosing and treating any causes for lower levels.

2. Avoid traumatic procedures and be cognizant of the presence of potential causes for hemorrhage.

3. Watch the condition of the uterus constantly after the birth of the infant.

4. Do not resort to placental expression until the fundus rises, indicating that the placenta has become completely separated. Premature attempts at expression are a frequent cause of partial separation, thus increasing bleeding.

5. There is a tendency toward relaxation of the uterus after prolonged labor, operative deliveries, general anesthesia, the birth of *twins* and in *hydramnios* and *placenta previa*. When hemorrhage is anticipated, start an infusion of glucose in water late in the first stage of labor and add 10 to 50 units of oxytocin to the bottle *(not into the tubing)* after delivery of the infant. Keep the uterus elevated out of the pelvis and maintain firmness with massage. Observe the patient in the delivery room or recovery room for at least an hour post partum.

6. If any remnant of placenta has been left, immediate removal should be done whether or not bleeding supervenes. It will occur sooner or later.

7. Thorough inspection of the cervix and vagina with immediate repair of all lacerations should be performed after *every* delivery.

Active. In the presence of hemorrhage the active treatment varies according to whether the placenta has been expelled.

1. If the placenta is in the uterus:

(a) It should be expressed at once by fundal pressure if possible.

(b) If expression fails, remove the placenta manually.

2. If the placenta has been delivered:

(a) Reinspect the cervix and vagina for overlooked lacerations. Palpate the uterine interior for retained placental fragments and for myometrial defects.

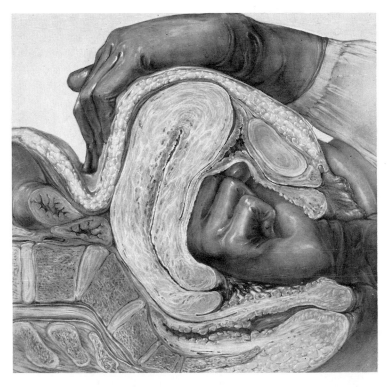

Fig. 26-1. Bimanual compression of postpartum uterus to control hemorrhage. (From Eastman and Hellman: Williams obstetrics, New York, Appleton-Century-Crofts, Inc.)

(b) If there are retained remnants, they should be removed manually.

(c) If uterine rupture has occurred, laparotomy should be performed and the uterus should be removed or repaired.

(d) If the hemorrhage is caused by atony:

(1) The uterus should be vigorously kneaded.

(2) Oxytocin, 10 units, followed by 0.2 mg. of ergonovine, should be given intramuscularly or intravenously. (Transabdominal instillation of 10 units of oxytocin directly into the anterior uterine wall may also be considered.)

(3) If these measures fail, bimanual compression and massage of the uterus should be tried (Fig. 26-1). Pull the uterus toward the symphysis with the hand on the abdomen and massage the anterior surface with the other fist in the vagina. This effects compression of venous sinuses.

(4) Packing the uterus with gauze no longer is considered desirable by most authorities because it distends the very sinuses that are bleeding, and it often leads to infection.

(5) Blood for transfusion should be obtained promptly and administered if over 500 ml. of blood appears to have been lost and the flow is continuing.

(6) If in spite of all measures bleeding continues, the uterus should be removed.

RETAINED PLACENTA

Retained placenta means failure of placental delivery within the first 30 minutes after the birth of the infant. Its cause is not known, but it occurs in at least 1% of deliveries.

Manual removal of the placenta is the obvious treatment of this condition. There is much difference of opinion as to whether a half hour should elapse before it is carried out, and certainly many capable obstetricians routinely interfere manually at a much earlier time.

Manual removal requires strict asepsis. The vulva should be cleansed, and fresh sterile gloves must be worn. After peeling the placenta away from the uterine wall, the entire mass should

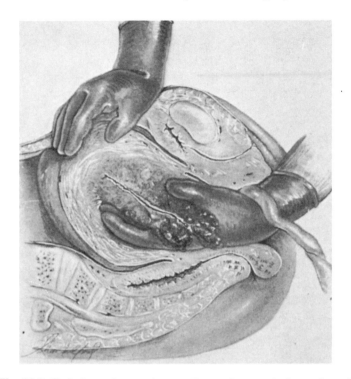

Fig. 26-2. Technique of manual separation and removal of an adherent, retained placenta. (From Willson: Management of obstetric difficulties, St. Louis, The C. V. Mosby Co.)

be grasped in the hand and gradually withdrawn during a uterine contraction. The free hand exerts counterpressure on the uterus through the abdominal wall (Fig. 26-2).

Placenta accreta (Fig. 26-3) is the condition in which:

1. The placenta is *inseparably attached* to the uterine wall.

2. Because of insufficient development of the decidua, villi come into immediate association with the uterine muscle. Varying degrees of placental association with the myometrium have been described and labeled. *Placenta accreta* is the condition in which there is simple direct contact of villi with uterine muscle;

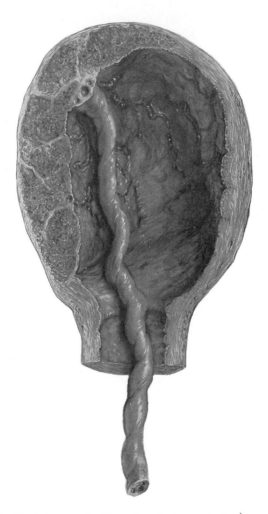

Fig. 26-3. Placenta accreta. The placenta has actually grown into the myometrium, with no line of cleavage, so that it cannot be separated. (From Titus: The management of obstetric difficulties, St. Louis, The C. V. Mosby Co.)

placenta increta is the penetration of villi into the myometrium; and *placenta percreta* is the penetration of villi through the entire thickness of the myometrium to the serosal surface. All are rare. The attachment may involve part of the placenta or its complete surface.

3. In all forms, normal detachment is impossible, and manual separation is too dangerous to be justifiable because an attempt to separate the placenta mechanically from the uterine wall into which it has grown causes alarming hemorrhage and possible rupture of the riddled, thin muscularis.

In trying to remove a retained placenta, *if no line of cleavage is found, no further attempt should be pursued, but a hysterec-*

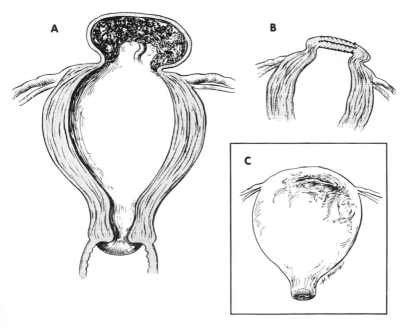

Fig. 26-4. A, Placenta trapped in the sacculated portion of the uterus. **B,** Immediately after surgical incision and repair. **C,** Later view of uterine wall scar, no muscular defect. (Courtesy Dr. Donald A. Dallas, San Francisco.)

tomy should be performed. On the rare occasion when the diagnosis of *complete* placenta accreta has been made, the bleeding is negligible, and the patient is *highly* desirous of a subsequent pregnancy, the placenta may be left undisturbed with the anticipation of spontaneous resorption. Usually, however, the accreta is only partial and bleeding from the area of detachment is furious.

A rare but potentially disastrous entity is *sacculation of the uterus* with the placenta trapped in the sacculation (Fig. 26-4). Laparotomy may be required to liberate the placenta, depending on the size of the opening into the distended portion of the uterine wall.

INVERSION OF UTERUS

Inversion of the uterus is an extremely rare but potentially very dangerous cause of shock after delivery. Many obstetricians with large practices have never seen a patient with uterine inversion. On the other hand, it is much more frequently noted in the practice of midwives and careless physicians.

With incomplete inversion, the fundus is at or through the os uteri, whereas in complete inversion the entire uterus is turned inside out and is outside the vulva. The placenta not infrequently remains attached to the uterus.

Etiology
1. Laxity and thinness of the uterine walls
2. Pressure from above too strenuously applied
3. Traction upon the cord
4. Sometimes occurs spontaneously but is usually attributable to violence, either too vigorous Credé maneuver or traction on the cord
5. Fundal insertion of placenta

Symptoms
1. Great and alarming shock associated with severe pain.
2. Profuse hemorrhage is common.
3. Mild symptoms may indicate incomplete inversion.

Prognosis. The prognosis is very good if the condition is promptly detected and if the uterus is replaced at once. If strangulation or gangrene occurs, the outlook is very grave.

Treatment
1. Treatment is by pressure under anesthesia by several

fingers upward in the vagina at the junction of the cervix and corpus and in the axis of the superior strait.

2. If the placenta is attached, do not separate it until the inverted uterus is replaced.

3. If much blood has been lost, one is advised to wait until after transfusion of blood or the use of other measures before reducing the inversion. Although it is preferable, there is no *absolute* need to restore the uterus to its normal form at once if the patient is in good condition. As long as shock, anemia, and infection are controlled, the decision about ultimate handling of the uterus may be postponed, if absolutely necessary, for days or even weeks, pending postpartum involution.

4. In chronic or long-standing inversion it is often necessary to employ combined internal (abdominal incision) and external (vaginal) maneuvers in order to replace the uterus.

27

Injuries to the birth canal

INJURIES TO VULVA AND VAGINA

Virtually every vaginal delivery produces some variety of physical trauma to the lower generative tract or vulva, and these injuries must be assessed promptly to determine the need for surgical repair. Consequently, the vagina and cervix should be inspected after every delivery.

Lacerations involving the perineum and vaginal mucosa should be repaired in the manner of an episiorrhaphy (Figs. 27-1 and 27-2). Tears of the vestibular mucosa lateral to the urethral meatus occasionally occur, often bleed vigorously, and require suturing as a rule. Isolated lacerations of the upper vaginal mucosa may occur with or without injury at a lower level. Exposure of the full extent of the laceration may be difficult at times and assistance is usually required for optimal repair. Vaginal lacerations most commonly occur as a result of forceps operations.

LACERATIONS OF CERVIX

Slight lacerations of the cervix occur in almost every patient, but they usually heal rapidly and rarely give rise to symptoms. Deep cervical tears may involve the vagina and extend into the lower uterine segment (Fig. 27-3).

Cervical tears are usually associated with tumultuous labor or operative deliveries, especially forceps rotations, or from injudicious attempts at delivery through an incompletely dilated os. They are likely to bleed profusely.

The cervix should be grasped with two or more sponge or

398

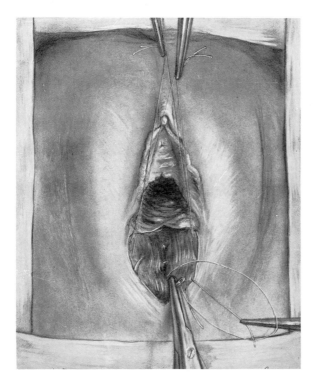

Fig. 27-1. Repair of second-degree perineal wound. Deep sutures are placed but not immediately tied. (From Titus: The management of obstetric difficulties, St. Louis, The C. V. Mosby Co.)

ovum forceps and its entire circumference inspected. Major lacerations should be repaired whether actively bleeding or not.

The cervix is brought into view by traction with the sponge forceps and if necessary by pressure upon the fundus, with the vagina being retracted by right-angled specula. (Fig. 27-4). Chromic catgut sutures are placed rather loosely to avoid necrosis in this already traumatized area.

Annular detachment is the separation of the entire vaginal portion of the cervix from the rest of the uterus. This usually

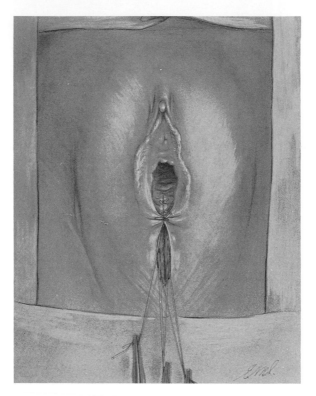

Fig. 27-2. Closing the superficial fascia and skin in repair of perineal wound. (From Titus: The management of obstetric difficulties, St. Louis, The C. V. Mosby Co.)

is observed only in excessively long labors or forced deliveries. Bleeding is often surprisingly minimal if thrombosis has occurred as a result of prolonged compression of the tissue but will usually be torrential if the cervix is acutely and traumatically avulsed.

RUPTURE OF UTERUS

Ruptures of the uterus (Fig. 27-5) are classified as follows:
1. Rupture at the site of an incisional scar

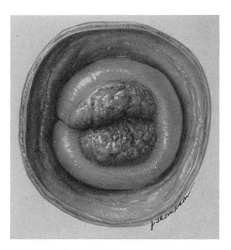

Fig. 27-3. Lacerated and everted cervix after postpartum involution. (From Richards: Surgery for general practice, St. Louis, The C. V. Mosby Co.)

2. Spontaneous rupture of the intact uterus
3. Traumatic rupture of the intact uterus

The incidence is about 1 in 2,000 deliveries. Approximately 5% of maternal deaths are attributable to uterine rupture.

Etiology. An incisional scar in the uterus, most commonly from previous cesarean section, myomectomy, or metroplasty, may spontaneously rupture either silently or with symptoms. The silent variety represents a dehiscence of the anatomically weak area and is most frequently discovered at the time of repeat cesarean section. If bleeding is negligible, the incision may be reapproximated and the uterus preserved. Approximately 1% or 2% of classical cesarean section scars rupture during subsequent pregnancy, about half of them prior to labor. The prognosis for scars from myomectomy and hysteroplasty is essentially the same. Only about 1 in 200 scars from previous transverse lower segment cesarean sections subsequently rupture, with the majority of these occurring during labor.

Spontaneous rupture of the intact uterus occurs most com-

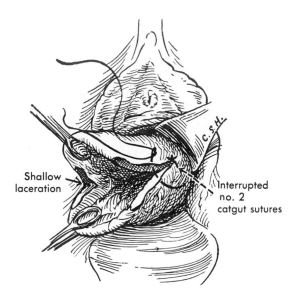

Shallow laceration

Interrupted no. 2 catgut sutures

Fig. 27-4. Repair of the torn cervix. Sutures must not be too tightly tied. (From Falls and McLaughlin: Obstetric and gynecologic nursing, St. Louis, The C. V. Mosby Co.)

monly in multiparas and is usually associated with protracted, effortful, and often neglected labor in cases of feto-pelvic disproportion. When a serious obstacle interferes with the progress of labor, the upper segment is stimulated to greater action. As it contracts it likewise retracts so that its lower margin, the contraction ring of Bandl, is drawn up, eventually occupying a much higher level than usual. As a result, powerful upper traction is exerted on the passive lower segment and it becomes thinner and thinner. In essence, the fetus is driven from the powerful and shrinking upper segment into the passive and stretching lower segment. If contractions persist and fetal descent is impossible, the lower segment must ultimately rupture. The injudicious use of oxytocin may also be incriminating. Such use may accentuate the above event or may produce a situation in which the normal resistances cannot be overcome with suf-

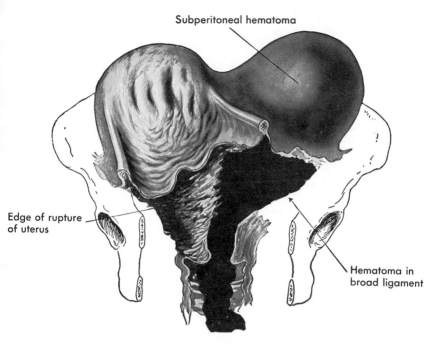

Fig. 27-5. Longitudinal rupture of the uterus. (From DeLee: Principles and practice of obstetrics, Philadelphia, W. B. Saunders Co.)

ficient rapidity to appease the excessively powerful and insistent uterine forces.

Impending rupture may be diagnosed by the presence of a distended lower uterine segment and a thick, high contraction ring often near or at the level of the umbilicus. The lower segment is usually tender and the contractions are strong and painful.

Traumatic rupture of the intact uterus may occur as a result of nonobstetric violence or injury but is most commonly produced by intrauterine manipulation, forceps operations, and inordinate fundal pressure during delivery.

Symptoms and diagnosis. The symptoms of uterine rupture may vary from only mild discomfort and minimal bleeding to dramatic, tearing pain and vascular collapse. Tenderness of the lower uterine segment rapidly develops.

If the rupture is complete and the fetus is expelled into the abdominal cavity, the contractions may cease, the patient's pain may be temporarily relieved, and a small hard uterus may be felt in the pelvis as a separate mass. The fetus usually succumbs unless immediate laparotomy is performed.

If the rupture is incomplete, the symptoms may be slight and labor may continue. Pain and abdominal tenderness usually persist and the development of shock may be insidious. The fetus is imperiled but may survive if delivery is effected before anoxia develops.

Incomplete ruptures in the lower uterine segment often extend into the broad ligament. A large subperitoneal hematoma slowly forms, which may secondarily rupture into the peritoneal cavity, accentuating symptoms.

Traumatic ruptures at delivery are commonly associated with more external bleeding than is seen in the other varieties. Diagnosis is made by manual intrauterine examination, which should be performed in all instances of operative delivery followed by intractable uterine bleeding.

Treatment

1. Intelligent care of the woman in labor should almost entirely eliminate spontaneous uterine rupture. Any obstacle to delivery should place the physician on guard for signs of impending rupture.

2. When rupture has occurred, laparotomy must be done at once. Occasionally it may be possible to repair the uterine defect, but in the main, hysterectomy will be necessary.

3. To control bleeding from a hematoma in the broad ligament it may be desirable to ligate the hypogastric artery if the uterine artery cannot be located promptly.

Prognosis. Fetal mortality has been 50% to 70% with spontaneous rupture of the intact uterus, and reported figures for maternal mortality have ranged from 20% to 40%. Maternal mortality after rupture of a cesarean section scar has been around 5%. Maternal mortality should be amenable to improvement by more immediate operation and adequate treatment of shock.

28

Puerperal infection

DEFINITION

Puerperal infection is a general term for any infection arising in the parturient canal, most commonly in the endometrium, soon after delivery. It may remain localized but often extends widely throughout the usual channels by which infections are disseminated. The severity of the illness depends on the character of invading organisms, the patient's resistance, and the speed and specificity of treatment. Infection is one of the three most common causes of maternal death.

It is reasonable to attribute every fever in the puerperium to puerperal infection unless fairly positive proof exists that it has resulted from another cause, such as urinary tract, respiratory, or venous infection.

ETIOLOGY

1. The introduction of bacteria into the genital tract by attendants is the prime cause of puerperal infection. The bacteria may come from an attendant's symptomatic or asymptomatic respiratory, nasopharyngeal, or skin infection, from the patient's own skin, vagina, or bowel, or from the infected tissues of another patient. They may be introduced directly by examining hands or instruments or indirectly by contamination of the patient's skin or bedding with subsequent self-inoculation. Their growth may be enhanced by chronic ill health and poor nutrition, prenatal anemia, long and exhausting labor, tissue damage, relative excess blood loss, prolonged membrane rupture, retained fragments of placenta and membrane, and other events permitting

405

prolonged or massive contamination or diminished patient resistance, or both.

2. *Infecting bacteria:*

(a) *Streptococcus,* in its various forms, is the most common infecting organism. The hemolytic streptococcus is the common cause of overwhelming infections and of the epidemic form of puerperal infection. But the most common cause of ordinary infections is the *anaerobic streptococcus.*

(b) *Staphylococcus, aureus* principally, *albus* and *citreus* rarely

(c) *Gonococcus* in pure or mixed cultures

(d) *Escherichia coli, Proteus vulgaris, Enterobacter aerogenes*

(e) *Pneumococcus*

(f) *Bacteroides* and other anerobes

(g) *Bacillus diphtheriae*

(h) *Clostridium perfringens (C. welchii)*

PATHOLOGY

Lesions vary from local inflammation of the episiotomy area, lacerated pelvic floor, vagina, or cervix to the infected open wound of the placental site, extending to the whole endometrium (endometritis). The infection, carried by the lymphatic system and bloodstream, often extends beyond the uterus to the adjacent parametrium and peritoneum and then becomes a general systemic bacteremia, with secondary infective lesions occurring almost anyplace. Fortunately, defensive forces attempt to limit the infection to the primary lesion by a protective barrier of leukocytes between the infected area and the healthy tissue.

TYPES
External genitalia

The common lesion is a localized infection in a repaired episiotomy incision or laceration. The edges of the wound become red and edematous, sutures give way, and the gaping wound exudes pus. Severe operative trauma to the vulva may create wounds that become infected and covered with an inflammatory exudate.

Cervicitis

The torn cervix is easily infected. Because of its deep clefts, it harbors bacteria a long time, and because of the exceedingly rich lymph drainage into the pelvic cellular tissue and nodes, it is the common source of pelvic cellulitis (parametritis).

Endometritis

Endometritis is the most common form of pelvic infection because of the easy entrance of bacteria into the open wound of the placental site. The entire endometrium quickly becomes involved due to the encouraging medium for bacterial growth offered by necrotic tissue and lochia.

Leukocytes appear in the underlying tissues to form a protective barrier, and presumably the local effusion of serum contains antibodies. There are great variations in the degree of necrosis and subsequent slough and thus in the vaginal discharge manifested by the patient.

Peritonitis

Peritonitis is a very grave complication that causes a majority of the deaths from puerperal infection. The infection reaches the peritoneum through the lymphatics or by escape of pus through the fallopian tubes.

The more virulent the bacterial organism, the less is the peritoneal reaction. Bacteremia is an almost inevitable accompaniment of widespread peritonitis.

Pelvic cellulitis (parametritis)

1. Pelvic cellulitis or parametritis is one of the most common complications. The bacteria reach the pelvic cellular tissue through the lymphatics, principally from the infected cervix and less often from the uterine cavity.

2. The cellulitis commonly does not spread beyond the confines of the broad ligaments, but it may extend laterally to the pelvic side walls and follow the loose connective tissue, beneath the peritoneum forward and around the base of the bladder to the abdominal walls and posteriorly into the uterosacral ligaments and around the rectum. When the loose connective tissue of the whole pelvis is involved, it has been called "plaster of paris pelvis" because of the stonelike hardness of the cellulitic infiltration.

3. The spaces in the loose connective tissue are filled with inflammatory exudate that often collects into small pockets of

purulence, which may become confluent and form large pelvic abscesses.

4. Pelvic cellulitis is most often unilateral and is very frequently accompanied by local thrombophlebitis.

Phlebitis (thrombophlebitis)

Two groups of veins may be involved in phlebitis or thrombophlebitis:

1. Uterine, ovarian, and hypogastric
2. Femoral, saphenous, and popliteal

The former constitutes *pelvic thrombophlebitis,* the latter, *femoral thrombophlebitis.*

Pelvic thrombophlebitis is the source of small emboli disseminated to various parts of the body, especially the lungs, kidneys, and heart valves. Large pulmonary emboli causing sudden death are uncommon. Ovarian vein thrombosis probably occurs more frequently than previously considered, and extension of the thrombus into the inferior vena cava has been described. Pelvic thrombophlebitis is present in at least half of the cases of fatal puerperal infection.

Femoral thrombophlebitis may arise locally or may be an extension from pelvic veins. Usually, however, it is not associated with puerperal infection but is initiated by venous stasis without an inflammatory etiologic component. The obstructed venous return classically produces swelling of the lower extremity, which may be accompanied by fever, pain, and local tenderness. Frequently, however, the entire process is silent until symptomatic embolization occurs. In other instances, mild temperature elevation may be the only evidence of its existence. Bilateral involvement is not uncommon and the threat of pulmonary embolism is significantly greater than with pelvic thrombophlebitis.

Phlebothrombosis (clot formation without inflammation of the vessel wall) may develop silently in pelvic veins and produce fatal pulmonary embolism without warning a week or more after delivery. The major etiologic factor is venous stasis. A clinical differentiation between thrombophlebitis and phlebothrombosis is often impossible because of the common asymptomatic nature of each. Pulmonary embolism has been discussed in Chapter 22.

Pyemia and bacteremia

The common source of the bacteria is from infected emboli broken from sinus thrombi of the placental site or thrombosed pelvic veins. Infected emboli create secondary inflammatory lesions in the heart, kidneys, lungs, brain, and joint spaces. Bacterial endotoxic shock with disseminated intravascular coagulation and a consumptive coagulopathy may also occasionally occur.

SYMPTOMS AND DIAGNOSIS

1. Any recently delivered woman who develops chills, fever, and rapid pulse presumably has puerperal infection unless another condition can be demonstrated. Fever above 100.4° F. on two successive days, excluding the first 24 hours after delivery, is defined as *puerperal morbidity* and is generally considered to be attributable to puerperal infection.

2. Cultures should be taken from the endometrial cavity and from any draining or erythematous wounds.

3. Blood cultures are valuable when positive, but many serious cases show no bacterial growth.

4. Subinvolution and tenderness of the uterus is common.

5. In pelvic cellulitis (parametritis) induration is found on either or both sides of the pelvis. Abscesses are likely to form, which may "point" in the posterior cul-de-sac or above Poupart's ligament.

6. Any suppuration with a fecal odor should suggest anaerobic organisms and special cultures should be obtained. *Escherichia coli* is odorless.

7. Any patient with a diagnosis of pelvic infection who continues to be severely febrile, despite apparently appropriate antibiotic therapy, should be suspected of having a pelvic thrombophlebitis. This may result from either aerobic or anaerobic organisms. A dramatic clinical response within 24 to 48 hours after the initiation of a trial of therapy with heparin would be strong confirmatory evidence of septic thrombosis.

8. If thrombophlebitis is suspected, the radioactive fibrinogen uptake test may be of use in establishing the diagnosis. After blocking the thyroid uptake of iodine with exogenous, nonradioactive iodine, radioiodinated fibrinogen is administered intra-

venously. It is anticipated that the radioactive fibrinogen will become incorporated in the fibrin matrix of the clot and allow diagnosis and localization by scintillation scanning.

9. The diagnosis of urinary tract infection (especially pyelitis) must be considered and may be established on the basis of urine culture. Mammary engorgement occasionally may be associated with a transitory elevation of temperature. Pneumonia, pharyngitis, and thrombophlebitis are sufficiently common to regularly require exclusion.

TREATMENT

Prophylaxis. Prevention is the key to reducing the incidence and mortality of puerperal infection. Infections elsewhere in the body should be eliminated prior to labor, anemia should be corrected, coitus should be forbidden after membrane rupture, and delivery should be accomplished within 24 hours thereafter, especially if uterine contractions occur and the pregnancy is beyond 34 weeks of gestation.

During labor and delivery. Infections occur so easily during labor that efforts to avoid contamination must be constant.

1. Any excrement passed during labor should be immediately removed from the bed, the perineum thoroughly cleansed and clean sheeting reapplied.

2. Vaginal examinations should be conducted with clean or sterile gloves, and contamination from the rectum must be avoided.

3. Intrapartum patients with known transmittable infections or with fever of unknown etiology should be isolated.

4. Personnel with upper respiratory or skin infections should not be permitted to attend patients in childbirth.

5. The duration of labor must be limited, and the patient maintained in a normal state of hydration and nutrition.

6. Blood loss must be replaced promptly if excessive.

7. The delivery must be as atraumatic as feasible.

8. The cervix and vagina must be inspected aseptically after delivery and, as with the episiotomy, any lacerations must be immediately repaired.

9. Placental fragments must not be left within the uterus.

After delivery. Perineal pads should be sterile and changed frequently. Use simple external washes and sitz baths for the vulva and perineum, but avoid deep entry of solutions into the vagina. Every potentially or actually infected patient must be isolated to protect others on the nursing unit.

Curative. Puerperal infection is treated with the antibiotic agent most effective against the organisms involved. When bacterial cultures are available, the choice of therapeutic agent is based on specific in vitro sensitivity tests. When cultures are not available, broad-spectrum antibodies to which all of the more common organisms are susceptible must be chosen. Some authorities advise prophylactic antibiotic therapy for all patients potentially infected by prolonged labor or difficult operative delivery. However, most bacteriologists decry the indiscriminate use of antibiotic agents lest too many resistant strains of bacteria be developed. Additionally, sensitization of the patient to the antibiotic or the production of a serious reaction from previous sensitization are also potential disadvantages.

Infected vulvar and vaginal wounds should be opened to secure adequate drainage. With endometritis, uterine drainage may be promoted by securing intrauterine material for culture.

Breast nursing may or may not have to be discontinued, depending on the severity of the infection and the time required for it to respond to treatment. Hemoglobin determinations should be made frequently and blood transfusions given when indicated.

Peritonitis is treated by massive antibiotic therapy parenterally, intravenous fluids, and continuous gastrointestinal suction.

In the presence of pelvic cellulitis, frequent examinations should be made to detect an abscess, and the latter should be opened abdominally or through the cul-de-sac.

The therapy of thrombophlebitis includes bed rest and the use of anticoagulants and antibiotics. Both heparin and warfarin (Coumadin) should be used initially. When Coumadin has become effective, 36 to 72 hours later, heparin may be discontinued. It is unlikely that spontaneous wound hemorrhage will occur but, in that eventuality, protamine sulfate and vitamin K may be used as antidotes for the heparin and Coumadin, respectively. In refractory cases it may be desirable to ligate the inferior vena cava and the ovarian veins to prevent pulmonary embolization and the spread of infected thrombi. When phlebitis involves the femoral vein, the affected extremity should be elevated and protected from external pressure until pain and fever disappear. For many months thereafter, an elastic support should be worn and positions that create venous stasis should be avoided.

29

Puerperal complications other than puerperal infection

SUBINVOLUTION OF UTERUS

Subinvolution of the uterus is the failure or retardation of the normal autolytic process of involution that ordinarily restores the uterus to its nonpregnant size and shape. It may result from various factors that interfere with myometrial contraction, such as retention of placental fragments, endometritis, or myomas in the uterine wall.

Symptoms and signs

1. Persistence of lochia
2. Leukorrhea
3. Backache and a sensation of weight in the pelvis
4. Uterus enlarged; softer than normal for a given period post partum
5. Occasionally profuse hemorrhage

Treatment

Ergonovine, 0.2 mg. every 6 hours, is given over a period of 3 to 4 days. When subinvolution of the placental site is associated with prolongation of postpartum bleeding or intermittent episodes of appreciable bleeding, curettage must be performed. Retained placental tissue may be recovered, but in many instances only meager fragments of vascularized material will be present. In either event, curettage usually is curative.

DISPLACEMENTS OF UTERUS

Retroversion and retroflexion. As soon as the uterus involutes sufficiently to reenter the pelvic cavity, retroflexion and retroversion may occur. During the early puerperium severe retro-displacements may cause imprisonment of the lochia—*lochiometra*. Retroversion often is associated with some mild degree of subinvolution. In the main, however, such retrodisplacements rarely cause symptoms or subsequent difficulties.

Prolapse of uterus. Women who have shown a moderate degree of prolapse of the uterus or *descensus uteri* (Fig. 29-1) before pregnancy often will show a recurrence of this condition during the puerperium. It is often associated with urinary stress incontinence. Operative procedures for correction of prolapse,

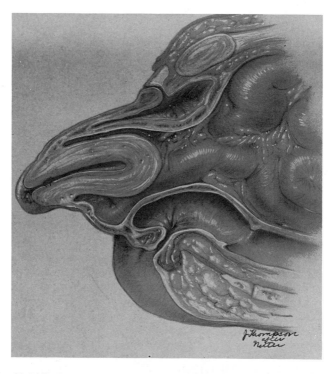

Fig. 29-1. Prolapse of the uterus with cystocele and rectocele, sagittal view. (From Richards: Surgery for general practice, St. Louis, The C. V. Mosby Co.)

cystocele, rectocele, and lacerations of the pelvic floor should not be undertaken until 3 to 6 months post partum. As a rule, plastic operations to repair minor degrees of these conditions are best postponed until after the childbearing period or until permission can be obtained for sterilization at the time of the plastic procedure.

VULVAR OR PUERPERAL HEMATOMAS

Vulvar or puerperal hematomas are tumefactions caused by escape of blood into the subcutaneous and paravaginal connec-

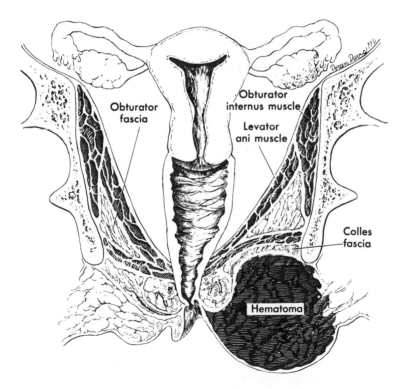

Fig. 29-2. Puerperal hematoma spreading through left ischiorectal fossa.

tive tissues of the perineum and ischiorectal fossa. The vascular rupture usually occurs during labor, and the delivery need not be operative. The hematoma forms gradually and may not be discovered until several hours after delivery, when the patient complains of severe perineal pain. If the torn vessel is above the pelvic fascia, the hematoma develops alongside the upper vagina and may spread into the broad ligament.

Large hematomas bulging perineally (Fig. 29-2) should be opened and hemostasis attempted. Primary repair is the treatment of choice whenever feasible although modest hematomas will usually resolve spontaneously. Often the cavity must be packed and counterpressure achieved by a vaginal pack. Blood replacement and antibiotic therapy are essential in the more severe cases and laparotomy may be required if broad ligament and retroperitoneal hematomas continue to expand.

OBSTETRIC PARALYSES

Cramplike pains or neuralgia in the legs may be due to pressure of the fetal head or obstetric forceps on branches of the sacral plexus. Grave lesions seldom follow, but paralysis of the muscles supplied by the external popliteal nerve—the flexors of the ankle and extensors of the toes—may occur. This is explained by the fact that the fibers of the popliteal nerve pass over the brim of the pelvis where pressure of the head may injure the nerve.

Rare cases of *neuritis* occurring after delivery have been reported and may be local or generalized. The symptoms depend on the particular nerve or nerves involved (for example, median or ulnar); the prognosis is good for the patient with localized paralysis and poor for the patient with generalized paralysis.

Pain simulating neuritis may be caused by a separated symphysis pubis or looseness of the sacroiliac joints.

Paralysis of central origin may result from the rupture of a normal or aneurysmal vessel, usually in hypertensive, but occasionally in normotensive, patients.

ABNORMALITIES AND DISEASES OF BREASTS
Abnormalities of nipples

Depressed nipples. Depressed nipples (invagination) are those in which lactiferous ducts open directly into a depression in the center of the areolae.

Flat nipples. Flat nipples are stunted nipples that scarcely project above the surface.

Normal suckling may be difficult and a nipple shield or breast pump may be required. Persistence in their use will occasionally succeed in developing functional nipples. Manual traction or other manipulation before or after delivery is seldom of any avail.

Fissures. Fissures (cracks), the result of injury by the baby's mouth, make nursing very painful and provide a pathway for infectious organisms. Scrupulous cleansing and the use of a nipple shield during nursing for 2 or 3 days is usually adequate therapy. Discontinuation of nursing is rarely required.

Abnormalities of mammary secretion

There is great individual variation in the amount of milk secreted in normal women; this does not always depend on the size of the breasts—large ones may be very inefficient and small ones very efficient.

Agalactia. Agalactia is complete absence of secretion. This condition is rare.

Polygalactia. Polygalactia is excessive secretion. Milk is so abundant that it is constantly escaping from the nipple.

Galactorrhea (Chiari-Frommel syndrome). Galactorrhea is a condition in which lactation and amenorrhea continue indefinitely post partum, sometimes for years. The cause is assumed to be blockade of the prolactin-inhibiting center in the hypothalamus by an agent as yet unknown. Some therapeutic success has been achieved with clomiphene citrate and more specifically with L-dopa and ergot alkaloids. The latter have been noted to cause cessation of galactorrhea, resumption of menses, and a fall in serum prolactin levels to normal in the majority of patients in whom they have been used. Chronic administration is required.

Engorgement of breasts. Engorgement of the breasts, referred to by the laity as "caked breasts," often occurs at the beginning of the establishment of lactation, about the third day of the puerperium, and disappears in 12 to 48 hours. It is caused by venous and lymphatic stasis. Sometimes the engorgement may be excessive and painful, but ordinarily it is not accompanied by an elevation of temperature. Symptomatic treatment with breast support, ice packs, and analgesics are occasionally required.

Drying up breasts. Drying up the breasts may be accomplished simply by leaving them absolutely alone. If engorgement becomes painful, ice bags and analgesics may be used for relief. Secretions usually disappear in less than a week. The use of a breast pump in this situation is self-defeating. The use of estro-

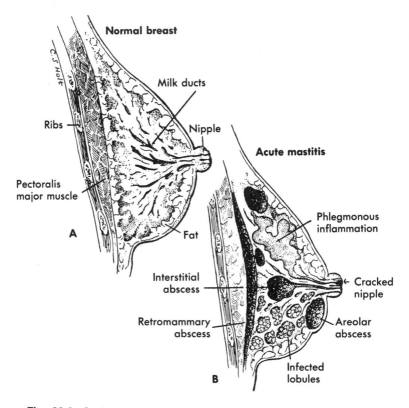

Fig. 29-3. Sagittal sections of normal, **A,** and infected, **B,** puerperal breasts. (From Falls and McLaughlin: Obstetric and gynecologic nursing, St. Louis, The C. V. Mosby Co.)

gens alone or in combination with androgens is often successful if employed immediately after delivery, especially if long-acting agents are used. It is not uncommon, however, for delayed engorgement to occur.

Inflammation of breasts

Mastitis is fairly common in the puerperium (Fig. 29-3). Engorgement often precedes the onset of true inflammation. The inflammatory process frequently may be stopped in its early stages by the use of antibiotics. If the inflammation persists for longer than 2 or 3 days, suppuration with abscess formation is the more usual occurrence.

Mastitis seldom occurs prior to the end of the first week after delivery and often is seen for the first time 3 or 4 weeks post partum. The usual symptoms are mild chills, fever, and breast soreness. Soon erythema develops over the infected and indurated segment of the breast. Tender, ipsilateral, axillary adenopathy is common.

Etiology. The infecting organism is most often a staphylococcus. The infection usually arises from organisms in the infant's nose and throat and may enter either through the milk ducts or through a nipple abrasion or fissure. Those occurring in the hospital or very shortly after dismissal should be suspected of being nosocomial in origin and caused by coagulase-positive staphylococci. Colonization of personnel and other infants in the nursery should be investigated if this organism is recovered from either the infant or the infected mother.

Treatment

Prophylactic. Prophylactic treatment consists simply of frequent soap and water cleansing of the breasts and nipples and prompt attention to cracks and fissures.

Curative

1. Suppuration usually may be aborted by the prompt administration of antibiotics in substantial dosage.

2. Nursing from the infected breast should usually be discontinued during treatment. A breast pump may be employed to prevent painful engorgement. The milk should be offered to the infant only if cultures show it to be sterile, which is not commonly the case.

3. Local heat should regularly be employed and analgesics used as required.

4. An abscess should be opened under anesthesia as soon as fluctuation can be demonstrated. Incisions should be made radially, like spokes of a wheel, the nipple being the hub. If the abscess is small, a single incision may be sufficient; but if large, the gloved finger should be introduced and the walls between pockets broken down so that there will be only one cavity to drain. A counter stab wound at the most dependent point of the abscess cavity favors drainage. Drainage may be maintained by loose gauze packing or by a rubber drainage tube.

Galactocele

Galactocele is a collection of milk held back by a clogged duct. Erythema, axillary nodularity, and fever do not usually occur. Spontaneous resolution can be anticipated. Local heat and analgesics may be used to diminish symptoms. Puncture of a galactocele is not necessary.

Supernumerary breasts

These small structures tend to occur in pairs on the anterior thoracic and abdominal walls, sometimes in the axillae, and rarely in the groin or on the thigh. Engorgement of an axillary breast may produce much discomfort. Regression usually occurs promptly, and no special treatment is necessary.

PUERPERAL PSYCHOSES

A puerperal psychosis appears, usually within 2 weeks after delivery, about once in 500 to 1,000 deliveries. Half of the patients show schizophrenic features, 40% are manic-depressive, and the remainder usually are affected by various psychoneuroses. Primiparas and multiparas are equally affected, and psychotic episodes may be repeated in subsequent pregnancies. Puerperal psychosis is not a distinct clinical entity. Delivery and the new problems that it uncovers are precipitating factors that disrupt the personality structure.

These patients often require hospitalization. Some puerperal psychotic breaks may be prevented by suitable therapy during pregnancy, and the obstetrician should develop an ability to detect prenatal patients with serious personality difficulties. Postpartum "maternity blues" should not be mistakenly dismissed as unimportant because in some instances they may presage further psychiatric difficulties.

AMNIOTIC FLUID EMBOLISM

After the membranes have ruptured and particularly just before or after delivery, amniotic fluid may gain access to venous sinuses in the uterine wall and travel to pulmonary vessels. The hair, vernix, and other material in the fluid may form small emboli in the lungs, causing sudden pain, dyspnea, pulmonary edema, and cyanosis. The presence of meconium in the embolic fluid is particularly lethal. Numerous instances of profound shock and *sudden death* from this phenomenon have been reported. The true frequency of this accident of childbirth has not been determined, as the diagnosis is essentially impossible to establish except on postmortem examination.

It tends to occur in rapid labors with powerful contractions and often in conjunction with the use of oxytocin for stimulation. Disseminated intravascular coagulation with resulting incoagulability of the blood (Chapter 18) may develop. Although the fatality rate has been close to 100%, an occasional patient may be saved by prompt action with oxygen, assisted ventilation, blood transfusion, and treatment of the shock. The central venous pressure must be carefully monitored during infusion therapy to avoid cardiac failure and pulmonary edema.

30

Injuries and diseases
of the newborn infant

PERINATAL MORTALITY

When one discusses perinatal mortality, it is customary to differentiate fetal mortality from neonatal mortality. Fetal mortality means the death of fetuses before or during labor in pregnancies of more than 20 weeks' duration (or fetuses weighing over 500 grams). Fetal mortality may be subdivided into antepartum and intrapartum categories. If an infant shows any sign of life at birth but then dies, the death is called "neonatal," as is any death during the first month of life. Perinatal mortality is the summation of fetal and neonatal mortality, which usually are of about equal magnitude in large samples.

The mortality for infants is greater during the first 3 days of life than it is for the entire remainder of the first year. Three fourths of neonatal deaths occur in premature infants, and the most common single cause in Potter's study was hyaline membrane disease, or respiratory distress syndrome. The other major causes are malformations, infection, intrauterine hypoxia, and cerebral hemorrhage.

Injuries and disorders that are not lethal presumably lead to cerebral palsy, defective mentality, and other neurologic problems. Much research is now being directed along these lines, and there is a vast national effort in progress to reduce perinatal mortality and morbidity in the United States.

APNEA OR ASPHYXIA OF THE NEWBORN

Apnea is the major objective manifestation of *asphyxia of the newborn*. Asphyxia is characterized by hypoxia, acidosis, and an elevated tension of carbon dioxide in the blood and tissues. The normal oxygen saturation of fetal arterial blood at birth is about 60%, but in severe degrees of asphyxia the blood oxygen is reduced to one fifth or one tenth of normal. The following situations may lead to asphyxia:

1. Compression of prolapsed cord
2. Premature separation of the placenta
3. Tetanic contractions of the uterus
4. Cord around the neck or body
5. Short cord
6. Pressure on the brain in difficult labors or operative procedures, leading to vagus irritation and slowing of the fetal heart.
7. Intracranial hemorrhage resulting from cerebral compression, especially when the vessels have been rendered additionally susceptible to trauma by hypoxia
8. Narcosis from maternal drugs in the absence of effective artificial respiration. (Narcotized premature infants respond less well to artificial respiration and varying degrees of hypoxia or asphyxia may persist despite treatment.)

Diagnosis. It is important to watch for signs of intrauterine anoxia. Their recognition often affords the indication for operative delivery.

The production of hypoxia in experimental animals has shown the following sequence of events:

1. Increased respiration and cardiac rate as an initial compensatory reaction to overcome the anoxemia and tissue hypoxia
2. Loss of consciousness
3. Cessation of respiration
4. Acidosis
5. Sharp reduction in cardiac rate
6. Cardiac arrhythmia
7. Hypotension
8. Blanching of skin
9. Skeletal muscle paralysis
10. Smooth muscle paralysis with relaxation of anal sphincter and discharge of rectal contents

11. Cessation of heartbeat

The process is reversible within the first few minutes but irreversible thereafter if anoxia is complete. If anoxia is mild or intermittent, the process can be protracted or remitting. Authorities believe that these changes are typically reproduced with intrauterine fetal hypoxia in the human.

These signs form the basis for the Apgar scoring system used in assessing the condition of the infant after delivery (such as respiratory effort, cardiac rate, skin color, muscle tone, and reflex irritability). (See Chapter 14.)

To the extent that it is currently possible, they also form the basis for assessing the condition of the fetus in utero. The fetal heart rate may be monitored, the fetal scalp blood may be sampled for determination of pH, and the existence of meconium may be detected by amnioscopy, amniocentesis, or direct observation. These measures have been described previously in Chapter 12.

Every effort should be made to detect and to attempt to alleviate intrauterine fetal hypoxia during labor. If this can be accomplished by placing the patient on her side, administering oxygen, correcting maternal hypotension, or reducing the intensity and duration of uterine contractions, or if the process is mild or only intermittent, vaginal delivery can be awaited. If the hypoxia is severe and nonremitting, and these measures fail, the situation can be corrected only by extrauterine resuscitation. Surgical extraction of the fetus from the uterus is required.

Whenever the amniotic fluid is yellowish green and contains particles of meconium, the infant is in potential danger and should be delivered as promptly as is compatible with the safety of the mother. In *breech* presentations, the expulsion of meconium does not have this degree of significance.

One should understand, however, that the diagnosis of fetal distress by changes in fetal heart rate and appearance of meconium in amniotic fluid is not infallible. Consequently, considerable clinical judgment and intuition must be applied in the interpretation of this data and the handling of each situation.

Parenthetically, in difficult breech extractions, when delay is experienced in delivering the aftercoming head, efforts of the infant to breathe may be seen or felt. A similar phenomenon may be occasionally observed in vertex presentations when the head is arrested on the pelvic floor and movements of the mouth are seen or felt through the thinned perineum. Very exceptionally, if air gains access to the fetus (for example, when the hand or an instrument is introduced into the vagina), the fetus may give utterance to sounds while still within the uterus (*vagitus uterinus*).

Prognosis. Profound anoxemia is always serious. The prognosis is more favorable when caused by mechanical interference with placental circulation and less favorable when caused by brain injuries, for example, hemorrhage, fractures, and depression of the skull. Usually it is impossible to distinguish at first between apnea of the newborn infant caused only by anoxia and that caused by cerebral hemorrhage. However, most apneic infants do not have cerebral hemorrhage, and this fact provides the keynote for treatment. (See Chapter 14.)

The late effects of cerebral hypoxia are enormously variable. Although some infants show only a delay in normal behavior, others exhibit convulsive states, mental deficiency, spastic paralysis, speech disorders, ataxia, and other neurologic problems.

MECONIUM ASPIRATION SYNDROME

In approximately 10% of deliveries, meconium is present in the amniotic fluid and may be aspirated by the fetus. This can produce a mechanical obstruction of the respiratory tract leading to an air block syndrome with hyperacration and a roentgenologic appearance similar to emphysema. Tissue irritation and reaction are not commonly noted.

One third of the infants from these deliveries demonstrate at least some degree of respiratory difficulty, and 50% of the group require active treatment. The mortality for those requiring ventilatory care is 5% to 20%. Pneumothorax and pneumomediastinum are often complicating events.

The prognosis is not well correlated with the infant's Apgar score. In fact, vigorous respiratory activity by the infant who has aspirated meconium is probably detrimental in that it allows deep inspiration of the obstructive material. Infants with respiratory depression, on the other hand, will frequently have had resuscitative aspiration of the meconium prior to their initiation of deep breathing.

Recent evidence reveals that the syndrome is nearly completely preventable. This may be accomplished by routine endotracheal intubation and suction of *all* infants with meconium staining. This should be done whether the presenting part was breech or vertex and regardless of the degree of initial respiratory activity.

INJURIES

Fractures. Fractures of the clavicles or humerus may occur when the shoulders are delivered in head presentations or when the extended arms are freed in breech presentations. Treatment of a fractured clavicle is simple: outward and backward rotation of the arm above the child's head. The humerus may be splinted by the hand-on-hip position and held by a Velpeau bandage. Femur fractures are rather rare, but they may occur by careless freeing of the leg in breech delivery. The simplest treatment is laying the baby on his back and suspending the leg to the ceiling (or a frame), letting the baby's weight supply the traction to the fractured bone. These measures, however, should be handled by a trained orthopedist.

Muscle injury. The sternocleidomastoid muscle may be injured by excessive lateral traction on the neck when the shoulders are delivered under the symphysis pubis. The blood extravasation will disappear in a few weeks without special treatment.

Intracranial hemorrhage. Intracranial hemorrhage formerly ranked high among the causes of stillbirths. The worst hemorrhages are caused by rupture of large vessels in the falx or tentorium, which is likely to occur in difficult labors, for example, in contracted pelves, forceps or breech deliveries, and internal versions. The incidence may be reduced by avoiding fetal hypoxia, by careful observance of proper indications for versions and forceps deliveries, and by meticulous adherence to a technique that avoids pressure upon the occipital bone during the delivery of the head under the symphysis pubis.

Symptoms include feeble cry, pallor, vomiting, and convulsions. Oxygen, vitamin K, and lumbar puncture may be helpful. Residual motor disturbances and mental deficiency are not uncommon. Recent studies indicate that traumatic delivery only rarely can be linked with cerebral palsy. The most common cause of cerebral palsy is prematurity, but the precise mechanisms responsible have not been discovered.

Obstetric paralyses. As the result of a nerve injury inflicted during a difficult extraction, *Erb-Duchenne paralysis* may affect the deltoid, infraspinatus, and flexor muscles of the forearm and cause the entire arm to fall close to the side of the body, at the same time rotating inward with the forearm extended on the arm. The mobility of the fingers usually is not affected. Such a paralysis is produced by a lesion involving the fifth and sixth roots of the brachial plexus. The brachial plexus is put under extreme tension as a result of pulling obliquely on the head in order to flex it toward the other shoulder in an attempt to deliver a shoulder in a vertex presentation. Therefore, in extracting the shoulders care must be taken not to bring about too much lateral flexion of the neck. In breech presentations this sort of paralysis may be caused by the Prague maneuver in which two fingers of one hand grasp the shoulders from below; this may cause the clavicle to compress the brachial plexus.

The *prognosis* is fair, with many infants recovering spontaneously. Some of them, however, may resist all ordinary treatment. Hence, the infant should be placed at once under the care of a competent orthopedic surgeon since intelligent postural treatment will ensure a useful arm even if degenerative changes occur in the nerves and muscles. In infants in whom the nerves have been badly torn, suture of the nerve has given good results; this necessity is very rare.

Damage to the cord may be associated with many kinds of infantile palsy, and these have been seen after difficult breech extractions. *Facial paralysis* occasionally is noted at birth but is not always the result of damage from obstetric forceps. Spontaneous resolution is common.

RESPIRATORY DISTRESS SYNDROME (HYALINE MEMBRANE DISEASE)

This syndrome originally was called hyaline membrane disease because alveoli of the partially atelectatic lungs were lined at autopsy with acidophilic hyaline-like membranes. It is a frequent cause of death of prematurely born infants and occasionally of term babies.

Clinically the infants develop respiratory distress soon after birth and die in 4 to 48 hours. The lungs are atelectatic and contain distended alveoli and alveolar ducts lined by eosinophilic hyaline membranes. The membranes are composed primarily of fibrin and resemble a plasma clot; the material presumably is a capillary transudate. The condition apparently results from lack of surfactant—a group of surface tension–reducing phospholipids. If alveolar surface tension cannot be overcome, alveolar expansion cannot be maintained. Lecithin is the principal surface active component and the biochemical pathways for its synthesis in required quantities are not ordinarily developed until late in pregnancy (Chapter 4).

Most infants with this disorder develop tachypnea, chest retraction, cyanosis, dyspnea, and expiratory grunting. Hypoxia, hypothermia, hypotension, and acidosis are usually present. A diffuse, granular pattern is seen in the lung parenchyma by x-ray.

Treatment varies in different clinics, and currently there is no known specific remedy. About two thirds of the newborn infants with this syndrome recover, showing rapid improvement after 3 to 4 days of treatment with oxygen, wetting agents, antibiotics, and other drugs. Positive-pressure ventilation may be required.

High concentrations of oxygen can injure pulmonary tissue and produce what has been called *bronchopulmonary dysplasia.* In the ventilator-dependent infant, evidences of excessive mucosal necrosis can be demonstrated by chest x-ray and cytologic examination of pulmonary secretions. These toxic effects can be minimized by reducing the concentrations of therapeutic oxygen.

FETAL SYPHILIS

Syphilis in the fetus is an uncommon entity, occurring in fewer than 1 in 5,000 newborns. It is transmitted from the mother through the placenta, but, for unknown reasons, this rarely occurs before the eighteenth week of gestation.

Serologic screening of all prenatal patients and antibiotic treatment during pregnancy of those with a positive serologic test virtually eliminates the potential for this disease in the fetus at birth. Both the mother and the intrauterine fetus may be treated simultaneously at essentially any time in pregnancy,

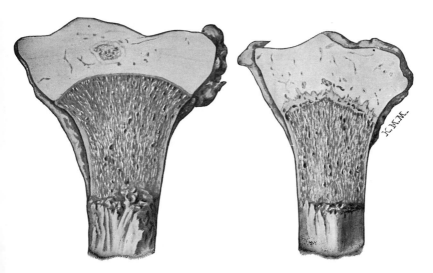

Fig. 30-1. Normal (left) and syphilitic (right) fetal long bones. Note sharp, narrow line of Guerin in the normal bone and jagged, broad line in the syphilitic bone. (From Stander: Williams obstetrics, New York, D. Appleton-Century Co.)

since penicillin, the preferred antibiotic, crosses the placenta readily.

Occasionally, however, a stillbirth resulting from congenital syphilis may still be seen. The placenta is large and thick. At autopsy, characteristic interstitial changes in the lungs, liver, and pancreas are frequently noted. Positive diagnosis is made by finding the *Spirochaeta pallida* (treponema) in these organs.

One characteristic pathologic sign of syphilis is the typical change of Guerin's line, where the epiphysis joins the bone. Normally this is a narrow, white line, whereas in syphilitic osteochondritis it is two or three times wider than normal, yellowish, and irregularly saw-toothed (Fig. 30-1). It is a most valuable diagnostic sign, being visible to the naked eye at autopsy and easily revealed by x-ray examination, especially at the distal end of the femur.

HEMOLYTIC DISEASE (ERYTHROBLASTOSIS)

Hemolytic disease affects about 1% of newborn infants. A few are decidedly edematous, have huge placentas, and fit the older designation of "general dropsy of the fetus." Others show minimal to major degrees of anemia, jaundice, hepatomegaly, and splenomegaly. The disorder results from blood group differences between the mother and the fetus, and once the pattern of events has been established, it tends to be repetitive. That caused by Rh incompatibility is by far the most common.

There are six common Rh antigens. In the American (Wiener) system of nomenclature these are designated Rh_0, rh', rh'', Hr_0, hr' and hr''. The British prefer Fisher's scheme, using the letters, D, C, E, d, c, and e, respectively. Each of these antigens may stimulate the production of its equivalent antibody. The relationship of the members of these pairs, for example C and c, is that of genetic allelomorphism. In other words, a chromosome can carry C or c, but not likely both; likewise, a chromosome may carry D or d, but not both. Since each cell has a double set of chromosomes, the genetic constitution may be designated simply by stating the nature of the gene in each chromosome and combining the symbols, as CC, Cc, or cc. D and d and E and e behave similarly. The three genes (C or c, D or d, and E or e) are close together or probably adjacent on the same chromosome. The partnerships of such linked genes seldom are broken up by the phenomenon of crossing-over.

From the above it is apparent that there are *eight* theoretical Rh phenotypes produced by different combinations of the elementary antigens, each representing a single Rh chromosome (such as CDE, cde, cDE). Each cell contains two such chromosomes, and consequently 36 different combinations or genotypes are possible (such as CDe/cde, CDe/cDe). Actually, the situation is somewhat more complex than this because other allelomorphs at the C and D loci have been discovered, such as C^w, D^u, E^w, and e^s. Though one need not be concerned with these unusual allelomorphs in obtaining an elementary understanding of the topic, it is of considerable importance in occasional clinical situations. For example, the D^u variant is of clinical significance because cells with this antigen may not agglutinate with anti–Rh_0 (D) sera, and the blood will appear falsely to be Rh_0 (D) negative.

The D^u antigen is found in 1% to 2% of American whites, often along with C and E, and is capable of isoimmunizing an Rh-negative person.

The various factors diminish in their antigenic capacity in the following order: D, C, E, c, e, d. Inasmuch as Rh_0 (D) is the most important Rh antigen clinically and was the first to be discovered, it has become common practice to use the term "Rh positive" to mean the presence of the Rh_0 (D) antigen and "Rh negative" to mean the absence of Rh_0 (D). For simplicity, this terminology will be perpetuated here with the understanding that it could equally apply to any of the other Rh antigens.

The Rh factor (Rh_0 [D]) is present in the red blood cells of about 85% of white persons, 93% of black persons, and nearly 100% of Orientals. When introduced into the blood of Rh-negative persons, it will stimulate the production of Rh antibodies. These will agglutinate and hemolyze any red blood cells containing the antigen.

Such antibodies occasionally are formed in women by:

1. Transfusion of Rh-positive blood to an Rh-negative recipient
2. Intramuscular injection of Rh-positive blood into an Rh-negative person
3. Passage of erythrocytes of an Rh-positive fetus across the placental barrier and into the bloodstream of an Rh-negative woman

The last may occur at any time during pregnancy but most commonly occurs at time of labor and delivery. In subsequent pregnancies, circulating maternal Rh antibodies may cross the placenta and hemolyze fetal red blood cells containing the Rh antigen. (Rh-negative fetuses are not at risk.) The dangers to the fetus include anemia, hyperbilirubinemia, hydrops, circulatory failure, and death.

Detection of Rh antibodies is accomplished by means of the Coombs' test, a standard procedure in hematologic laboratories. *Quantitation* of antibodies may be accomplished by testing serial dilutions of the serum. The Rh antibody *titer* is the highest dilution that causes agglutination in a 2% to 3% suspension of Rh-positive cells.

Because of the distribution of the antigen among white persons in the United States, it is probable that 13% of marriages between whites are incompatible matings in the sense that an Rh-negative woman is married to an Rh-positive man. Nonetheless, the woman has only a small chance of becoming sensitized to the Rh antigen and bearing children with hemolytic disease. If the father is homozygous (genes for the D antigen in both members of the pair of chromosomes), he must transmit the D gene to every child and all of his children will be Rh positive. If he is heterozygous (Dd), there is only a 50% chance that the D gene will be transmitted. The mother, being Rh-negative, will pass along the d gene to every child, and half the children may be expected to be Rh negative (genotype dd). Roughly 60% of Rh-positive men are heterozygous, so that one would expect 70% Rh-positive and 30% Rh-negative children in random matings of negative women with positive men. Thus, of 100 children taken at random, there would be 10 Rh-positive children whose mothers are Rh-negative. But the incidence of the Rh type of hemolytic disease is about 1 in 200 pregnancies, not 20 in 200 as might be predicted from the calculations just given. In other words, about 1 in 20 children born to Rh-negative women may be expected to show some degree of hemolytic disease. Actually, Potter found that among 7,000 pregnant women at the Chicago Lying-In Hospital the incidence of hemolytic disease among children of Rh-negative women was 1:37, the fatal form having an incidence of 1:56.

Pathologic findings. Pathologic findings in the severely affected infant include pronounced subcutaneous edema, ascites, hydrothorax, cardiomegaly, enlargement of the liver and spleen, erythroid hyperplasia of bone marrow, extramedullary hematopoiesis in the spleen and liver, pulmonary hemorrhages, and yellowish pigmentation of the basal nuclei in the brain (kernicterus). Serious neurologic abnormalities result from this bilirubin staining of basal nuclei. The hydropic infant may die in utero at essentially any time in pregnancy.

The placenta may be decidedly edematous with prominent cotyledons. The villi are large and show persistence of Langhans' cells and areas of erythropoiesis.

Clinical picture. The living hydropic fetus is pale, limp, and has a large spleen and liver and scattered petechiae. Cyanosis and death may occur in a few hours. Some nonhydropic infants may appear normal at birth but develop jaundice in 1 or 2 days. Still others exhibit only anemia, and their disease may not be discovered without routine immunologic and hematologic studies.

Usually the delivery of a sick infant is anticipated on the basis of maternal history and blood studies. A long piece of cord should be left attached to the infant to allow subsequent access to the umbilical vein. Samples of cord blood are examined for Rh status, ABO group, hemoglobin level, Coombs' reaction, reticulocyte count, and the numbers of nucleated red cells in the smear.

Treatment. Treatment consists of exchange blood transfusions plus general supportive measures. Hemoglobin values and serum bilirubin levels are guides to be followed in determining whether exchange transfusion should be performed. This is typically undertaken if the infant's hemoglobin is below 14 gram % or the serum bilirubin level approaches 20 mg%. The goal is prevention of the impact of anemia and hyperbilirubinemia by replacement of the infant's blood with fresh, Group O, Rh-negative blood, which cross matches with the maternal serum.

Clinical management

1. Determine the Rh status of every pregnant woman at the time of her first prenatal visit and screen her serum for atypical antibodies regardless of her Rh type. This screening will detect and identify antibodies induced by transfusion or by fetal cell transfer in a previous pregnancy. When such an antibody is detected, its identity should be established with panels of group O cells with known antigenic characteristics.

2. If no antibodies are found and the patient is Rh-negative, the Rh antibody screening test should be repeated at 26, 32, and 36 weeks of gestation. If no Rh antibodies are detected, the pregnancy should be managed in the routine fashion without regard to the Rh-negative status.

3. If antibody is noted at any of these examinations, the titer should be determined and repeat determinations should be obtained at regular intervals thereafter. If the antibody titer is stable at 1:8 or less, consideration should be given to elective termination of the pregnancy at 36 to 38 weeks' gestation. If the titer is over 1:8, and especially if it is rising, transabdominal amniocentesis (Fig 30-2) and spectrophotometric scanning of the amniotic fluid for products of hemoglobin degradation should be performed.

4. Spectrophotometric analysis will allow a computation of

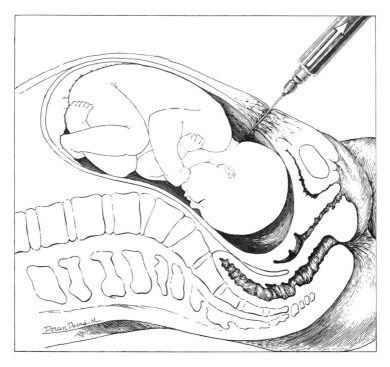

Fig. 30-2. Technique of amniocentesis.

the difference in optical density (ΔOD) at 450 mμ between the amniotic fluid sample and that anticipated for normal, unaffected amniotic fluid. Absorption of light at this wave length is attributable to bilirubinoid pigments, and the higher the ΔOD, the greater the concentration of blood breakdown products and the more severe the hemolytic process. Repeat amniocenteces and ΔOD determinations are required to follow the course of the fetal disease.

5. Predictive charts have been formulated for use in interpretation of these spectrophotometric readings. Figs. 30-3 and 30-4 are flow sheets recommended for use in the management of Rh-negative women in pregnancy.

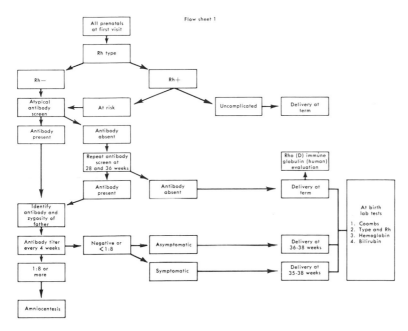

Fig. 30-3. Flow sheet for clinical management of prenatal patients regarding Rh isoimmunization. (From Technical Bulletin no. 17, American College of Obstetricians and Gynecologists, Chicago.)

6. *Fetal transfusion in utero.* It is possible to transfuse packed red cells into the peritoneal cavity of the fetus in utero. The fetal abdomen is radiographically localized after ingestion by the fetus of contrast material injected into the amniotic fluid. The fetal peritoneal cavity is then entered with a needle inserted through the maternal abdominal wall. A conduit is maintained with a catheter threaded through the needle. Group O, Rh-negative, packed red cells that cross match with the maternal serum are administered in small quantities. The relatively large percentages of adult hemoglobin found at birth in infants so treated suggests that red cells are absorbed via the peritoneal lymphatics. Fetal demise in response to the procedure is not uncommon. Intra-

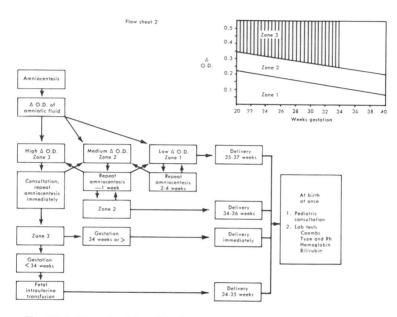

Fig. 30-4. Flow sheet for clinical management of sensitized Rh-negative prenatal patients requiring amniocentesis. (From Technical Bulletin no. 17, American College of Obstetricians and Gynecologists, Chicago.)

uterine transfusion is futile if fetal hydrops has occurred, as red cell absorption is negligible.

Prevention of Rh isoimmunization in the mother. It has been demonstrated that Rh_0 (D) immune globulin will suppress Rh sensitization if given intramuscularly to an unsensitized Rh negative and D^u-negative woman within 72 hours after delivery of an Rh-positive or D^u-positive infant. The major transfer of fetal Rh-positive blood to the maternal system occurs during labor, particularly at the time of placental separation. Fetal Rh-positive cells are eliminated from the circulation by the antigen-antibody reaction before they can stimulate an innate and permanent maternal antibody response. The passive immunity is temporary.

The D^u status of the mother should be known because it is unwise to give Rh_0 (D) immune globulin to a person who is D^u-positive. Maternal isoimmunization may be produced when the immune globulin reacts with D^u-positive antigen, and the result is similar to that occurring after transfusion of mismatched blood.

Women who abort or deliver stillborn infants should also be protected from Rh isoimmunization. The prevention of maternal immunization in this manner is of enormous importance and the universal application of this principle will virtually eliminate hemolytic disease of the newborn.

Isoimmunization by other blood antigens. Some cases of hemolytic disease of the newborn infant result from incompatibility of blood groups A and B. Antepartum diagnosis is difficult because A and B antibodies occur normally, and the maternal titers may not be impressively high. Most instances have been seen in group O mothers carrying fetuses with type A or B blood.

Apparently fetal blood cell antigen will stimulate in the mother formation of immune antibodies small enough to traverse the placenta, whereas the naturally occurring anti-A and anti-B isoagglutinins are macroglobulins that do not enter the fetal circulation. However, because the smaller antibodies appear to combine weakly with fetal cells, hemolysis is not extensive and the fetal hemolytic disease is relatively mild.

After delivery of a group O mother, the infant's blood should be typed. When the infant is type A or B, further evaluation of the infant's hematologic status is indicated (for example, hemoglobin, bilirubin, reticulocyte count) so that appropriate treatment may be started as early as possible.

Although ABO hemolytic disease can be severe, it usually is milder than that associated with Rh factors, but it may, of course, occur rather often in the offspring of primigravidas. Jaundice appears within 24 hours, as well as anemia, reticulocytosis, and increased fragility of red cells. Exchange transfusion with group O blood may be necessary.

There have been a few cases of hemolytic disease in association with the Kell, Duffy, Kidd, and MNSs systems of antigens. Antibodies of the P, Lutheran, and Lewis systems seem to cause very little red cell destruction in the fetus.

REACTIONS TO LEUKOCYTE AGGLUTININS

Febrile reactions simulating those of puerperal infection may occur after the transfusion of incompatible leukocytes in women with isoagglutinins for human leukocytes. These unpleasant responses can be prevented by removal of leukocytes from the blood to be transfused. Leukoagglutinins have developed in pregnant women in the absence of previous transfusions or injections of blood, and presumably the provoking antigens are fetal leukocytes. Usually two pregnancies are required to produce leukoagglutinins, and they tend to persist for many years after sensitization. There is no established disease of the newborn infant from isoimmunization of the mother by fetal leukocyte antigens.

EPIDEMIC DIARRHEA

Epidemics of diarrhea in newborn infants have been prevalent in hospital nurseries in recent years. The etiology is not established, although several bacterial organisms and viruses have been implicated. Numerous watery, yellowish green, and sometimes blood-tinged stools are noted to appear 2 or more days after birth. The affected infants must be isolated at once, and no new infants should be placed in the contaminated nursery until it has been thoroughly cleaned. Because epidemic diarrhea can become an extremely serious problem, with mortality ranging up to 50%, elaborate and rigid precautions must be taken as soon as there is the merest suggestion of impending trouble.

For treatment of this disorder, the reader is referred to textbooks of pediatrics.

PREMATURITY

There is general agreement that a body weight of 2,500 grams marks the upper limit of prematurity. The lower limit is less well defined, although most authorities have agreed on 400 grams, since no fetus weighing less than this has been known to survive. Actually, the probability of survival if the birth weight is under 1,000 grams is quite small, and it is helpful statistically to group such fetuses under the heading "immature infants."

Prematurity is the principal cause of death in the neonatal period. Prematurity is associated with multiple gestation, maternal disease requiring terminating of pregnancy, maternal disease that leads to spontaneous onset of labor, and congenital abnormalities. However, about one half of all premature births are not explainable on the basis of current knowledge.

Prematurely born infants suffer from lack of functional maturation of certain organs and enzyme systems necessary for extrauterine adaptation. The more mature these systems, particularly those related to cardiopulmonary and thermoregulatory activities, the greater the potentiality for survival.

Most deaths of premature infants occur during the first 24 hours. Respiratory distress with alveolar hyaline membrane formation (p. 427) is the most common cause of death.

Survival may be associated with pulmonary as well as neurologic sequelae. Retrolental fibroplasia, an ophthalmologic sequela, may also occur. This is characterized by the formation of opaque tissue behind the lens and is found usually in infants weighing under 3 pounds at birth; this tissue develops gradually during the first few months of life, leading to partial or total blindness. It is caused by the sustained administration of a high concentration of oxygen (over 40%) for more than 24 to 48 hours and is a preventable disease.

INTRAUTERINE GROWTH RETARDATION

Infants weighing less than 2,500 grams at birth are not uniformly premature. Some of them, as well as others weighing somewhat more, are small for gestational age. They presumably have suffered from chronic intrauterine growth retardation from inadequate intrauterine nutrition, congenital abnormalities, or intrauterine infection.

The malnourished infant will appear emaciated and generally undersized although the growth of the head and brain are often unaffected. Clinically such infants appear more mature than those of similar weight, but learning problems and neurologic sequelae may occur. They do not commonly achieve normal growth and continue to lag behind their peers throughout life.

POSTMATURITY

Postmaturity is a controversial syndrome defined as prolongation of pregnancy beyond 42 weeks, a situation supposedly detrimental to the fetus because of the limited life-span of the placenta. This is not a rule, however, as some fetuses appear to continue to thrive and show no appreciable effect from prolonged gestation. Others fail to grow and are believed to have become inadequately nourished as a result of late gestational placental insufficiency. Long nails, pale skin with epithelial desquamation, reduced vernix, excessive scalp hair and oligohydramnios are believed to be signs of postmaturity. Dehydration and hypoglycemia may also occur. The presence of meconium augments the diagnosis and is associated with an increase in fetal mortality.

The reality of postmaturity in any specific instance is related to the reliability of the menstrual history, dates of coitus, and time of ovulation. These data often are not well documented, and therefore many clinicians have been reluctant to induce labor or perform cesarean section to prevent death of a fetus whose life may not really be at risk. Use of the current methods for assessment of placental insufficiency (Chapter 12) and fetal maturity (Chapter 7) should be helpful in resolving such a dilemma.

31

Obstetric surgery

THERAPEUTIC ABORTION

Therapeutic abortion is the intentional termination of pregnancy prior to fetal viability for the purpose of improving the physical or mental health of the mother, or of prevention of the birth of an infant with an undesirable inherited anatomic or metabolic defect. Unlike other surgical operations, abortion is regulated by legal statutes that differ widely in various states and countries. Recently (January 1973) the United States Supreme Court ruled that antiabortion laws are unconstitutional, but suggested that a state might establish regulations applicable after the first trimester, with a view to preserving and protecting maternal health. They judged that a state's interest in the mother was negligible during the first trimester because at that early stage of pregnancy mortality from abortion is less than mortality from normal delivery at term. This decision has led to the removal of restrictions against early abortion virtually everywhere except in Catholic hospitals, but it is unlikely that all legal interest in regulating therapeutic abortion has ended.

In addition to the simple desire of a pregnant woman to have her pregnancy interrupted, because of socioeconomic factors, other indications may be classified as medical (such as cardiovascular, renal, or pulmonary disease), psychiatric, or fetal. The fetal indications include potential malformation after maternal viral disease early in pregnancy, after the use of teratologic drugs or radiation therapy, or for inheritable defects.

Techniques

1. Dilatation of the cervix and evacuation of uterine content

with ovum forceps and curet used to be the common procedure in the first trimester. *Great care must be taken to avoid uterine perforation.* The completeness of the evacuation may be checked digitally.

2. *Uterine aspiration* has gradually replaced curettage for first trimester abortions. After the usual cervical dilatation a transparent plastic cannula attached by flexible tubing to a vacuum pump is inserted into the uterine cavity until the gestational sac is encountered. Suction then is started and, as the cannula is advanced toward the fundus, the gestational material is sucked into a collection bottle. Generally this method is speedier and attended by less loss of blood than sharp curettage. Preliminary dilatation of the cervix with a *laminaria tent* (made from the root of *Laminaria digitata,* a seaweed) inserted 8 to 18 hours before curettage greatly facilitates entry into the uterus. Cervical laminaria tents are cylindric devices 5 to 6 cm. long, available in various diameters ranging from 3 to 10 mm., and they swell

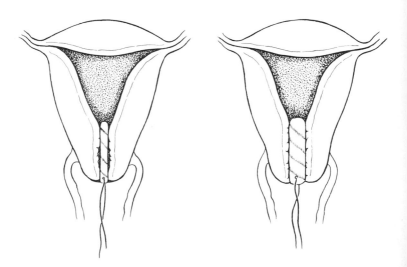

Fig. 31-1. Left, Laminaria tent inserted through narrow cervical canal beyond internal os. Right, Cervix dilated 12 to 24 hours later.

considerably in a moist environment (Fig. 31-1). The largest size that can easily be inserted is chosen, or two small tents may be placed side by side.

3. *Injection of hypertonic sodium chloride solution* through the abdominal wall into the amniotic fluid is feasible in the second trimester. From 100 to 300 ml. of amniotic fluid are removed and replaced with an equal volume or at least 200 ml. of 20% sodium chloride. Contractions begin within 8 to 48 hours and are augmented with oxytocin. Reinjection occasionally may be required to initiate uterine action. Presumably the hypertonic solution interferes with placental endocrine function and thus terminates the progesterone blockade (Csapo).

4. *Abdominal hysterotomy* should be performed if the pregnancy has advanced beyond the twelfth week of gestation and the saline method fails. This procedure affords an opportunity for simultaneously effecting tubal ligation (sterilization).

5. In selected multiparas *abdominal hysterectomy* has obvious advantages over hysterotomy.

6. *Vaginal hysterotomy* may be performed if there is an impelling reason to avoid a transabdominal operation (Fig. 31-2).

7. *Menstrual extraction,* or the aspiration of endometrial tissue with a slender cannula, is feasible in a woman whose expected menstrual bleeding has been delayed a week or so and who may possibly be pregnant. Obviously the widespread application of this technique results in the disruption of considerable numbers of endometria in women who are not actually pregnant.

8. *Prostaglandins* have been investigated extensively as a means of terminating midtrimester pregnancies. However, a maximally effective dose schedule, with an acceptable incidence and severity of complications (vomiting, pain, diarrhea, and fever), remains to be demonstrated for the intra-amniotic use of these substances.

STERILIZATION

Most serious medical disorders justifying therapeutic abortion are indications also for permanent interruption of childbearing. After multiple cesarean sections (three or more) sterilization commonly is advised to avoid the dangers of repeated laparotomies, as well as the problem of rupture of the uterine scar. A small

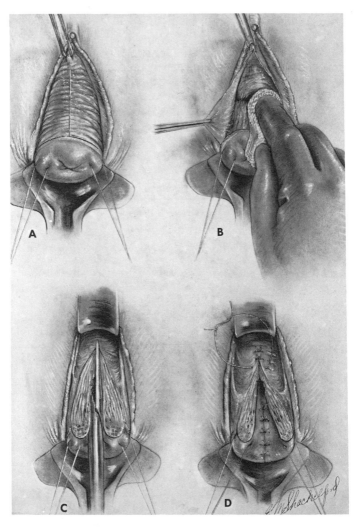

Fig. 31-2. For legend see opposite page.

number of women who are sterilized will regret, for one reason or another, having submitted to the procedure and will return asking for tuboplasty procedures to restore fertility.

There is very little logic in performing a major operation on a nonpregnant woman *solely* for the purpose of preventing a pregnancy that may never occur even with patent tubes. Therefore interval surgical sterilizations of nonpregnant women rarely are justified, particularly because the risk of laparotomy or even culdotomy is not negligible. If standard contraceptive measures should fail, consideration may be given early in the subsequent pregnancy to combining therapeutic abortion and sterilization.

Sterilization usually is effected by one of several common procedures that involve ligating and excising portions of the uterine tubes (Fig. 31-3). Such operations are not foolproof, and the failure rate is about 1 in 200. Puerperal sterilization may be done within 24 hours after vaginal delivery when there are good reasons for preventing further pregnancies. Although great multiparity (eight or more deliveries) has been widely recognized as a valid indication in itself for sterilization, some authorities now question this because of the alleged hazards of the operation (for example, pulmonary embolism and subsequent tubal pregnancy).

The tubes may be approached either through an abdominal incision or an incision in the posterior vaginal fornix. Metallic clips have been placed on tubes after identifying them through a *colposcope*. The *laparoscope* is widely used to electrocoagulate and excise small segments of tubes, and electrocoagulation of the cornual ostia of tubes through a *hysteroscope* has been accomplished by a few investigators. Others are attempting to perfect methods for injecting liquified plastics that will solidify and plug the tubes. Failure rates for these instrumental techniques have not yet been determined, but it seems inevitable that major

---

Fig. 31-2. Vaginal hysterotomy. **A,** An inverted T-incision is made through the mucosa. **B,** The bladder is then dissected from the cervix and pushed upward. **C,** The cervix is incised through the internal os, and a similar incision may be made through the posterior cervical lip if more room is required. **D,** If the posterior lip is incised, it should be repaired before attempting to repair the anterior lip. (From Titus: The management of obstetric difficulties, St. Louis, The C. V. Mosby Co.)

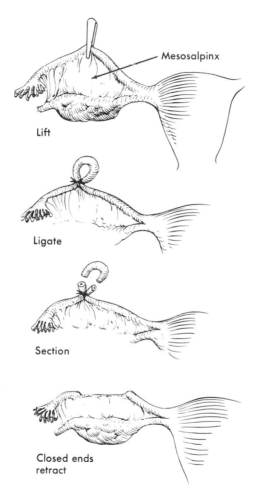

Mesosalpinx

Lift

Ligate

Section

Closed ends
retract

Fig. 31-3. Pomeroy method of surgical sterilization (tubal resection). (From Benson: Handbook of obstetrics and gynecology, Los Altos, Calif., Lange Medical Publications.)

surgical procedures to effect sterilization of the female will soon be abandoned.

INDUCTION OF LABOR

1. Intravenous oxytocin, 5 units in 500 ml. of 5% glucose in water, given at the rate of 0.5 unit in 30 minutes usually is effective. The rate of flow should be gradually increased from zero, and it is desirable to use an infusion pump to regulate the flow in accordance with uterine response. If labor has not begun after 8 to 10 hours, the medication is discontinued, but induction may be attempted again the next day or even on a third consecutive day.

2. *Rupture of the membranes* may be done if the cervix is soft, patent, and partially effaced. This is a simple procedure that may be done with the patient on an ordinary bed. A suitable instrument is slipped along a gloved finger that has been inserted through the cervix, and after the membrane has been punctured, the fetal head is displaced upward slightly to allow a large amount of amniotic fluid to escape. An unfavorable cervix may be converted to a structure that makes membrane rupture feasible by giving a course of intravenous oxytocin, as described above.

3. Occasionally just *stripping the membranes* away from the lower uterine segment provides sufficient stimulus to induce labor. This may be tried in selected patients when the criteria for rupture of membranes are not fulfilled.

Induction of labor without medical indication is permissible in selected multiparas with rapid labors who live far from a hospital. But *elective* induction merely for the convenience of the patient or physician may be associated with various hazards—prematurity, intrapartum infection after a prolonged latent period, or prolapse of the cord.

Intra-amniotic injection of hypertonic sodium chloride, as described above for therapeutic abortion, is an efficient means of inducing labor in the second half of pregnancy, provided that the fetus is dead or anencephalic.

FORCEPS DELIVERY

The obstetric forceps is a double-bladed instrument intended for extracting the head of the infant, whether the head is fore-

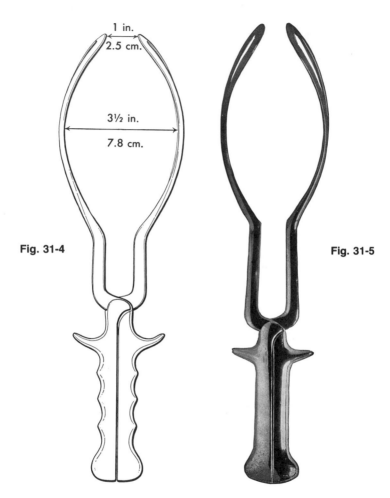

Fig. 31-4. Braun-Simpson forceps. The forceps designed by Sir James Y. Simpson is the most popular forceps used. Carl Braun's modification by widening the cephalic curve from 3 to 3½ inches (7.8 cm.) was a distinct improvement because it avoids too much pressure upon the infant's head and grasps the head more accurately.

Fig. 31-5. Simpson forceps, showing the pelvic curve. Note that the cephalic curve is narrow, only 3 inches (From DeLee: Principles and practice of obstetrics, Philadelphia, W. B. Saunders Co.)

coming or aftercoming (as in breech presentation). Forceps were devised at the end of the sixteenth century by a member of the famous Chamberlen family of England (Figs. 31-4 and 31-5).

The ordinary forceps has two curves: the cephalic to fit the head and the pelvic for accommodation to the pelvic axis. The function of the forceps in general is to terminate labor when the second stage is unduly prolonged (dystocia) and when the mother or the baby is endangered. The use of regional block anesthesia (spinal or caudal) has greatly increased the need for outlet or low forceps delivery because a very high percentage of women thus anesthetized are unable to exert the voluntary muscular action needed to complete the second stage of labor.

The principal maternal indications for delivery by forceps are dystocia, medical complications demanding elimination of second stage labor, and regional anesthesia. The fetal indication is circulatory embarrassment denoted by tachycardia (over 160 per minute), bradycardia (less than 100), or distinct irregularity of the heartbeat.

Forceps operations may be subdivided into two major groups: *elective* and *required.* These terms may be added to the other designations, as, for example, in the phrase "elective low forceps"—meaning a low forceps delivery not absolutely necessary as a lifesaving measure.

The incidence of forceps deliveries in any area is related to the prevalent modes of analgesia and to the philosophy of the practitioners involved.

Many varieties of obstetric forceps are available, each with its own minor peculiarities of construction. The operator should become proficient in the use of a standard model (choice of fenestrated or solid blades), a rotational instrument (no pelvic curve), and an axis traction device.

Prerequisites

Prerequisites for the use of forceps are as follows:

1. *The cervix must be completely dilated.* Even a narrow rim of cervix may offer great resistance to traction and result in extensive cervical lacerations.

2. *The head must be engaged,* preferably deeply engaged.

3. *The fetus must present by the vertex, or by the face with the chin anterior.*

4. *The membranes must be ruptured* to permit a firm grasp on the head.

5. *The position of the head must be known* precisely so that proper rotation can be effected if necessary.

6. There must be *no disproportion* between the size of the head and the available space at midpelvis or outlet levels.

The bladder should be emptied by catheter only if a midforceps delivery is to be undertaken. *Episiotomy* generally is advisable and may be performed just before application of the blades or when traction on the head begins to distend the perineum. The latter is commonly preferred because undue loss of blood will be prevented if there is delay in properly adjusting the blades.

Application

Application is designated according to the station of the head (Fig. 31-6).

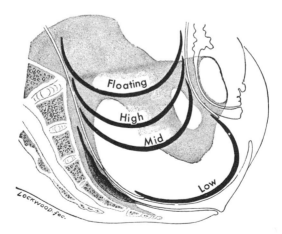

Fig. 31-6. Diagram showing station of the head in high, mid, and low forceps applications. Forceps must not be applied to the floating head. (From Stander: Williams obstetrics, New York, D. Appleton-Century Co.)

High forceps. In high forceps application the vertex of the head is above the ischial spines. A head floating above the pelvic brim is a contraindication to the use of forceps and high forceps are rarely justifiable.

Midforceps. In midforceps application the vertex is between the ischial spines and tuberosities.

Low forceps. In low forceps application the head is on the pelvic floor (deeply engaged) with the sagittal suture in the antero-posterior axis.

Although many forceps deliveries of patients under caudal or spinal anesthesia do not technically qualify as low forceps, they are generally classed as such because of the ease with which extraction is effected. To code them all as midforceps would suggest erroneously an enormous incidence of rather difficult deliveries.

Outlet forceps. In outlet forceps application the head distends the introitus considerably. Forceps delivery from this position is usually not indicated unless fetal distress appears when the baby is about to be born.

Adjusting blades

Cephalic application, that is, the blades applied to the sides of the fetal head, should be made whenever possible.

Pelvic application implies application along left and right sides of the maternal pelvis without reference to the position of the fetal head. Thus the head would be grasped properly only when the sagittal suture is oriented anteroposteriorly. Pelvic applications may injure the fetus and should be avoided.

If the fetal head lies transversely in the pelvis, cephalic application can be made only by placing one blade beneath the maternal bladder and the other in the sacral concavity. This should *not* be done with standard forceps that have a pelvic curve. Special forceps lacking the pelvic curve, such as the Kielland or Barton models, may be used to rotate a transversely arrested head into the anteroposterior axis in order to make delivery possible.

Technique of introduction for simple cephalic application (head in O.A., L.O.A., or R.O.A.)

1. Grasp the handle of the left blade in the left hand like a violin bow.

2. Introduce two fingers of the right hand alongside the head and inside the cervix if it has not yet slipped over the head.

3. Gently push the blade between the fingers and head.

4. In the same manner introduce the right blade.

5. Lock the blades without undue force.

6. If the fetal head lies in the L.O.A. or R.O.A. position, rotate it to the O.A. position before applying traction. A gentle trial pull determines that the blades are not likely to slip off the head and that the cervix has not been trapped between the blade and head (Figs. 31-7 to 31-9).

7. Delivery is then accomplished by alternately pulling and

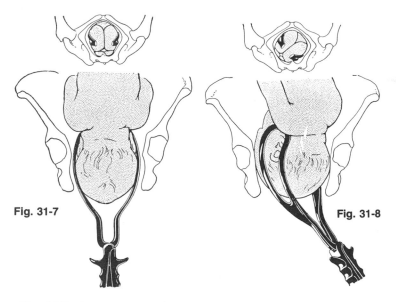

Fig. 31-7

Fig. 31-8

Fig. 31-7. Cephalic forceps application when the head is completely rotated. Visualized from the front and from below. (Redrawn from Bumm.)
Fig. 31-8. Oblique application of forceps in the L.O.A. position before the head has rotated. Visualized from the front and from below. (Redrawn from Bumm.)

resting, always exerting force in the axis of the pelvic canal, at first horizontally and gradually elevating the handles until the pull is perpendicular. The pull must be only with the arms; no use of body weight or bracing of the feet is permissible.

8. Essentially the same technique may be used if one deliberately elects to deliver from O.P., L.O.P., or R.O.P. positions (Fig. 31-10). After the sagittal suture is clearly in the anteroposterior diameter of the maternal pelvis, traction is made horizontally until the roof of the nose has been brought down to the level of the symphysis pubis. The handles then are gradually elevated until they are almost perpendicular and the occiput is slowly de-

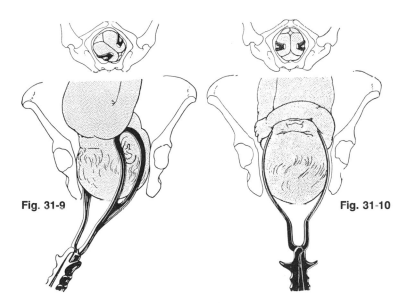

Fig. 31-9. Oblique application of forceps in the R.O.A. position. (Redrawn from Bumm.)
Fig. 31-10. Application of forceps when occiput has rotated directly posterior into the hollow of the sacrum. (Redrawn from Bumm.)

livered over the perineum. Then a downward tipping of the handles will cause the forehead, nose, mouth, and chin to appear from under the symphysis.

Tears are more frequent when the directly posterior occiput is delivered; they can be minimized by slow, careful delivery or by wide episiotomy.

Application in transverse arrest. There are several possible solutions to the problem of delivery from the R.O.T. or L.O.T. positions.

1. Rotate digitally or manually to at least an obliquely anterior position, maintain the new position with counter-pressure

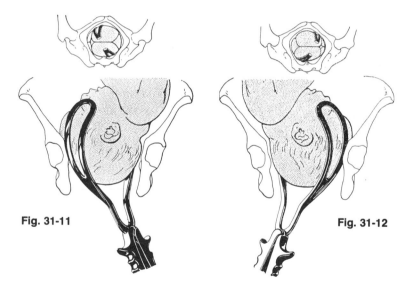

Fig. 31-11   **Fig. 31-12**

Fig. 31-11. Application of forceps when the head lies transversely. Visualized from the front and from below. Note that one blade lies over one cheek and the other slightly behind the opposite ear. (Redrawn from Bumm.)

Fig. 31-12. Application of forceps in the right transverse position. Visualized from the front and from below. Note one blade over one cheek and behind the opposite ear. (Redrawn from Bumm.)

through the lower uterine wall, and apply forceps as for simple cephalic position.

2. Apply standard forceps over one cheek and behind the opposite ear (Figs. 31-11 and 31-12) and try to rotate the head 45 degrees into an obliquely anterior position. Then readjust the blades to a perfect cephalic application and proceed as above.

3. Apply special forceps lacking pelvic curvatures (for example, Kielland or Barton), rotate to O.A., remove blades, and use standard instrument for extraction. The reader is referred to larger textbooks for details of use of special forceps. One should not attempt to use such devices without having had special instruction and practice on an obstetric manikin.

Rotation with forceps from R.O.P. or L.O.P. When the occiput lies obliquely posterior, it usually rotates to the front spontaneously. When rotation fails and delivery is urgent, manual rotation certainly should be tried first. When this fails, forceps may be used by the *Scanzoni maneuver* (double application):

1. A cephalic application is made just as in an anterior position.

2. The head is slowly rotated to the anterior position, not by

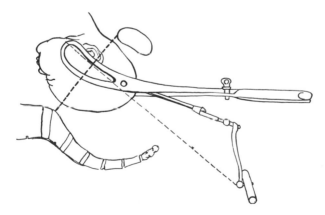

Fig. 31-13. Axis-traction forceps. Pulling on the handle of the right-angled arm ensures traction along the broken line from the head to the handle, that is, in the axis of the pelvis. (From Titus: The management of obstetric difficulties, St. Louis, The C. V. Mosby Co.)

twisting the shank but by rotating the handles in a wide, sweeping arc until the pelvic curve of the forceps is reversed (upside down).

3. The instrument is now removed and reapplied as in an occiput anterior position, and the baby is delivered.

Axis-traction forceps. Axis-traction forceps were devised by Tarnier (1877) to ensure traction constantly in the axis of the pelvis. They should be used for all difficult midforceps deliveries. The same instrument without the traction rods and bar may be used for simpler extractions (Fig. 31-13).

Application in face presentations

1. A cephalic application is made with the blades applied along the mento-occipital diameter (chin anterior) (Fig. 31-14).

2. The handles are kept loose, raised, locked tightly, and then depressed. This maneuver will increase the desired extension of the head.

3. The pull is downward until the chin emerges under the symphysis pubis.

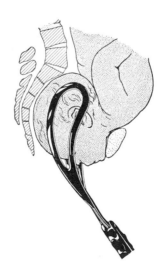

Fig. 31-14. Application of forceps in a face presentation, chin anterior. (Redrawn from Bumm.)

4. Then by an upward pull, the face passes over the perineum (the nose, eyes, brow, and occiput appearing in succession).

Kielland forceps may be effective for rotation from the mentoposterior position. Tarnier axis-traction forceps may be preferable to classical instruments in mentoanterior positions.

Application to aftercoming head. Application of forceps to the aftercoming head, using the ordinary or especially designed Piper forceps, must be undertaken when the Smellie-Veit-Mauriceau maneuver is difficult or impossible. (See Chapter 24.)

1. The baby's body is suspended in a towel and lifted upward slightly by an assistant.

2. The forceps are then applied underneath the body and to the sides of the head.

Vacuum extractor. The vacuum extractor is a metal suction cup to be applied to the fetal scalp as a substitute for forceps. It has the advantage of occupying less pelvic space than obstetric forceps, but it produces minor trauma of the scalp and distortion of skull bones. It has been widely used in Scandinavian countries but is not currently used to any great extent in the United States.

The extractor may be helpful in terminating certain positional arrests not easily corrected by conventional forceps, or in overcoming uterine inertia unresponsive to oxytocin with virtually complete cervical dilatation in a multipara. A rare additional indication is the need for instrumental delivery when general or conduction anesthesia is unavailable or deemed undesirable. Prolonged use and multiple applications are not justified because of potential damage to the fetus. If forceps have failed, a vacuum extractor will not be helpful.

The extractor may obviate the need for cesarean section occasionally, but unfortunately neither the instrument nor operators skilled in its use are generally available in American hospitals.

Trial forceps. Trial forceps means attempting midforceps delivery with the realization that it may fail and that delivery may have to be accomplished by cesarean section. If the application is satisfactory but several firm pulls produce no descent of the fetal head, the effort should be abandoned because it may be lethal to the infant.

Failed forceps. Failed forceps is a term that usually implies much more of an effort to deliver than does trial forceps. Such failures are related to disproportion, lack of full cervical dilatation, or malpositions of the fetal head. Cesarean section should be done if the infant is alive and craniotomy if it is dead.

BREECH EXTRACTION

It is customary to distinguish between three types of breech delivery:

1. *Spontaneous breech*—entire infant expelled without any manipulation (except support of the baby) (see Chapter 24)

2. *Partial breech extraction*—operator extracts infant after umbilicus has passed the vaginal outlet

3. *Complete breech extraction*—entire infant delivered by manipulations of the operator

Breech extraction has already been covered to some extent in discussing the mechanism of labor in breech presentations (see Chapter 24).

1. Extraction is required as soon as the umbilicus appears because of the danger of compression of the cord between the head and pelvis, extension of the arms, and possible separation of the placenta by the pull upon the cord. A short portion of umbilical cord must be drawn down to avoid later tension and compression of the cord. If no slack is available, it should be clamped between hemostats and cut.

2. The resistance of the pelvic floor should be minimized by "ironing out" the pelvic floor digitally or by performing episiotomy.

3. When the breech appears, pull upward until it is delivered. Then disengage the legs.

4. Grasp the femurs with the fingers of each hand, with the thumbs over the sacrum. As the grasp is made successively higher, avoid pressure above the iliac crests upon the abdomen to avoid injury to the abdominal organs. Continue traction until the scapulae are seen.

5. While these procedures are in progress, an assistant should press upon the fundus of the uterus (always in the axis of the pelvis). The purpose of this pressure is only to keep the head flexed or the arms from extending above the head. *It should not be forceful* but merely sufficient for the purpose. A little later stronger pressure may be needed to aid in descent of the head.

6. At this juncture, *Bracht's method of assisted breech delivery*

may be tried. When the infant's body is lifted toward the mother's abdomen, the arms usually deliver spontaneously. Suprapubic pressure then forces the head into the pelvis, whereupon the chin, nose, and brow emerge from the vagina.

7. If this simple maneuver fails, *partial breech extraction* is required. Wrap the infant's trunk in a towel and, with a combination of traction and rotation, bring the bisacromial axis into the antero-posterior diameter of the pelvis. Then either the anterior or posterior arm and shoulder are delivered manually. To deliver the posterior shoulder first, grasp both ankles in one hand and elevate the baby laterally over the mother's groin opposite the baby's back. This brings the posterior shoulder to or beyond the perineum. The arm and hand may then drop out. If they do not, they may be gently released with a digital maneuver.

8. Then the anterior arm may be delivered:

(a) Depress the baby's body until the shoulder is under the pubic arch. If the arm does not spontaneously drop out, it may be gently delivered manually.

(b) Or when the posterior arm has been delivered, the anterior shoulder may be rotated until it is posterior to facilitate delivery.

9. When an arm becomes extended above the fetal head, it may be disengaged by two fingers over the shoulder pressing the arm across the chest, with the fingers always being kept as nearly parallel to the humerus as possible to avoid injury to the arm. A finger should never be hooked around the arm because of the danger of fracture.

10. Delivery of the aftercoming head is best accomplished by the following:

(a) The *Smellie-Veit-Mauriceau maneuver* (Fig. 24-5) begins by laying the baby astride the operator's arm. Two fingers of the other hand are placed over the shoulders, with the palm on the infant's back. Downward traction brings the occiput under the symphysis, and delivery is completed by raising the baby's body toward the mother's abdomen.

Lacerations of the pelvic floor are more likely to occur with delivery of the aftercoming than with the forecoming head. Therefore, a deep midlateral episiotomy or an even deeper Schuchardt incision is advisable.

(b) *Forceps to the aftercoming head* is seldom necessary if the physician has mastered the manual maneuver. However, Piper designed a special forceps for the aftercoming head, and its use has become quite popular, being preferred by many to any other method. (See Fig. 24-6.)

When by rare chance the back (and therefore the head) does not rotate to the front, it may be made to do so as follows:

(1) By making stronger traction upon the leg that should naturally rotate anteriorly.

(2) If this does not succeed by the time the hips appear, the back can be rotated forward by stepping to the side of the patient and pulling laterally on the leg. It is surprising how easily the back and head rotate to the front by this maneuver. If despite every effort the shoulders are born and the back is posterior, the head may be rotated manually by internal manipulation or delivered with the occiput posterior. However, extensive lacerations are likely to occur.

11. *Complete breech extraction* may be required for delivery of a frank breech presentation or for other varieties of breech if fetal distress appears in the second stage of labor. In frank breech presentation the problem is complicated by mechanical difficulty in securing the feet for traction. Three approaches are possible:

(a) Traction with the index finger hooked into the anterior fetal groin; the trunk flexes laterally to permit insertion of the other index finger into the posterior groin. Use of a blunt hook for this purpose is permissible only when the fetus is dead.

(b) Disengage the feet and legs manually, pushing the fetus upward into the pelvis if necessary to provide working space. Pinard's maneuver is used on the anterior extremity to create a single footling and then on the posterior leg so that both legs may be used for traction. After a leg is identified by palpation in utero, pressure on the popliteal space will shorten the hamstring muscles and flip the foot down against the operator's fingers. He grasps the foot and draws it down beyond the breech. It is most desirable to bring down both feet before proceeding with traction.

(c) If a frank breech is deeply engaged but cannot easily be moved along by the finger-in-groin maneuver, application of forceps over the hips may be considered. In the main, however, this procedure is condemned because the forceps blades tend to slip off the presenting part and to traumatize soft tissues.

VERSION

Version is a maneuver designed to change the position of the fetus within the uterus in order to facilitate delivery. Most commonly, version is used to change a transverse lie to a breech or head presentation.

1. *Cephalic version* is changing a breech or transverse lie to a head presentation by *external* manipulation.

2. *Podalic version* creates a breech presentation by *internal* manipulation.

Combined versions employ external and internal manipulations simultaneously.

External or cephalic version

Theoretically external version, if successful, should lessen perinatal mortality by eliminating undesirable breech deliveries. However, there is a small risk to the fetus from placental and cord accidents associated with the necessary manipulations; external version under anesthesia is particularly dangerous, except in the most expert hands. Often the vertex presentation will revert to a breech before labor starts. In other instances spontaneous version of a breech to a vertex position may occur during the third trimester.

Prerequisites

1. The breech must not be deep in the pelvis.

2. There must be no disproportion between the pelvis and the infant.

3. Preferably the membranes should not have been previously ruptured. Certainly sufficient amniotic fluid must remain to permit free turning of the baby. A dry uterus is a positive contraindication.

4. The uterus must not be irritable. Version during labor seldom succeeds because the manipulations stimulate contractions.

Technique

1. Accurately recheck the position and presentation.

2. With one hand at each pole gently (always gently; strong force is dangerous) push (or draw) the breech laterally out of the pelvis.

3. The head is manipulated simultaneously in the opposite direction.

4. Listen to the fetal heart tones frequently.

5. Suspend manipulation during contractions of the uterus.

6. Finally, when the head presents, try to push it into fixation and hold it for a time. Do not persist when the version is very difficult and when two attempts have failed.

Internal or podalic version

Internal version is a procedure performed in the second stage of labor, under deep anesthesia, to effect prompt delivery of a fetus in either head or transverse (shoulder) position. The objective is to grasp one or preferably both feet, turn the fetal body within the uterus, and complete the delivery by breech extraction (Fig.31-15).

Indications

1. When the fetus lies transversely or obliquely.

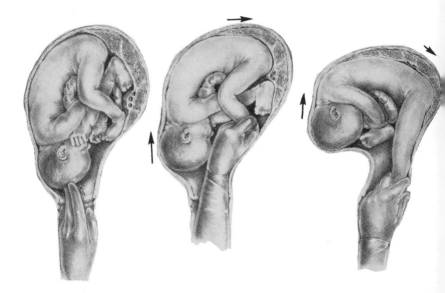

Fig. 31-15. Internal podalic version. Note successive steps of technique. (From Titus: The management of obstetric difficulties, St. Louis, The C. V. Mosby Co.)

2. In certain cephalic presentations when rapid delivery may be secured better by version than by forceps delivery. For example:

(a) Brow presentations

(b) High face presentations when the condition of the mother or baby requires prompt delivery

(c) Floating head of a second twin, if delivery is urgent

(d) Prolapse of the cord if the cervix is fully dilated

Contraindications

1. Hydrocephalus

2. Contracted pelvis (unless very moderate)

3. Undilated cervix

4. Tetanic uterus

5. Contraction ring of Bandl

Technique of internal or combined version

1. Recheck the diagnosis of presentation, size of pelvis, and condition of the baby.

2. Secure complete dilatation of the cervix.

3. Introduce the hand and arm until near the feet before rupturing the membranes.

4. Grasp both feet if possible. Otherwise grasp one foot, the left when using the right hand and vice versa. This technique tends to bring the back to the front, which is very desirable.

5. Make traction until the other foot can be grasped.

6. The version may be facilitated by pushing the head upward with the free hand (combined version). When the knees are visible, the turning is finished.

7. Complete the delivery as described under breech extraction.

In transverse lie when the back is anterior, grasp the lower foot, but when the back lies posterior, seize the upper foot. Observation of these precautions will bring the back to the front.

(See the discussion of breech extraction for details of delivery of the aftercoming head.)

Bipolar or Braxton Hicks' version

Bipolar version is a rarely used maneuver to reverse the fetal position in utero when the cervix is only *partially dilated* and is applicable to either podalic or cephalic version. The entire hand is placed in the vagina and two fingers are used within the cervix to displace the presenting part upward. The opposite fetal pole is manipulated through the abdominal wall with the other hand,

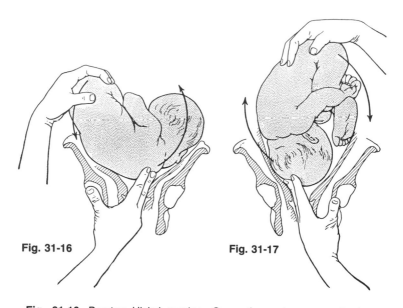

Fig. 31-16. Braxton Hicks' version. Converting a transverse lie to a longitudinal lie and a breech presentation. (Redrawn from Bumm.)
Fig. 31-17. Braxton Hicks' version. Converting a cephalic to a breech presentation. (Redrawn from Bumm.)

which tries to push the superior pole down toward the pelvis (Figs. 31-16 and 31-17).

The only remaining indication for this procedure is the rare instance of desperate need for tamponade of placenta previa in a primitive setting. Presumably one should be able to bring down a fetal foot and apply traction to it while cervical dilatation is completed.

CESAREAN SECTION

Cesarean section is the delivery of a fetus through incisions in the abdominal and uterine walls. Because incising the uterus is the cardinal feature of the operation, the term "cesarean section" should not be used to describe removal of a fetus from the abdominal cavity in a case of uterine rupture or abdominal pregnancy. The word "caesarean" was derived from the Latin verb *caedere*, 'to cut,' and section is from the Latin *secare*, also meaning 'to cut.' In the United States it is customary to omit the *a* in the *ae* ligature of "caesarean."

Removal of an infant through an incision in the abdominal wall and uterus was a disastrous procedure until very modern times. Because of the appalling number of deaths from infection, Porro in 1876 advocated removal of the body of the uterus and suture of the cervix into the abdominal wall. The mortality was lessened only slightly by this procedure. Sänger revolutionized the use of cesarean section when he insisted in his epoch-making paper (1882) that the uterine incision must be sutured.

Although deaths from infection were greatly reduced, the mortality was still considerable. Then Frank of Cologne in 1907 proposed the extraperitoneal route as a safeguard against infection. The mortality again decreased.

The next step in perfecting the operation was the contention of Krönig in 1912 that safety of the extraperitoneal operation was attributable more to the placement of the incision in the lower segment than to avoiding the peritoneal cavity. This idea was widely accepted, and from it has developed the modern lower segment cesarean section.

Indications

1. Potentially weak uterine surgical scar from previous cesarean section, myomectomy, or unification operation

2. Pelvic contraction and/or fetopelvic disproportion

3. Primary or secondary uterine inertia (prolonged labor despite uterine stimulation)

4. Placenta previa

5. Abruptio placentae

6. Malpresentation (shoulder, breech, brow, or mentoposterior)

7. Fulminating preeclampsia

8. Ruptured uterus

9. Obstructing pelvic tumor

10. Previous colporrhaphy or repair of genital fistula

11. Fetal distress, actual or potential (maternal diabetes, isoimmunization, prolapse of cord, or unexplained hypoxia)

Occasionally a cesarean section may be indicated because of

several minor indications that are additive in arriving at the decision to operate. The only indication in approximately half of all cesarean sections is the presence of a previous cesarean section scar. Such operations are called "repeat sections" and are justified on the basis that the scar may rupture during labor.

Incidence. In the United States 4% to 6% of deliveries are accomplished by section. However, the incidence varies among hospitals according to types of patients treated and local policies, particularly in regard to almost routinely repeating cesarean operations. In some institutions cesarean section rates for private patients are 9% to 10%, and invariably the rate is higher than that for clinic (staff) patients. In western European countries the incidence of cesarean section tends to be much lower (1.5% to 3%).

Types of operation. Space will not permit descriptions of each type of operation. The reader is referred to larger textbooks that give details of each type of procedure.

1. The classical operation of Sänger, although rarely done now, is useful (a) when adhesions block access to the lower segment, (b) when the fetal shoulder presents, (c) when a placenta previa is located on the anterior uterine wall, and (d) when speed is important (Fig. 31-18).

2. The low cervical or "lower segment" section, preferably through a *transverse* uterine incision, is the favored procedure for most purposes. The incisional area in the uterus is protected by the bladder and a peritoneal flap, adhesions to the scar are prevented, and blood loss usually is minimal in the thin lower segment musculature unless anterior placenta previa is encountered (Fig. 31-19).

3. Cesarean hysterectomy, with either total or subtotal removal of the uterus, usually is a combination of cesarean section followed at once by extirpation of the uterus (Fig. 31-20). If fetal death and intrauterine infection have occurred, the uterus may be removed unopened. Cesarean hysterectomy is done either to remove a defective uterus (for example, ruptured uterus or uterus with placenta accreta) or as an elective procedure to eliminate myomas or simply to effect surgical sterilization after several cesarean sections. This latter indication remains debatable because of the high morbidity and relatively great blood loss often requiring transfusions. Occasionally there is difficulty in identification of the

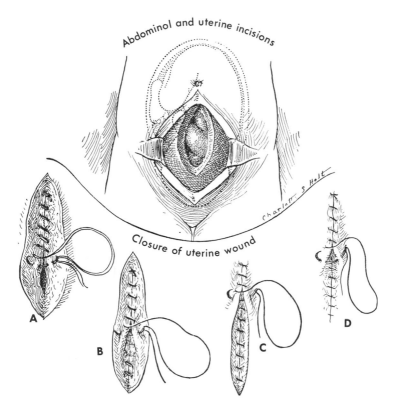

Fig. 31-18. Classical cesarean section. **A,** Suture uniting muscle close to but not penetrating the endomotrium. **B,** Suture uniting muscular wall. **C,** Approximating the serosa. **D,** Uniting the peritoneal surface by folding it over the deeper layers. (From Falls and McLaughlin: Obstetric and gynecologic nursing. St. Louis, The C. V. Mosby Co.)

lower limit of the cervix and some portion of this structure remains in situ.

4. Extraperitoneal cesarean section formerly was used in frankly infected patients to avoid spillage of infected fluid into the peritoneal cavity. Because of technical difficulties, it has been very largely supplanted by lower segment section and antibiotic ther-

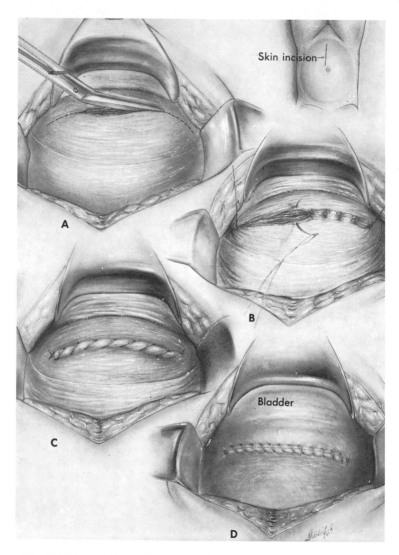

Fig. 31-19. Technique of transverse lower segment cesarean section. **A,** Making curved uterine incision. **B,** Interrupted closure of first layer. **C,** Continuous closure of second layer. **D,** Peritoneal flap resutured. (From Titus: Management of obstetric difficulties, St. Louis, The C. V. Mosby Co.)

Skin incision→

Bladder

apy. A paravesical (Latzko) or retrovesical (Waters) incision through the lower uterine segment avoids the peritoneal cavity and the bladder.

5. *Postmortem cesarean section.* When maternal death is imminent in a pregnancy of more than 28 weeks, preparation for a postmortem operation should be made. Although permission is desirable, it may not be essential in every instance. Some authorities believe that failure to try to obtain a living infant might be

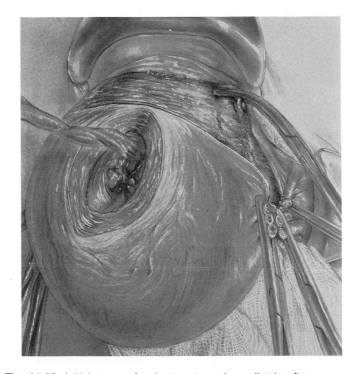

Fig. 31-20. Initial steps of a hysterectomy immediately after cesarean section. The placenta may be left in the uterus during the operation if the physician so chooses. (From Titus: Management of obstetric difficulties, St. Louis, The C. V. Mosby Co.)

grounds for a lawsuit on the basis of negligence. Though the outlook for the infant is notoriously poor, a few surviving normal children have been reported when removal was accomplished within 2 to 10 minutes after maternal death.

Morbidity and mortality. For the mother, morbidity and mortality depend on the indication for cesarean section, duration of labor and of ruptured membranes, the effectiveness of antibiotics, and the type of operation. The maternal mortality in large hospitals in the United States is now 0.1% to 0.2%, but it may be much higher in less favored areas. There is still an excessive number of preventable deaths after cesarean section.

The infant mortality is several times what it is in vaginal delivery. This is not the result of the method but of (1) prematurity, (2) abruptio placentae, (3) prolapse of the cord, (4) poor choice of anesthesia, and (5) other situations that are harmful to the infant. In a large series of electively repeated cesarean sections, however, the total perinatal mortality was 0.9% and for term infants 0.85%. One must avoid the error of performing elective cesarean section so early that prematurity becomes a factor in survival of the infant.

Management of subsequent pregnancies. If the indication for the initial cesarean section persists, the operation is repeated at term or at the onset of labor. A patient with a scar from a *classical* section should be delivered again by section, irrespective of persistence of the original indication, to avoid the rather high risk of rupture of the uterus.

When the indication for the original lower segment cesarean section no longer exists, there is a choice between (1) repeating the cesarean operation electively or (2) permitting a trial of labor and ultimately vaginal delivery unless symptoms of impending rupture develop. If the latter course is chosen, the physician must personally observe the progress of labor and preparations must have been made for immediate operation and blood transfusion.

Surgical sterilization commonly is recommended after two or three cesarean sections to avoid the risk of a potentially weak uterine scar and the hazards of repeated major abdominal operations.

PUBIOTOMY AND SYMPHYSIOTOMY

Pubiotomy (hebosteotomy) is division of the pubic bone near the symphysis with the Gigli saw to enlarge the contracted pelvis.

Symphysiotomy is division through the pubic joint. For all practical purposes these operations have been abandoned in the United States. The maternal complications are excessive, and cesarean section is safer.

These operations are still done in Africa when it seems likely that the patient cannot be followed in a subsequent pregnancy. In such an instance, a woman delivered by cesarean section for contracted pelvis may die from rupture of the uterus in her next pregnancy, whereas symphysiotomy may enlarge the pelvis sufficiently to permit vaginal delivery.

CRANIOTOMY

Perforation of the infant's head (Fig. 31-21) is done to decrease its size preparatory to delivery by the cranioclast, basiotribe, or forceps.

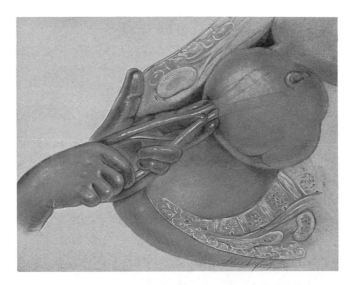

Fig. 31-21. Craniotomy. Perforating the head. Note that the perforator is kept in the axis of the pelvis to avoid possible injury to the mother. The aftercoming head may be similarly perforated. (From Titus: The management of obstetric difficulties, St. Louis, The C. V. Mosby Co.)

Indications
1. Hydrocephalus
2. An aftercoming head that cannot otherwise be delivered

Contraindications
1. A pelvis with an absolute contraction
2. A living baby

Technique. The operation consists of:

1. Perforation of the skull, preferably through a fontanel with Smellie's scissors

2. Breaking up the contents and evacuation with a sterile douche or vacuum aspirator

3. Application of the cranioclast with the solid blade within the skull and the fenestrated blade over the face (Fig. 31-22)

4. Delivery as with forceps

It is not always necessary to apply the cranioclast. The collapsed skull may permit spontaneous expulsion; delivery may be accomplished by hooking a finger in the opening. Forceps may be ap-

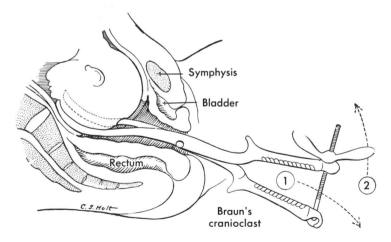

Fig. 31-22. Application of the cranioclast. The solid blade is within the skull and the fenestrated blade is over the face. (From Falls and McLaughlin: Obstetric and gynecologic nursing, St. Louis, The C. V. Mosby Co.)

plied, or even a tenaculum to grasp the skull may suffice. The *basiotribe*, a combination of a perforator and a forcepslike grasping instrument, is preferred by some authorities.

To make sure that the baby does not breathe after delivery, the upper part of the medulla may be destroyed. To avoid any chance of breathing, it may be desirable to submerge the perforated baby's head downward in a large vessel of water that has been made ready in advance.

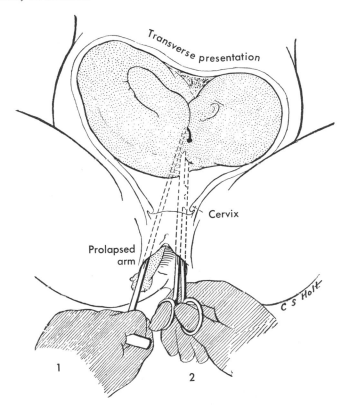

Fig. 31-23. Decapitation. Braun's blunt hook around the neck, embryotomy scissors cutting soft tissues. (From Falls and McLaughlin: Obstetric and gynecologic nursing, St. Louis, The C. V. Mosby Co.)

EMBRYOTOMY

Evisceration. Perforation of the abdomen or thorax to remove viscera may (very rarely) be required with certain monstrosities or shoulder impaction in neglected transverse lie.

Decapitation may be indicated for an impacted transverse presentation of a dead fetus. The neck is held by a blunt hook while the head is severed with a long-handled scissors (Fig. 31-23). The torso may be delivered by traction on one arm if the cervix is dilated; otherwise a fillet may be applied to a foot until dilatation and delivery are accomplished.

If the head is not easily expelled by pressure from above, it may be grasped with a tenaculum or held with a finger in the fetal mouth while the skull is perforated, decompressed, and delivered.

Cleidotomy. When necessary to reduce the shoulder diameter, the clavicles may be cut through with strong curved scissors.

At the present time there is only rarely a real indication for any type of destructive operation, and the graduates of most obstetric training programs have had no practical experience in the use of such instruments as cranioclasts and basiotribes. In the main, the seriously neglected obstetric labor with a dead fetus and an infected uterus is best handled by cesarean hysterectomy.

32

Contraceptive methods

Contraception refers to the prevention of pregnancy by some means other than permanent surgical sterilization. Because it is desirable for every woman capable of reproduction to space her pregnancies in such a way that care of her children is not an excessive burden for her, the obstetrician should volunteer to assist with appropriate planning in the immediate postpartum period. Furthermore, the threat of excessive growth of the world's population makes it imperative that women be indoctrinated into the concept of voluntary limitation of family size.

Although the postpartum patient is the obvious candidate for contraceptive planning, there is also much need for effective contraception among general medical patients who have not just completed a pregnancy but who have life-threatening diseases or undesirable hereditary problems. Far too often such patients are merely admonished not to become pregnant, but no specific advice or prescription is provided, and as a result of such neglect many of these women later must face the ordeal of therapeutic abortion.

Currently available methods of contraception fall into four broad categories:

1. *Biologic maneuvering:*

(a) *Rhythm method,* in which intercourse is restricted to an arbitrary number of days before and after the presumed day of ovulation. Because of uncertainties about the time of ovulation and the duration of sperm viability, this is not a reliable procedure unless the period of restriction on intercourse is so lengthy as to be rather impractical.

(b) *Coitus interruptus (withdrawal)*, though widely practiced, cannot be recommended because of the presumed likelihood of some degree of seminal emission prior to complete removal of the penis. Inasmuch as valid data on the use of this method are not available, its effectiveness cannot be assessed.

2. *Medicinal suppression of ovulation and of endometrial development (oral contraceptives):* Various combinations of progestogens and estrogens are used chiefly to suppress the production of pituitary gonadotropins and thus, in turn, to prevent ovulation. In addition, the progestational components of at least some of these preparations eventually create regressive histologic changes in the endometrium and presumably minimize the possibility of implantation of a fertilized egg.

These drugs are exceedingly effective when properly used. Unfortunately they produce undesirable symptoms in a small percentage of users. These symptoms include nausea, breakthrough spotting or frank bleeding, weight gain, chloasma, and headache. It is alleged that prolonged use of these steriods may be associated with increased risk of thromboembolic disease, neurologic and ophthalmic disorders, hypertension, and a prediabetic state. A recent study indicated that the use of oral contraceptives is much more common in women 15 to 44 years of age who have thrombotic strokes than it is in matched controls. There is no evidence of a higher risk of breast cancer in oral contraceptive users.

Many oral contraceptives have been approved for marketing in the last decade. The person who wishes to prescribe such medications must familiarize himself with the available products and with the various dosage combinations that are designed to minimize side effects and to provoke desirable amounts of withdrawal bleeding at the conclusion of a treatment cycle.

Most of the products are combinations of an estrogen and a progesterone, but some are packaged with a sequence of 15 or 16 estrogen tablets alone, followed by six doses of a combination. These so-called sequential dosage arrangements supposedly mimic the normal output of ovarian steroids, but almost invariably the withdrawal bleeding they provoke is appreciably greater than that seen after a cycle of combination tablets. Another choice is the use of rather small amounts of progestogen alone administered without interruption. Presumably this regimen interferes with penetrability of cervical mucus rather than blocking ovulation, and thus the effectiveness of this method is somewhat less than that of standard combinations. Furthermore, there is a significant incidence of irregular and unpredictable endometrial bleeding, which many women find intolerable.

Complete physical examination, including careful inspection of the cervix uteri and a cervicovaginal cytologic smear, must be done before prescribing these potent drugs. The cervix is particularly susceptible to stimulation by ovarian steroids and may develop pronounced ectropion. It may be desirable, at least psychologically, to interrupt the use of oral contraceptives once every 1 or 2 years and permit normal menstruation to occur. Frequently there may be at least a minor delay (1 to 3 weeks) in the onset of the anticipated menstrual bleeding, and during this time an alternative method of contraception must be used.

Estrogen-progestogen combinations are useful for regulation of uterine bleeding in women who have no need for contraception but who have dysfunctional bleeding. Regularly recurring endometrial bleeding can be provoked as a replacement for irregular and unpredictable bleeding in the woman who is anovulatory and thus lacking progesterone. Occasionally the regressive changes in the endometrium that are engendered by synthetic progestogens may minimize menstrual bleeding that tends to be profuse in the untreated woman. On the other hand, if heavy bleeding occurs in a myomatous uterus, estrogen-progestogen combinations usually are contraindicated because estrogen often stimulates growth of myomas.

3. *Physical devices:*

(a) *Vaginal diaphragm:* A dome-shaped rubber cup with a flexible metal rim that is inserted digitally into the vagina to cover the cervix prior to intercourse. A spermicidal jelly or cream is applied to its surfaces, and it is left in the vagina 6 to 8 hours after use. This is the standard device for intelligent, highly motivated women and is exceedingly effective when meticulously used. The patient must be provided with a diaphragm precisely the right size for her vaginal canal, and the size should be checked after each delivery.

(b) *Cervical cap:* A device that fits snugly over the cervix alone but does not cover the entire anterior vaginal wall, as does the diaphragm. It is useful in certain multiparas who cannot use a diaphragm effectively because of vaginal relaxation, particularly cystocele.

(c) *Condom:* A widely used device that is particularly suited to the intelligent, highly motivated male who will use a reputable brand of sheath and who will apply it before intromission. This method of contraception is especially useful as a temporary expedient while oral contraceptives are being withheld to permit resumption of physiologic function, or as a supplement to the use of a modified rhythm method in which unprotected intercourse is permitted only during the premenstrual week.

(d) *Intrauterine device* (IUD): There are numerous plastic or metal coils, spirals, rings, and T-shaped devices that may be placed more or less permanently in the endometrial cavity via the cervical canal by means of special inserting devices. The precise mechanism by which such a foreign body prevents pregnancy is not known. Fertilization may occur, but increased tubal motility perhaps results in delivery of the zygote to the endometrium before implantation is feasible. Direct interference with implantation also may be a factor. The disadvantages are uterine perforation during insertion, spontaneous expulsion, bleeding and cramping, and pelvic inflammatory disease. Furthermore, in women who tolerate the device satisfactorily, the incidence of pregnancy is 2% to 3%. Thus, for the individual patient an IUD is less protective against conception than an oral contraceptive, but obviously less of a metabolic risk and far less costly (Fig. 32-1).

The addition of a progesterone coating or a copper-wire wrapping on intrauterine devices to affect the endometrium directly and thus make them more reliable is being investigated with extensive clinical trials. Another experimental device is a small plastic bag that is inflated with sterile saline solution after insertion in the uterine cavity.

4. *Vaginal medications and douches:* Numerous spermicidal substances are available for intravaginal use in the form of jellies, creams, suppositories, foaming tablets, and aerosol creams. These are applied 1 to 10 minutes before intercourse and, in addition to destroying spermatozoa, may provide some degree of mechanical barrier at the external cervical os. They are not as effective as the combination of diaphragm with a spermicidal agent but are widely

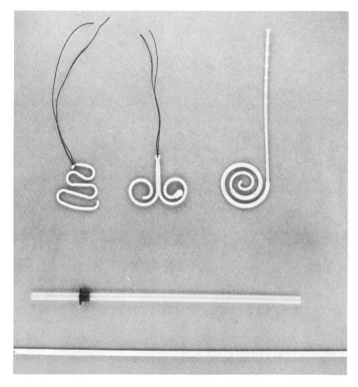

Fig. 32-1. Various types of plastic intrauterine contraceptive devices, with an inserter tube and plunger. Left, Lippes loop; center, Saf-T-Coil; right, Margulies spiral.

used by women who for one reason or another find the use of a diaphragm distasteful.

Vaginal douching, with water or medicated solutions, immediately after intercourse is widely employed, but it is the least dependable method of contraception. Semen enters the cervix promptly after ejaculation and often is well beyond the reach of any liquid introduced from below under low pressure. Postcoital douching is generally a waste of time and effort.

The ideal method of contraception has not yet been discovered, but an enormous effort is being expended to develop better ways of controlling fertilization and implantation because of widespread concern about the world's population problem and about the incidence of induced abortion. Much basic research in reproductive biology is being sponsored by both governmental and private agencies, with the hope that fuller understanding of the processes involved will lead to mechanisms for their artificial manipulation. Many pharmacologic products, particularly long-acting steriods, are being tested clinically in women, and various chemicals that interfere with spermatogenesis are being tried in males, but at the moment a thoroughly reliable and absolutely safe contraceptive medication is not available for universal use.

Contraceptive methods currently available are, however, enormously effective when intelligently applied, and every physician must assume the responsibility for providing each of his patients with the knowledge and physical materials suitable for her particular situation. And additionally, opportunities to substitute permanent surgical sterilization (particularly in the male) for temporary contraception should not be overlooked.

CONTRACEPTIVE PLANNING FOR THE PREMARITAL PATIENT

Contraception usually is a major concern of the patient who seeks a premarital examination, and the physician should introduce the subject during the preexamination interview. Advantages and disadvantages of the various methods should be explained, and specific written instructions should be provided for the method ultimately chosen because patients tend not to remember large segments of information transmitted verbally and rapidly.

Frequently a rather small vaginal introitus precludes proper fitting and use of a vaginal diaphragm. Assuming the introitus is at least adequate for intercourse, or will be made adequate by digital stretching carried out by the properly instructed patient herself, the use of condoms for a few weeks will greatly facilitate the later use of a diaphragm. Care must be taken to avoid prescribing a diaphragm that is one size too large because the discomfort thus generated may lead to unnecessary rejection of the method. The rim of a properly fitted diaphragm should slip easily out of sight behind the symphysis pubis, and the patient should be unaware of its presence in the vagina because the vaginal walls above the level of the introitus are extraordinarily distensible in a relaxed person. Either the physician or his nursing assistant must instruct the patient meticulously in the technique of insertion of a diaphragm and then check the diaphragm's position after the patient has performed the insertion herself. The size should be redetermined after each delivery or after any plastic operation on the vagina.

Most premarital patients need and appreciate an explanation of the ovarian-endometrial cycle, along with the pertinent facts about fertilization and implantation. Such knowledge will assist them in combining biologic rhythm with use of a mechanical device during those days of the cycle when protection is mandatory.

The widespread demand for oral contraceptive medications makes it essential that the physician be conversant with the ever-increasing numbers of prescription products and the presumed advantages of the specific combinations and dosages of estrogens and progestogens. No longer is it feasible to prescribe the same trade product for every user, and a certain amount of shifting from one product to another in successive treatment cycles may possibly eliminate undesirable side effects. It is essential to impress the patient with the fact that she is artificially manipulating her endometrial function when she takes these medications and that her intrinsic menstrual cycle and physiologic bleeding have been deleted. Furthermore, she must understand that interruption of medication at any time is almost certain to be followed in 24 to 72 hours by an episode of uterine bleeding. And last, she should know that a reasonable amount of variation in the pattern of pill taking, designed to precipitate bleeding ahead of schedule or to delay it a bit, is perfectly permissible from time to time if it is planned intelligently, with a calendar in full view.

Index